ILLUSTRATED CLINICAL CASES

Anaesthesia

MAGNUS A GARRIOCH
MB ChB (Birm), FRCA, FRCP (Glas), FFICM
Consultant (Attending) in Anaesthesiology and Critical Care
Manchester Royal Infirmary
Central Manchester University Hospitals NHS Trust
Manchester, UK

W BOSSEAU MURRAY
MB ChB (Pretoria), FRCA (Lon), MD (Stellenbosch)
Professor of Anesthesiology
Department of Anesthesia
Pennsylvania State University
Hershey, USA

CRC Press
Taylor & Francis Group
Boca Raton London New York

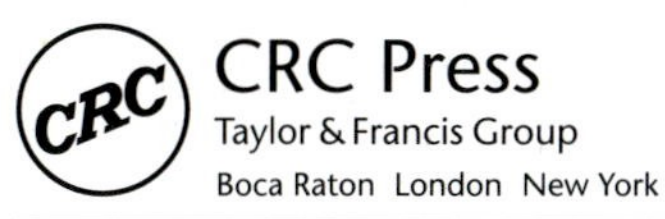

CRC Press is an imprint of the
Taylor & Francis Group, an **informa** business

CRC Press
Taylor & Francis Group
6000 Broken Sound Parkway NW, Suite 300
Boca Raton, FL 33487-2742

Printed and bound in India by Replika Press Pvt. Ltd.

Printed on acid-free paper
Version Date: 20140917

International Standard Book Number-13: 978-1-84076-077-4 (Paperback)

Visit the Taylor & Francis Web site at
http://www.taylorandfrancis.com

and the CRC Press Web site at
http://www.crcpress.com

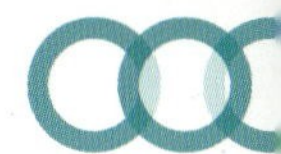

CONTENTS

PREFACE

The learning principles of this *Illustrated Clinical Cases* series of books lend themselves perfectly to the subject of anaesthesia. This book stimulates thought and enhances knowledge for both the novice and the experienced anaesthetist/anaesthesiologist alike. The reader becomes an active learning participant by considering questions based on the visual images presented and then immediately gaining access to the relevant answer on the following page.

The two authors, with their comprehensive trans-Atlantic clinical and teaching experience, have provided a wide breadth of subject matter that is directly related to the knowledge required to excel in anaesthesia. Many years of practical, hands-on teaching experience and of using actual patient cases to instruct trainees and colleagues have equipped them to produce this book. Their experience was particularly useful when thinking about how to phrase this collection of questions and answers.

Subjects are presented in a random fashion, in a similar way to which a practicing clinician encounters real clinical issues with patients, physicochemical concepts and anaesthesia equipment. By completion of the book, the reader will have gained much insight into most aspects of anaesthesia practice. Case reports are an integral part of learning, and by having to recall the facts related to a specific case, the reader will be able to recognise areas where more in-depth reading would be advisable.

A strong emphasis is also placed on the knowledge and comprehension required by both the Royal College of Anaesthetists and the North American examining boards to promote a deeper understanding of complex concepts, rather than just a simple list of facts. Readers will hopefully also be tempted to use some of the questions for their personal revision or the teaching of others. This book can be used again and again.

What is not intended is to provide a rigorous and detailed diagnosis and treatment of each disease as found in standard textbooks. The questions provided build upon one another to cover a broad scope of anaesthesia subjects presented in such a way as to be both varied and interesting.

Written with the needs of trainee doctors in anaesthesia in mind, we intend that the book might also be useful for experienced anaesthetists/anaesthesiologists with limited diversity of practice or for those who have become very specialised. These practitioners may not encounter such cases on a regular basis, but they might occasionally be required to deal with them. The book should also be useful for operating department practitioners and anaesthesia nurses in the UK and advanced Certified Registered Nurse Anesthetist (CRNA) students and experienced CRNA practitioners in North America.

Finally, we wish to acknowledge the numerous high-quality contributions from Dr David Fehr in the USA and Dr Alan McLean in the UK.

We also wish to thank our partners, James Allen and Janette Murray, for their love, patience and support, without which this book would not have come to fruition.

We sincerely hope you find this book both a useful and enjoyable read.

Magnus Garrioch
Bosseau Murray

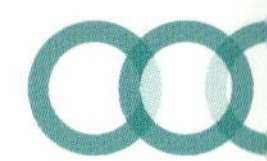

CONTRIBUTORS

Keith Anderson FRCA
Consultant Anaesthetist
Glasgow Royal Infirmary
Glasgow, UK

Dougal Atkinson FRCA, FFICM
Consultant in Anaesthesia and Critical Care
Manchester Royal Infirmary
Manchester, UK

Mark A Boustred MD
Assistant Professor of Plastic and Reconstructive Surgery
Pennsylvania State University College of Medicine
Hershey, Pennsylvania, USA

Colin Campbell FRCR
Consultant Radiologist
Southern General Hospital
Glasgow, UK

David Fehr MD
Associate Professor of Anesthesiology
Pennsylvania State University College of Medicine
Hershey, Pennsylvania, USA

Kevin Holliday FRCA
Consultant in Anaesthetics and Intensive Care
Raigmore Hospital
Inverness, Scotland, UK

Riyad Karmy-Jones MD, FRCSC, FRCSC(CT), FACS, FCCP, FAHA
Clinical Director of Trauma
Legacy Emanuel Medical Center
Portland, Oregon, USA

Stephen Kimatian MD, FAAP
Professor of Anesthesiology and Pediatrics
Cleveland Clinic
Cleveland, Ohio, USA

David Kissinger MD, FACS
Chief of Surgery
South Sacramento Kaiser Permanente Medical Center
Sacramento, California, USA

Donald Martin MD
Professor of Anesthesiology
Pennsylvania State University College of Medicine
Hershey, Pennsylvania, USA

Gavin McCalum FRCA
Consultant in Anaesthetics and Chronic Pain
Southern General Hospital
Glasgow, UK

John McGowan MSc, DIMC, RCSEd
RN Resuscitation Officer
Southern General Hospital
Glasgow, UK

Alan McLean FRCP
Consultant in Spinal Injuries
Southern General Hospital
Glasgow, UK

Regina O'Connor FFARCSI
Consultant Anaesthetist
Southern General Hospital
Glasgow, UK

Charles Palmer MD
Professor of Neonatal and Perinatal Medicine
Pennsylvania State University College of Medicine
Hershey, Pennsylvania, USA

Robert Prempeh FRCS(Ed), FRCS(Glas)
Consultant in Neurological Rehabilitation
Forth Valley, UK

Lester T Proctor MD
Professor of Anesthesiology
University of Wisconsin Medical School
Madison, Wisconsin, USA

Artur Pryn FRCA
Consultant in Anaesthetics
Inverclyde Royal Hospital
Greenock, UK

Puneet Ranote FRCA
Consultant in Anaesthetics
St George's Healthcare NHS Trust
London, UK

Urmila Ratnasabapathy FRCA
Consultant in Neuroanaesthetics
Southern General Hospital
Glasgow, UK

Kevin Rooney FRCA
Consultant in Anaesthesia and Intensive Care Medicine
Royal Alexandra Hospital
Paisley, UK

Kathleen R Rosen MD
Professor of Anesthesiology
Case Western Reserve University
Cleveland, Ohio, USA

Douglas Russell FRCA
Consultant Anaesthetist
Southern General Hospital
Glasgow, UK

John E Tetzlaff MD
Professor of Anesthesiology
Cleveland Clinic
Cleveland, Ohio, USA

Lars Williams FRCA
Consultant in Anaesthetics and Chronic Pain
Southern General Hospital
Glasgow, UK

Liz Wilson FRCA, FFICM
Consultant in Anaesthesia and Intensive Care
Royal Infirmary of Edinburgh
Edinburgh, UK

Margaret M Wojnar MD
Professor of Pulmonary and Intensive Care Medicine
Pennsylvania State University College of Medicine
Hershey, Pennsylvania, USA

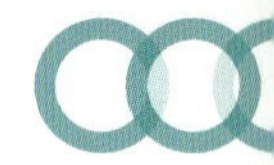

FOREWORD

The author Henry David Thoreau once said that "a truly good book teaches me better than to read it. I must soon lay it down, and commence to living on its hint". This is such a book. I doubt that anyone who reads it will not find an educational 'hint' on virtually every page. As such it is a tome that brings you up to date, stimulates your mind and encourages diagnostic and strategic thinking.

The specialty of anaesthesia is not simply a technical service. It is increasingly the case that the anaesthesiologist/anaesthetist is recognised as an overarching term for those with further skills in perioperative medicine and as physicians in intensive care and pain medicine.

The scope of this book is enormous and it covers all the specialty areas that anaesthesiologists/anaesthetists should recognise as their area of practice. It will stimulate you. Some readers will enjoy the revision in the fields of physics and clinical measurement. Others will be pressed by the physiology and pharmacology cases and others by the anatomical and statistical questions. However, all should enjoy the unique way that the scope of medical practice of relevance to anaesthesia is introduced within these pages. Learn from the proposed management given for the clinical scenarios; that is the future of our specialty, and this book will be an excellent read for all trainee anaesthesiologists/anaesthetists and more senior colleagues who aspire to that role.

Peter Nightingale MBBS, FRCA, FRCP, FFICM
Consultant in Anaesthesia and Intensive Care Medicine
University Hospital of South Manchester
Manchester, UK

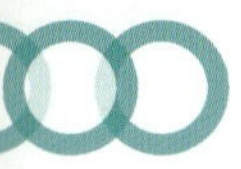

LIST OF ABBREVIATIONS

ACE	angiotensin-converting enzyme
AF	atrial fibrillation
APTT	activated partial thromboplastin time
ATLS	advanced trauma life support
AV	atrioventricular
BP	blood pressure
bpm	beats per minute
BSA	body surface area
CBC	complete blood count
CNS	central nervous system
CO_2	carbon dioxide
COPD	chronic obstructive pulmonary disease
CPET	cardiopulmonary exercise testing
CPR	cardiopulmonary resuscitation
CSF	cerebrospinal fluid
CT	computed tomography
CTPA	computed tomography pulmonary angiogram
CVP	central venous pressure
CXR	chest X-ray
D&C	dilatation and curettage
D&E	dilatation and evacuation
ECG	electrocardiogram
ECMO	extra-corporeal membrane oxygenation
EEG	electroencephalogram
EMG	electromyogram
ESR	erythrocyte sedimentation rate
ET	endotracheal (tube)
FBC	full blood count
FIO_2	fraction of inspired oxygen
GA	general anaesthesia
GCS	Glasgow Coma Score/Scale
GI	gastrointestinal
Hb	haemoglobin
HCG	human chorionic gonadotropin
Hct	haematocrit
I:E	inspiratory:expiratory (ratio)
ICP	intracranial pressure
ICU	intensive care unit
INR	international normalised ratio
IV	intravenous
LA	local anaesthesia
MAC	minimum alveolar concentration
NSAID	non-steroidal anti-inflammatory drug
O_2	oxygen
PaO_2	partial pressure of oxygen dissolved in arterial blood
P_AO_2	partial pressure of alveolar oxygen
PEEP	positive end-expiratory pressure
PO_2	partial pressure of oxygen
PT	prothrombin time
SIRS	systemic inflammatory response syndrome
SLE	systemic lupus erythematosus
TEG	thromboelastogram
TOE	transoesophageal echocardiogram/ echocardiography
U+E	urea and electrolytes
V/Q	ventilation/perfusion (ratio)

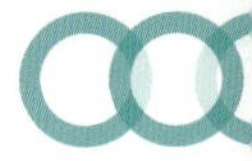

QUESTION 1

1 This 32-year-old lady presented with a diffuse swelling on the left side of her neck (**1a**). Over the past 3–4 months she had become slightly hoarse. The patient is scheduled for a partial thyroidectomy. A radiograph of her chest is shown (**1b**).

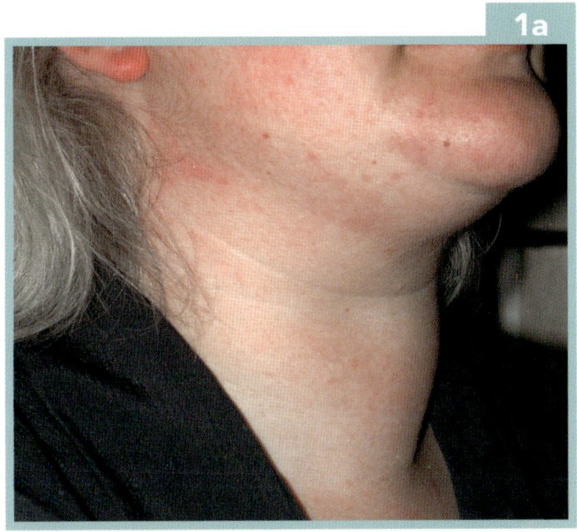

1a

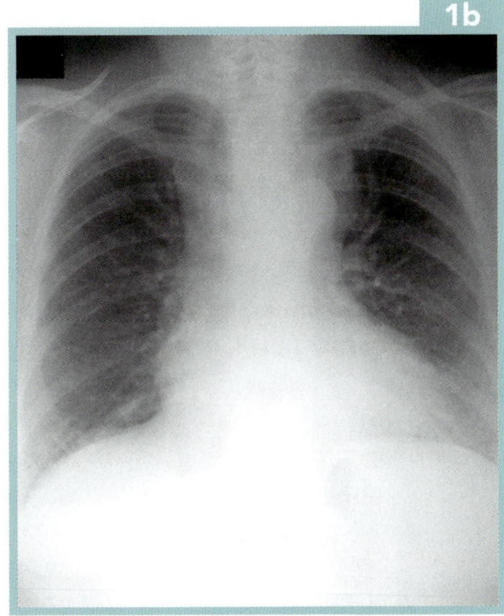

1b

i. What is this diffuse swelling likely to be?

ii. What other symptoms and signs may she mention or exhibit?

iii. What are the indications for partial thyroidectomy?

iv. Why should a CXR be done as a routine in this type of patient, and what does this radiograph show?

v. How would you manage this case at anaesthetic induction and at extubation?

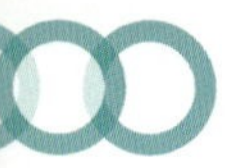

Answer 1

1i. A goitre. Goitres can be described as uninodular, multinodular or diffuse. In the developed world the commonest causes of goitre are Hashimoto's thyroiditis, an autoimmune destruction of the thyroid with hypothyroidism or an enlarged thyroid gland producing excess thyroid hormone and signs of hyperthyroidism. Patients with uncontrolled myxoedema or hyperthyroidism, presenting as an emergency, are at considerable risk of cardiovascular collapse.

ii. Hypothyroidism/myxoedema results in cold intolerance, fatigue, weight gain, constipation, dry skin, depression, muscle cramps and joint pain. Signs are bradycardia, hypothermia and slow speech, which in extreme cases can progress to coma. Hyperthyroidism causes nervousness, irritability, anxiety, excess perspiration, heat intolerance, palpitations, tremor and difficulty sleeping. Signs are weight loss, tachyarrythmias, hypoglycaemia, polyuria, delirium and pretibial myxoedema. New onset atrial fibrillation should always prompt investigation of thyroid function.

iii. Thyroidectomy may be needed for hyperthyroidism that is unresponsive to medical management or secondary to thyroid malignancy. Other indications are:

- Multinodular goitre, especially when compressing nearby structures.
- Graves' disease, especially with associated exophthalmos.
- Thyroid nodule, if fine needle aspiration results are unclear.
- Retrosternal goitre (even without airway obstruction).
- Recurrent hyperthyroidism.
- Cosmetic reasons.
- Anxiety (patients may insist on having a small goitre removed).

iv. A CXR excludes coincident pathology but also allows examination of the lower airway (i.e trachea and below). Goitres may occur retrosternally and on this film the goitre deviates the trachea to the right, with the possibility of tracheal collapse and lower airway obstruction. Hoarseness may indicate airway obstructive symptoms or compression of the recurrent laryngeal nerve.

v. Large goitres may present difficulty at intubation, particularly if they produce tracheal deviation or retrosternal extension. An inhalational induction is safest with inspection of the airway with laryngoscopy under GA. If the airway obstructs, then the inhalational agent wears off rapidly, enabling return of a patent airway. If airway inspection is straightforward, a relaxant can be given and the airway intubated with a smaller than usual endotracheal tube. Erosion of tracheal rings may cause airway collapse postoperatively and surgical stenting may be needed for such an airway. Good collaboration between the surgical and anaesthetic teams is essential.

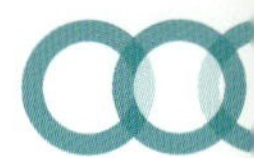

QUESTION 2

2 A capnogram is shown (**2**).

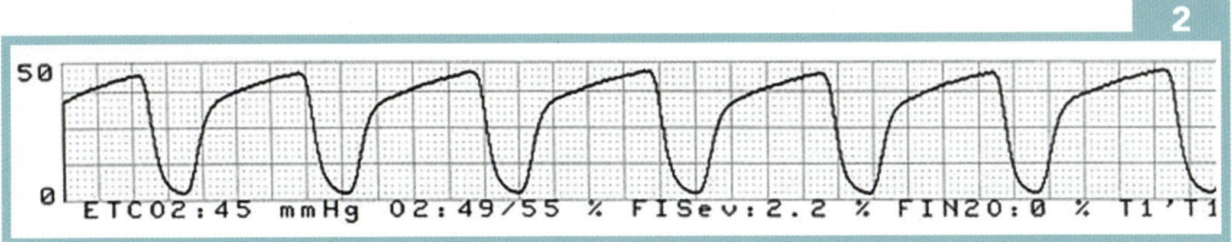

i. Identify the abnormality in the 'plateau' portion of the capnogram.

ii. Why might such an abnormality occur as a result of patient factors?

iii. What is the time constant of an alveolar unit, and why is it important to appreciate the meaning of the term time constant with an upsloping capnogram?

iv. Describe why a prolonged inspiratory pause would help to better match ventilation and perfusion in this patient.

Answer 2

2i. There is an exaggerated upslope in the plateau phase that is indicative of partial obstruction to flow and is a consequence of different time constants.

ii. This could either be patient generated (physiological – obstruction occuring in the smaller airways of patients with airway disease such as asthma and/or COPD) or equipment generated (physical – for example an obstacle [or resistance] to flow in the breathing circuit due to a kinked ET tube).

iii. It is the time it takes for an alveolus to empty or fill. Alveolar units (alveolus plus the conducting airways leading to the alveoli) in normal lungs have different time constants and can be relatively fast or slow. The time constant is rarely so long as to obstruct flow. In diseased lungs, abnormally long time constants can affect pathological alveolar units, which are difficult to fill with air. Two consequences result, normal ('fast') alveolar units have less obstruction, fill faster compared with abnormal units, receive more ventilation (hence lower CO_2 concentration), become overstretched and have a higher internal/alveolar pressure. Such alveoli will be overstretched, with 'too much' ventilation, and hence represent alveolar dead space (high V_A/Q ratio = lower CO_2 concentration.) They are also more likely to burst, causing a pneumothorax. Alveolar units with longer time constants have more obstruction in their conducting airways, receive less ventilation (hence higher CO_2 concentration), become less stretched and have a lower internal/alveolar pressure. These alveolar-capillary units are underventilated and contribute to shunt (low V_A/Q ratio = higher CO_2 concentration). The 'fast' alveoli (higher pressure with lower CO_2 concentration) will empty first, while the slower alveoli (lower pressure, higher CO_2 concentration) will empty last, thereby creating the upsloping capnograph trace.

iv. Increasing the duration of the inspiratory pause improves gas exchange by allowing alveolar units with fast time constants to equilibrate with those with slow time constants. Overstretched units have time to redistribute their air into underventilated units and better matching of ventilation and perfusion results.

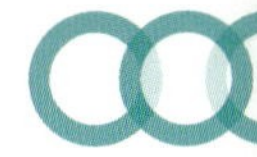

QUESTION 3

3 The hands of a woman in her late thirties, who is mentally slow and has been reluctant to seek medical advice, are shown (**3**). She has a history of many years of cold hands and complains of a feeling that her fingers are tight and turn white when they become cold. She presented to the hospital with concern about her fingers. She suffered severe pain in both hands approximately 3 weeks prior to presentation after being outside in cold weather for approximately 5 minutes without gloves. She lives in a temperate climate.

i. What condition does this patient have?

ii. What other symptoms and signs could be expected for this condition?

iii. What other associated conditions may be a source of concern for the anaesthesiologist?

iv. Would GA present a problem for this patient?

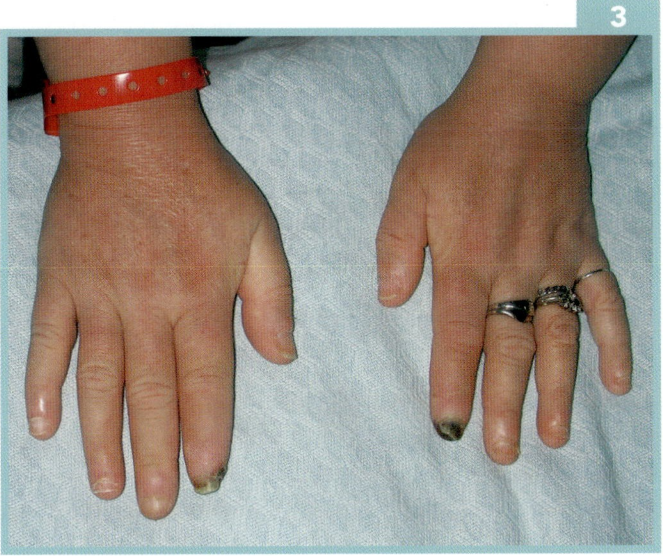

3

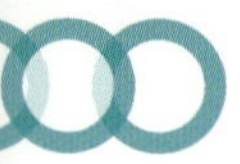

Answer 3

3i. Gangrenous fingertips. The duration of exposure to cold in a temperate climate is not long enough for frostbite and subsequent gangrene to have set in. The history of white fingers and cold hands for years suggests Raynaud's phenomenon.

ii. Spasm of the digital arteries and numbness, tingling and burning sensations predominantly in the fingers, but occasionally in the toes. Sensitivity to cold may be extreme and disabling. Colour changes in the digits occur and consist of three phases: pallor, due to vasospasm; cyanosis, due to sluggish blood flow; and redness associated with relaxation of the vasospasm and subsequent hyperaemia.

iii. The condition may be a manifestation of more serious connective tissue diseases such as scleroderma, SLE, rheumatoid arthritis, dermatomyositis, polymyositis, cold agglutinin syndrome, Ehlers–Danlos syndrome, anorexia nervosa, atherosclerosis, subclavian steal, Buergers syndrome, drug reactions (beta-blockers, some chemotherapeutic agents [bleomycin/cyclosporine]), occupational hazards (pneumatic drill operators, frozen food packers).

Ninety percent of patients with scleroderma experience Raynaud's phenomenon. It is also a component of the CREST (calcinosis, Raynaud's phenomenon, oesophageal dysmotility, sclerodactyly, telangectasia) syndrome. These patients have small vessel occlusive disease that may lead to digital pitting or ulceration. Later obliterative endarteritis may occur and result in thrombosis, ischaemic changes in the skin of the digits and nails, superficial necrosis and finally gangrene. Sudden onset renal failure or necrosis of the bowel may result from endarteritis. Rheumatology specialists should be consulted prior to a surgical procedure in a patient suspected of CREST syndrome.

iv. GA is not harmful but avoiding cold during operative procedures is important and vigilance is required for other preventable thrombotic problems. Stop smoking (or even use of a nicotine patch). Vasodilator therapy was started for this patient (calcium channel blocker, nifedipine). Infusions of prostaglandin E_1 or prostacyclin may be needed to treat severe digital ischaemia. In this case, surgical terminalisation of the fingers was not undertaken and the finger tips were left to slough off.

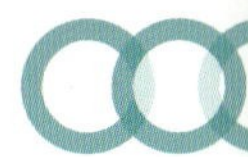

QUESTION 4

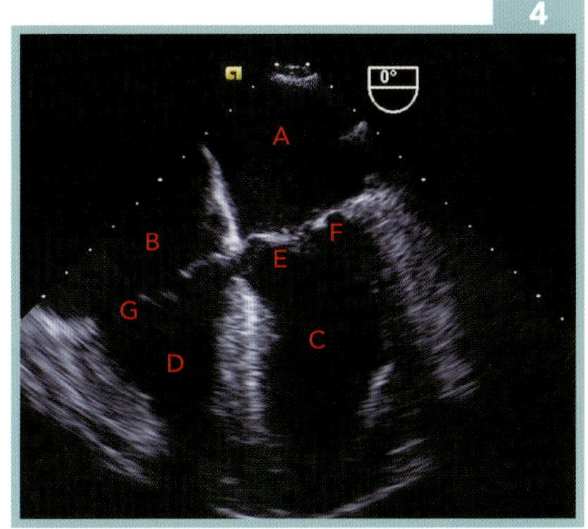

4 A TOE image is shown (**4**).

i. What is this view called?

ii. Which chambers are indicated by A, B, C and D?

iii. What structure is indicated by E and F? What subdivisions are indicated by E and F, respectively?

iv. What structure is indicated by G?

QUESTION 5

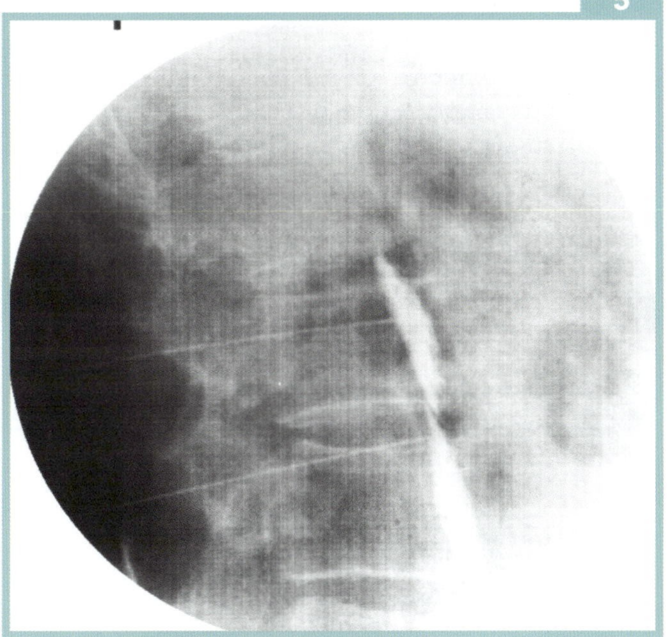

5i. What is shown in this image (**5**)?

ii. What are the likely causes of this condition?

iii. How do patients with this condition present?

iv. How can a patient be treated for the complications of this condition?

Answer 4

4i. The mid-oesophageal, four-chamber view.

ii. A = left atrium; B = right atrium; C = left ventricle; D = right ventricle.

iii. The anterior and posterior leaflets of the mitral valve.

iv. The tricuspid valve.

Answer 5

5i. It is a radiograph of a lumbar spine and demonstrates epidural fibrosis, shown by the poor spread of contrast injected into the epidural space, illustrating patchy fibrosis with loculation. There is occlusion around the nerve roots, in this case of L2/3.

ii. Likely causes of the occlusion include: congenital existence of fibrous raphes; failed back surgery (FBS) syndrome. FBS is a chronic pain syndrome that occurs after spinal surgery, including microdiscectomy, and can be caused by residual disc herniation, altered joint mobility with instability of the joint and chronic low level of disc content leakage or scar tissue at the site of operation; previous epidural anaesthesia; epidural infections including tuberculosis.

iii. The likely presentation of epidural fibrosis is with FBS syndrome. Symptoms are of a diffuse pain across the back and legs.

iv. FBS syndrome can be treated with: physiotherapy; NSAID (e.g. ibuprofen) and/or membrane stabilising (e.g. amitriptyline) medication; epidural steroids or local anaesthetic nerve root blocks; transcutaneous electrical nerve stimulation; intrathecal morphine pump; psychological support.

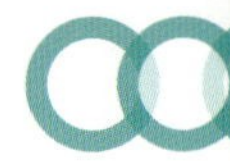

QUESTION 6

6 The man shown in **6a** fell heavily in a rural area and noted immediate, severe, left-sided chest pain, worsened by inhalation. At a rural hospital no fractured ribs or obvious pneumothorax were noted on CXR, but his O_2 saturations on air were 86%. Oxygen therapy was commenced, a chest drain was inserted at the left 5th intercostal space and he was airlifted to a trauma centre. The CXR performed on arrival at the trauma centre with the patient supine is shown (**6b**).

6a

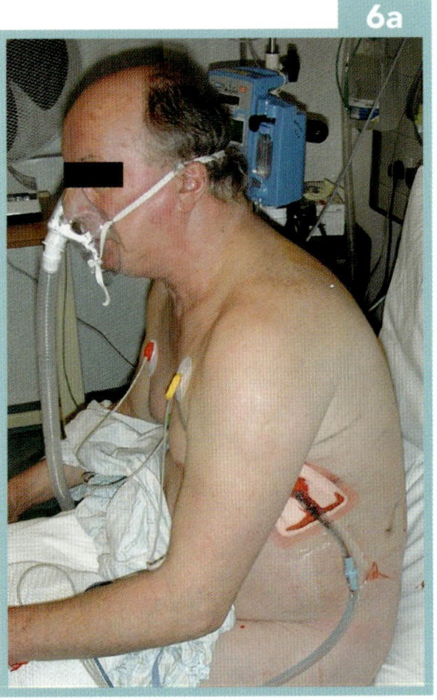

6b

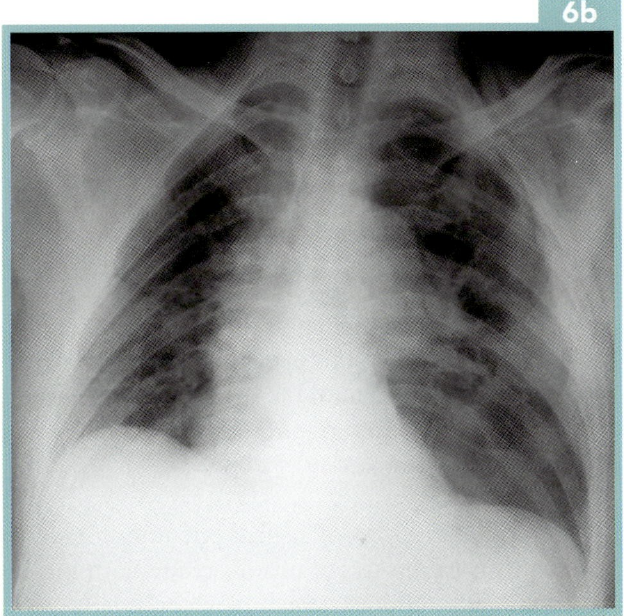

i. Does this man have a pneumothorax?

ii. What clinical sign is associated with the appearance of the CXR shown?

iii. Does the patient have a tension pneumothorax?

iv. What are the clinical signs of a tension pneumothorax?

v. Was it necessary to insert a chest drain before being transported by air, and if so why?

vi. Would GA also mandate a chest drain?

vii. Does the absence of rib fractures on the radiograph conclusively prove their non-existence?

Answer 6

6i. Yes, a pneumothorax is present but a supine film fails to show it.

ii. The radiograph shows subcutaneous emphysema, proving a communication between his lung and the underlying tissues; therefore, there must be a pneumothorax. Palpation around the chest wall reveals a crackling sensation.

iii. No, although the potential for one exists, especially after air transport.

iv. Tension pneumothorax is detected clinically by respiratory distress accompanied with the desire to sit up and forward, hyperresonance of the chest and absent breath sounds on the affected side. A deviated trachea on neck palpation (deviating to the opposite side from the lesion) is a late sign indicating marked mediastinal shift. Radiographic diagnosis is unnecessary and dangerous, as the patient may suffer cardiorespiratory arrest before the radiograph is obtained.

v. The pressure reduction associated with altitude may expand the pneumothorax, which may become clinically significant. The referring medical team correctly inserted a chest drain prior to air transport. A tension pneumothorax is life threatening and should be treated by decompressing the chest at the 5th intercostal space anterior to the mid-axillary line and positioning the chest drain cephalad within the thorax.

vi. Sudden expansion of a small pneumothorax is possible under GA. Positive pressure ventilation and use of nitrous oxide both increase the likelihood of expansion of the pneumothorax, which may 'tension'.

vii. The absence of rib fractures visible on a CXR proves nothing, especially if the CXR was taken in the supine position (typical for a trauma patient). The X-ray could have been taken when the rib ends were lying quite close together and the fractures are then not visible. This patient had very obvious fractures on palpation of the chest, but only one X-ray out of a series of five actually showed a fractured rib.

QUESTION 7

7 A 16-year-old 60 kg (132 lb) 180 cm (6 ft) patient is scheduled for scoliosis surgery with instrumentation from T4 to S1 (**7a**). The patient plays soccer at a competitive level and is a long distance runner. The surgeon has scheduled the surgery for 12 hours and has asked for a cross-match of 6 units of blood as well as for the cell saver. The surgery is completed (**7b**) and 4 units of blood plus 3 units of cell saver are transfused. Elective postoperative ventilation in an ICU is chosen because of swelling of the airways due to the prone position, prolonged surgery and the large fluid volumes needed for cardiovascular stability. Eight hours postoperatively the patient's back wound starts to bleed. Measured blood loss in the calibrated drains is 2,000 ml and blood replacement is in progress. The wound is still bleeding 2 hours later. Hb is 70 g/l (7 g/dl) and Hct 21%. The urine output was 0.5 ml/kg over the last hour. The surgeon requests emergency surgery to open up the wound to control the bleeding.

i. What are the letters ASA PS commonly used to classify in anaesthesia practice?

ii. Write down exactly what each class represents.

iii. What is the ASA classification of this patient preoperatively?

iv. What is the ASA classification of the patient 10 hours post surgery?

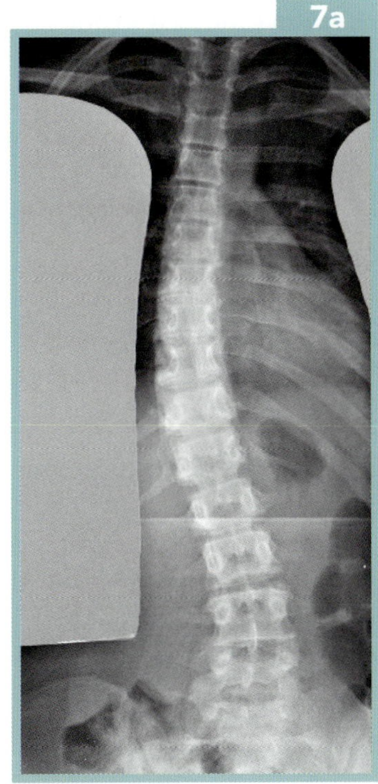
7a

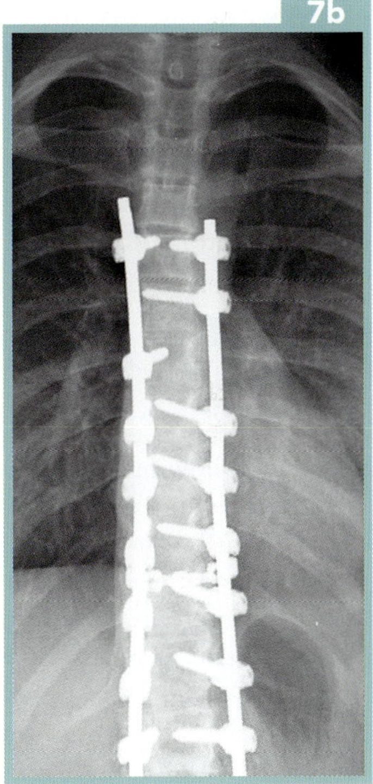
7b

QUESTION 8

8 What are the 10 indications for referral of a head injured patient to the neurosurgical unit?

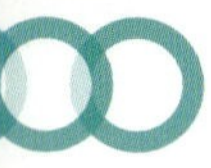

Answer 7

7i. American Society of Anesthesiologists Physical Status. The ASA classification was designed in 1963 in an attempt to classify patients according to their degree of abnormal physiology, with a scoring system known as the ASA Physical Status Index. It is used as an objective way of defining patient health before anaesthesia and surgery. It is also used as a means of retrospective review in patients who have either had a better than expected or worse than expected outcome from surgery.

ii. I = a normal healthy patient; II = a patient with mild systemic disease; III = a patient with severe systemic disease; IV = a patient with severe systemic disease that is a constant threat to life; V = a moribund patient not expected to survive without the operation; VI = a declared brain-dead patient whose organs are being removed for transplant purposes. The suffix E is added to indicate Emergency cases.

iii. ASA I. Note that the extent of the proposed major surgery does not have any bearing on the ASA status.

iv. ASA III E, by reason of the fact that the ASA status is worse than II, which is 'mild systemic disease', but the ASA status is not yet 'life threatening' as the urine output is still reasonable. The patient requires surgery as an emergency, hence the E designation.

Answer 8

8 The following 10 features in a patient with a head injury should be discussed with a neurosurgeon:

- A CT scan that shows a recent intracranial lesion.
- The patient fulfils the criteria for CT scanning but this cannot be done within an appropriate period.
- Persisting coma (GCS 8/15 or less) after initial resuscitation.
- Confusion that persists for more than 4 hours.
- A deterioration in the level of consciousness after admission determined by a deteriorating GCS. A sustained drop of one point on the motor or verbal subscales, or two points on the eye opening subscales of the GCS are sufficient. Neurosurgeons appreciate hearing the components of the score rather than a simple number. An accurate description of the GCS is ideal.
- Progressive focal neurological signs.
- A seizure without full recovery.
- Compound depressed skull fracture.
- Definitive or suspected penetrating injury.
- A CSF leak or other sign of a basal fracture (Battle's sign, bruising behind the ears or bilateral periorbital haematomas [Panda eyes]).

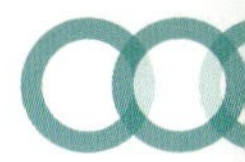

QUESTION 9

9 A patient is brought to the operating room for cardiac surgery with an intra-aortic balloon pump in place. The monitor displays the arterial wave form shown (**9a**).

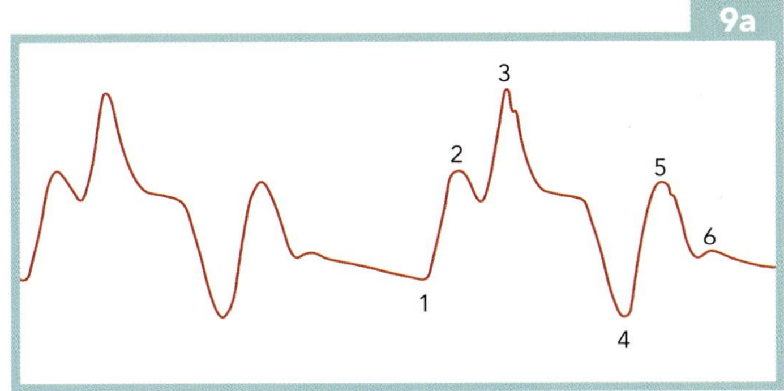

i. Match the following labels with the appropriate peak or trough on the trace: peak systolic pressure (PSP), assisted peak systolic pressure (APSP), dicrotic notch (DN), patient aortic end-diastolic pressure (PAEDP), balloon aortic end-diastolic pressure (BAEDP) and peak diastolic pressure (PDP).

ii. Identify which of the following parameters is improperly set: balloon inflation or balloon deflation?

iii. Also identify if the parameter is too early or too late.

iv. Identify the assist ratio.

v. What action should be taken? Explain your answer.

QUESTION 10

10 The Pin Index Safety System is shown (**10**).

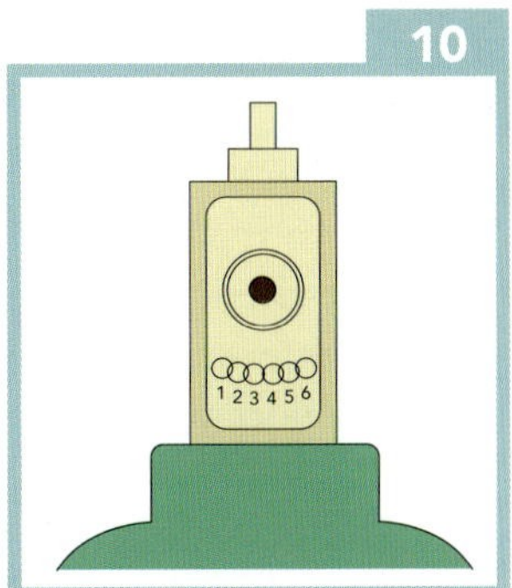

i. What is this?

ii. Using the numbers shown, what are the pin configurations for: O_2, N_2O, CO_2 and air?

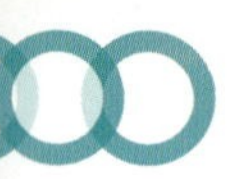

Answer 9

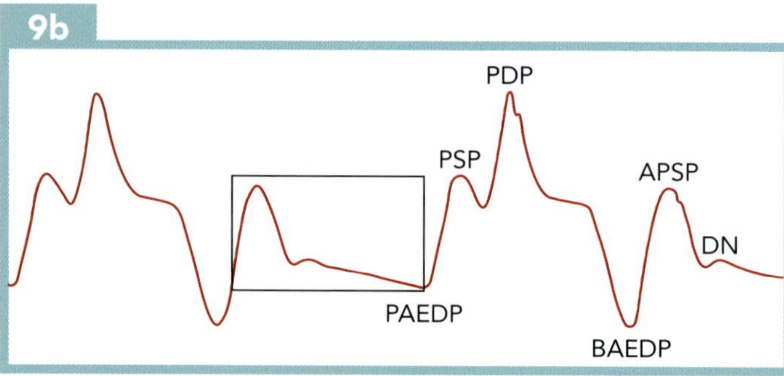

9i. The labels for each peak are shown (**9b**) and are as follows: 1 = PAEDP; 2 = PSP (produced by the patient's heart only); 3 = PDP; 4 = BAEDP; 5 = APSP (patient's heart, assisted by balloon pump); 6 = DN.

ii. Balloon inflation is improperly set.

iii. Balloon inflation is set too early.

iv. The arterial wave form (**9a**) demonstrates intra-aortic balloon pumping in a 1:2 assist ratio. The balloon cycles (inflation and deflation) once for every two patient systoles. This setting allows identification of landmarks on the patient's arterial trace to guide timing settings.

v. The appropriate action is to delay inflation until it occurs just prior to the DN. A normally timed balloon on 1:2 assist ratio is demonstrated in **9b**. The patient-generated arterial upstroke is shown in the boxed area. The PSP and APSP peaks are produced by the patient systolic ejection. PDP is a result of balloon inflation in diastole. BAEDP is a result of balloon deflation just prior to systole. Trace **9a** demonstrates early inflation of the balloon. The goal of balloon inflation is to produce a rapid rise in aortic diastolic pressure, thereby increasing oxygen supply to coronary circulation. Balloon inflation should occur just prior to the DN of the arterial wave. Properly timed inflation will result in a PDP greater than PSP. Early balloon inflation results in premature closure of the aortic valve. This reduces stroke volume and cardiac output.

Answer 10

10i. There is a specific pin configuration for each medical gas on the yoke of the anaesthetic machine. The matching configuration of holes on the cylinder valve block ensures that only the correct gas cylinder can be fitted in the yoke. The gas exit port will not seal effectively unless the pins and the holes are aligned.

ii. The pins are at the following positions for the gases shown: O_2 = 2 and 5; N_2O = 3 and 5; CO_2 = 1 and 6★; air = 1 and 5. (★ = no longer fitted to anaesthetic machines.)

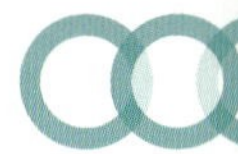

QUESTION 11

11 Draw an exponential process (e.g. the wash-out [clearance] of nitrogen from the lungs during preoxygenation).

i. Give a definition of the half-life of an exponential process.

ii. Give a definition of the time constant of an exponential process.

iii. For a given exponential process, which takes the longer time to reach: half-life or time constant?

iv. Give examples of exponential processes where half-life or time constants are relevant for:
- The cardiovascular system.
- The respiratory system.
- The hepatic system.
- The anaesthetic system.

QUESTION 12

12 A 64-year-old man presents for repair of an abdominal aortic aneurysm. He has previously undergone a cardiac surgery. Following uneventful induction of anaesthesia a TOE probe is inserted to monitor ventricular function. The four-chamber image obtained is shown (**12**).

i. What is the diagnosis?

ii. What should be done?

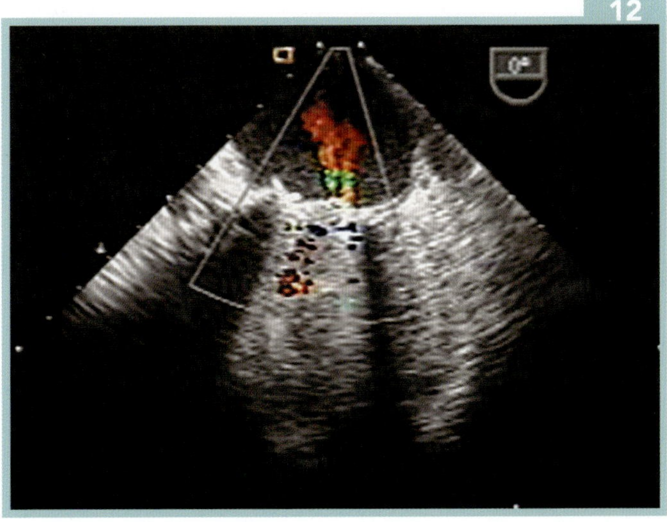

12

Answer 11

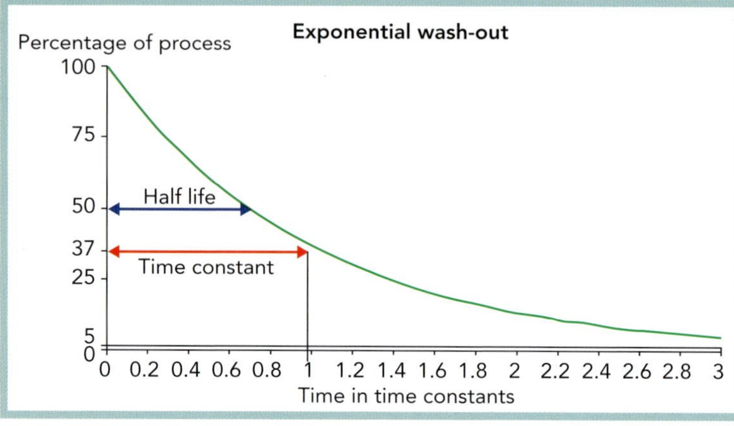

11 A diagram of an exponential process is shown (**11**).

i. The time it takes for the process to be 50% completed.

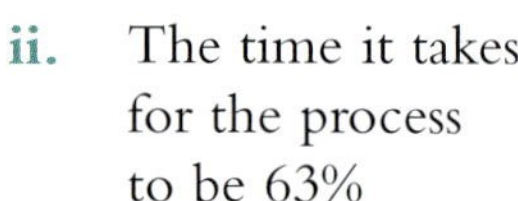

ii. The time it takes for the process to be 63% complete. A second definition is: the time the process would have been completed had the initial rate of change been maintained.

iii. The half-life takes only 50% of the process time, while the time constant needs 63% of the time to completion. The time constant is 1.44 times longer than the half-life.

iv.
- Cardiovascular: diastolic run-off, thermodilution and other cardiac output measurements, mixing of an injected agent with the blood.
- Respiratory: filling and emptying of the lungs during breathing, wash-in of volatile anaesthetic agents during induction, wash-out of nitrogen during pre-oxygenation.
- Hepatic: metabolism/clearance of medications and toxins from the blood.
- Anaesthetic system: wash-in of volatile agent into the circle breathing system.

Answer 12

12i. This is a transverse image obtained with an omniplane TOE transducer at 0°. The left atrium can be seen at the top of the image, with two posteriorly directed narrow colour Doppler jets. The left ventricular cavity is obscured. This patient has undergone a previous mitral valve replacement with a St. Jude bi-leaflet prosthesis. These valves normally have two small central regurgitant jets. Any regurgitant jets visible outside the sewing ring of the prosthetic valve would be abnormal and would indicate a perivalvular leak.

ii. No action should be taken since this image indicates normal prosthetic valve function.

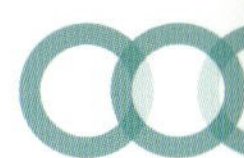

QUESTION 13

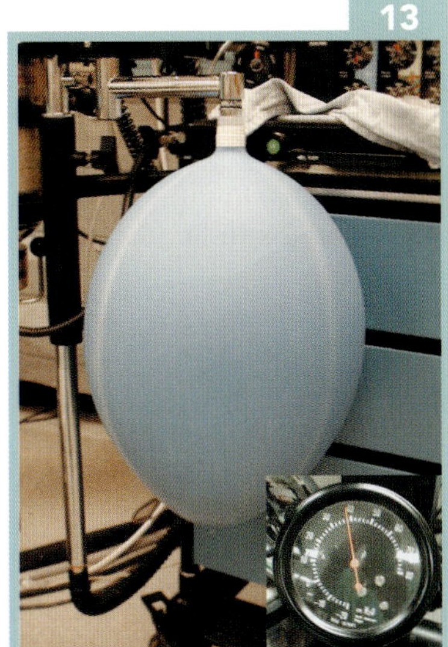
13

13 A patient has just been intubated. End-tidal CO_2 and bilateral breath sounds have been confirmed and the anaesthesia team is taping the endotracheal tube in position.

i. What should the anaesthesia team do next (two possibilities) to resolve this overinflation of the anaesthesia reservoir bag (**13**)?

ii. If the APL (adjustable pressure relief valve) ('pop-off valve') is set at 70 cmH_2O, what is the maximum pressure that can be generated in the breathing system?

iii. The anaesthesia reservoir bag is designed to allow only a certain maximum pressure to minimize barotrauma. What is this range of pressures?

iv. What is plastic deformation (in contrast to elastic deformation)?

v. List five functions of the anaesthesia reservoir bag?

QUESTION 14

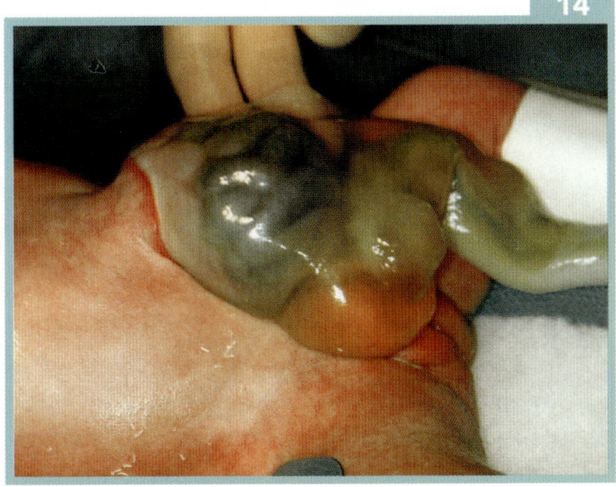
14

14 You are called to the neonatal ICU to evaluate this child (**14**) for surgery.

i. What is this neonate's diagnosis? Describe the embryology.

ii. How does this differ from gastroschisis?

iii. What are your anaesthetic concerns?

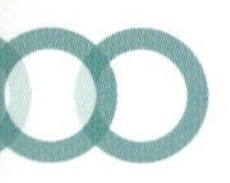

Answer 13

13i. Either leave the pop-off (APL) valve in a closed (high pressure) pop-off position, or do not switch to a mechanical ventilation mode on the anaesthesia machine.

ii. The maximum pressure inside the huge reservoir bag and breathing system is designed to be less than 60 cmH_2O. In this case it is 40 cmH_2O.

iii. The reservoir bag is designed to limit the pressure build-up to less than 50–60 cmH_2O.

iv. Plastic deformation is the phenomenon whereby the bag will increase in volume ('stretch') without significant increase in pressure. This is in contrast to elastic deformation (more common [e.g. rubber band or spring]) where continuously increasing recoil (pressure) is generated as the stretch (volume) increases.

v. It collects a continuous flow of fresh gas for intermittent use such as spontaneous breathing or controlled ventilation by hand; it allows continuous low fresh gas flow rates to be used for intermittent high-flow requirements; it enables controlled ventilation by hand; it gives a visual indication of spontaneous breathing: rate, tidal volume, pattern (I:E ratio, expiratory pause); it provides a safety factor against high pressures in the breathing system ('fail safe').

Answer 14

14i. This child has an omphalocele. An omphalocele results from failure of the gut to return to the abdominal cavity from the yolk sac. It presents at birth as an intestinal herniation covered by a membranous sac from which the umbilical cord arises.

ii. Intestinal herniation lateral to the umbilicus, secondary to occlusion of the omphalomesenteric artery, is called gastroschisis and does not have a membranous covering. An omphalocele, unlike gastroschisis, is often associated with other congenital defects, including Beckwith–Wiedmann syndrome (macroglossia, hypoglycaemia, polycythemia) and cardiac anomalies.

iii. A difficult intubation should be anticipated. ECMO will identify possible cardiac septal defects and/or shunting. IV fluid resuscitation must occur as dehydration is common. Cover the bowel in a plastic wrap to help maintain temperature and minimise insensible fluid loss. Induce anaesthesia with a rapid sequence induction or awake intubation. On reduction of the eviscerated bowel a dramatic increase in intra-abdominal pressure may occur, resulting in impaired ventilation and decreased perfusion to abdominal organs or lower extremities. A staged surgical reduction may have to be carried out with the bowels placed in a Silon pouch and reduced over a period of several days.

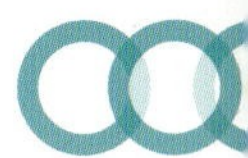

QUESTION 15

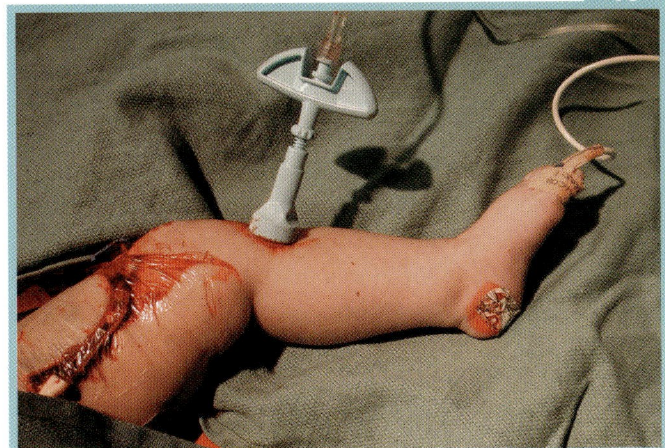
15

15i. What is this device (**15**)?

ii. What are the indications for its use, and who can it be used on?

iii. Name the preferred sites for cannulation.

iv. What tests can be performed on samples obtained from this route?

v. What fluids, blood products and medications can be administered via this apparatus?

vi. List the contraindications to its use.

vii. List some of the complications of its use.

QUESTION 16

16

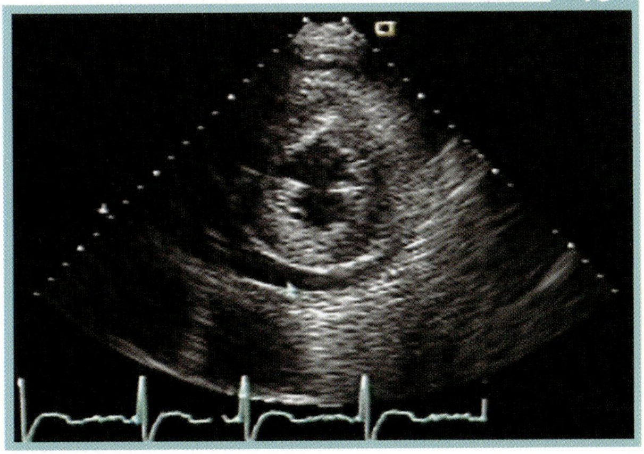

16 A 57-year-old female is scheduled to undergo a laparoscopic cholecystectomy. She complained of a recent viral illness. She has noted some mild shortness of breath, but has been afebrile. Upon induction of anaesthesia with propofol, her BP drops precipitously and is very difficult to support despite fluid boluses and vasopressor support. After stabilising the patient, a TOE is performed (**16**).

i. What is the diagnosis?

ii. What should be done?

Answer 15

15i. An intraosseous (IO) needle. The device is shown correctly placed. A femoral vein cannula has been added. Initially, the illustrated child was too shocked to obtain venous access and the IO needle was life saving.

ii. An IO needle is designed to administer resuscitative fluids if IV access is inadequate. Historically it was only used in children, but since 2005, improvements in the device characteristics have allowed IO access to become an acceptable, safe alternative to IV access in adults and is mentioned in ATLS guidelines.

iii.
- Proximal tibia: anteromedial surface, 2–3 cm below the tibial tuberosity.
- Distal tibia: proximal to the medial malleolus. **Note:** In a child, the IO needle must not be placed into the epiphyseal growth plate above the tibial tuberosity.
- Distal femur: midline 2–3 cm above the external condyles.
- Iliac crests may be used, although are not the preferred route. If possible, areas that are infected should be avoided.

iv. Bone marrow can be aspirated through the device and subsequently sent for FBC (CBC), cross-match and BUN and electrolyte concentrations. Laboratory staff must be informed that the sample is bone marrow, otherwise auto-analysing equipment may be damaged.

v. Crystalloid fluids, blood products and many drugs may be administered via the IO route. Fluids must be actively injected, as they will not run freely from a standard infusion giving set. Drugs reach the central circulation in less than 20 seconds.

vi. Contraindications include ipsilateral fracture and ipsilateral vascular injury, as injected fluids will extravasate from the injury site. Osteogenesis imperfecta is a rare contraindication where bone is deficient in osteocytes and fractures occur easily. Permanent deformities may result from IO needle placement in this condition.

vii. Complications include extravasation/subperiosteal infusion, osteomyelitis/local infection, skin necrosis, compartment syndrome and fat and bone microemboli.

Answer 16

16i. The TOE transgastric short-axis image of the left ventricle shows a large amount of fluid in the pericardial space (i.e. a large pericardial effusion). The ventricular cavity does not appear underfilled. The patient's BP fell following induction due to a decrease in ventricular preload and worsening tamponade.

ii. The cholecystectomy should be cancelled. Pericardiocentesis or a pericardial window should be considered in consultation with the cardiac surgery team.

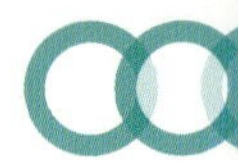

QUESTION 17

17 This image (**17**) shows the oxygen–haemoglobin dissociation curve.

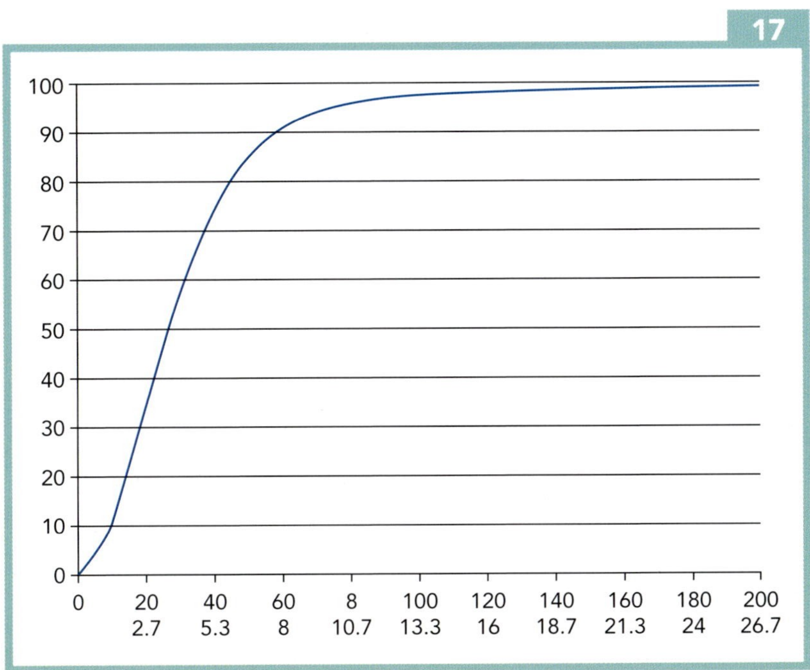

i. What values are on the x-axis (abscissa)?

ii. What values are on the y-axis (ordinate)?

iii. List four factors that will shift the curve to the right. Three of these factors are products of metabolism.

iv. Why would it be advantageous (useful) for these factors to shift the curve to the right?

QUESTION 18

18i. Define systemic inflammatory response syndrome (SIRS).

ii. Define sepsis.

iii. Define septic shock.

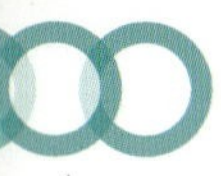

Answer 17

17i. Partial pressure of oxygen in mmHg/kPa.

ii. Saturation (0–100%). The y-axis might also be expressed as oxygen content. When the Hb level is 15 g/100 ml the scale runs from 0–20 ml oxygen/100 ml blood.

iii. Increases in H^+ (acidosis), CO_2, temperature and 2-3 di-phosphoglycerate.

iv. A right shift of the oxygen–haemoglobin dissociation curve increases O_2 release from haemoglobin molecules. Note that increased delivery (unloading) of oxygen is aided by products of increased metabolism so that local metabolism (see iii) increases O_2 supply without increasing cardiac output.

Answer 18

18i. SIRS is characterised by two or more changes in body temperature, respiratory rate, heart rate or white cell count precipitated by a pathological cause (see Table below).

Signs of SIRS	Precipitating causes
Any two or more of the following: • Hyperthermia >38.3°C (100.9°F) or hypothermia <36°C (96.8°F) • Acutely altered mental status • Tachycardia >90 bpm; tachypnea >20 bpm • Leukocytosis (>12,000 μl^{-1}) or leukopenia (<4,000 μl^{-1}) or >10% bands • Hyperglycaemia (>6.7 mmol/l [120 mg/dl]) in the absence of diabetes	Infection Intestinal endotoxin Ischaemia Multiple trauma Noxious substances Pancreatitis Shock Thermal injury

ii. Sepsis is SIRS caused by a documented (e.g. known bacteraemia) or highly suspected infection (e.g. appearance of intra-abdominal abscess on CT scan).

iii. Septic shock is sepsis complicated by organ failure (see Table below) and hypotension that is unresponsive to a fluid challenge.

Affected organ	Signs of organ failure
Brain	Confusion
Lungs	Hyperventilation (respiratory rate >20). Hypoxaemia (acute lung injury defined as PO_2/FIO_2 ratio <40 kPa/300 mmHg)
Heart	Heart rate >90 bpm
Circulation	BP <90 mmHg (or 20 mmHg below 'normal' for that patient) that is unresponsive to a 20 ml/kg IV fluid bolus
Kidneys	Urine output below 0.5 ml/kg/hour. Raised urea and creatinine

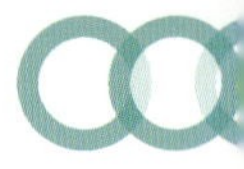

QUESTION 19

19 Pressure gauges for oxygen (**19a**) and nitrous oxide (N_2O) (**19b**) are shown.

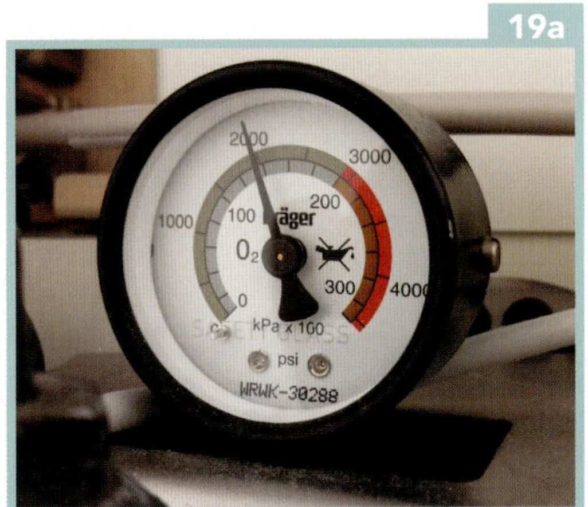

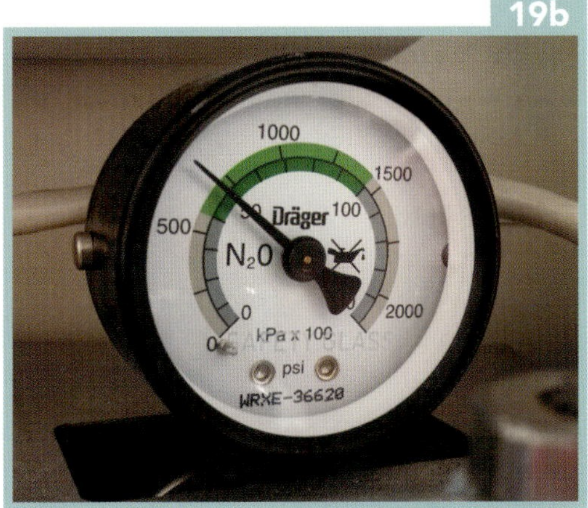

i. Is it possible for the oxygen and N_2O cylinders to both be 'full' even though the pressures differ?

ii. Why does a full N_2O cylinder (with a lower pressure) contain more molecules of gas/vapour than a full oxygen cylinder (with a higher pressure)?

iii. Do the pressure gauges indicate how much of the contents remain? Explain why or why not. The fact that N_2O is not an ideal gas at room temperature explains this. What is an ideal gas, and why is N_2O not ideal at room temperature?

iv. Will the cylinder pressures change with altitude and temperature?

v. What percentage of N_2O content remains when the delivered pressure starts to decrease?

vi. Will the N_2O cylinder explode (burst) when the cylinder temperature goes above 36.5°C (98°F)? Why/why not?

vii. What is special about the temperature of 36.5°C (98°F) in relation to N_2O?

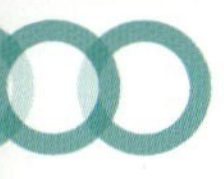

Answer 19

19i. Oxygen is a true gas at room temperature, N_2O is a vapour, so an oxygen cylinder is 'full' when filled to a pressure of 2,000 psi (13,700 kPa). The pressure inside a N_2O cylinder is determined by the saturated vapour pressure (SVP), which is 735 psi (4,400 kPa) at room temperature (21°C/60°F). The N_2O cylinder has to be weighed to determine when it is 'full' (typically about 75–90% of the internal volume is filled with liquid N_2O).

ii. The liquified N_2O (and N_2O vapour in the cylinder) is packed more densely than the gaseous oxygen.

iii. The pressure gauge on the oxygen cylinder gives a direct (accurate) measurement of the amount of oxygen remaining in the cylinder: when half the oxygen is used, the pressure will halve. Boyle's Law is applicable. Boyle's Law for an ideal gas is only applicable for a gas above its critical temperature and pressure. Boyle's Law states:

$$P1 \times V1 = P2 \times V2 \text{ at a constant temperature}$$

The pressure inside the N_2O cylinder is determined by the SVP. As long as there is a single drop of liquid N_2O remaining in the cylinder, the pressure will be constant (at 735 psi [4,400 kPa]). N_2O is below its critical temperature (50°C [122°F]) at room temperature. An ideal gas is one that obeys the 'ideal gas laws' of volume, pressure and temperature, therefore because at room temperature N_2O can be liquefied by pressure, it will not have a constant relationship of pressure and volume at this temperature and is not an ideal gas until it is heated above 50°C (122°F).

iv. With altitude, no; with temperature, yes. For oxygen, Charles' Law is applicable:

$$P1/T1 = P2/T2 \text{ for a constant volume}$$

For N_2O, SVP increases with increases in temperature in a non-linear fashion.

v. One-eighth (0.125%) of the contents of the N_2O cylinder remains when the pressure starts to decrease (after the last liquid drop of N_2O has vaporised).

vi. The N_2O cylinder will not burst when the temperature exceeds the critical temperature (when all liquid N_2O turns gaseous) because a gas or vapour close to the critical temperature and pressure does not follow ('obey') the ideal gas law and is much more compressible (due to Van der Waal's Forces on intermolecular attraction).

vii. N_2O has a critical temperature of 36.5°C (98°F) so it will be a mixture of liquid and vapour below this temperature. It will only be totally gaseous above the critical temperature.

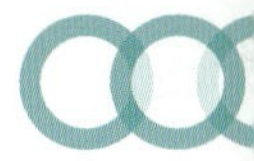

QUESTION 20

20 This 24-year-old man has presented in the emergency department with pain and swelling around his neck (**20**). He is confused and his BP is 75/40 mmHg. His white cell count is 23 × 10^9 cells/mm^3 and he has a temperature of 39°C (102.2°F).

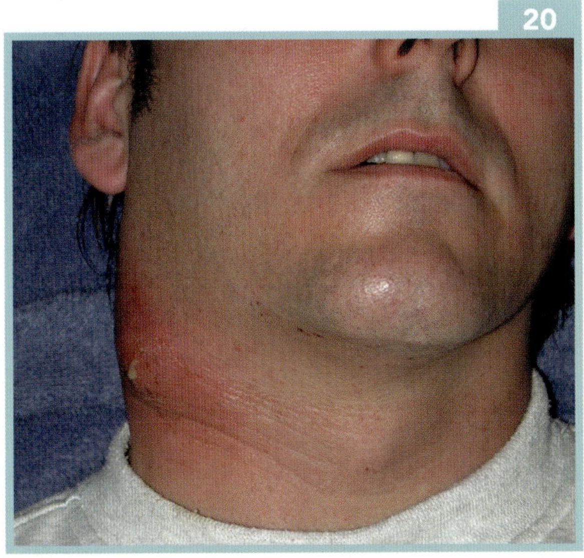

20

i. Would you define this man's condition as sepsis, severe sepsis or septic shock?

ii. What six tasks should occur within the first hour of presentation?

iii. Why is anaesthesia challenging for this patient?

iv. How would you anaesthetise him?

Answer 20

20i. He has sepsis because he has SIRS with infection. The sepsis is severe, as he has signs of organ failure (confusion), but there is insufficient information to say whether he has septic shock. If his BP is unresponsive to a 30 ml/kg bolus of crystalloid solution (e.g. Hartmanns solution) given over the first 3 hours of treatment, he has septic shock.

ii. The six tasks, known as the Sepsis Six (Survive™ Sepsis campaign), are: give high-flow oxygen; take blood cultures; give antibiotics; start IV fluid resuscitation (often large volumes, as much as 10–20 ml/kg are needed over the 1st hour); check haemoglobin level and venous lactate (Hb should be >70 g/l [7 g/dl] and lactate should be <4 mmol/l [36 mg/dl]); monitor accurate urine output.

iii. Anaesthesia is challenging in this patient for two reasons:

- The systemic effects of the abscess as a septic focus. Further resuscitation must be weighed against the urgency of taking the patient to the operating room. Until the abscess is drained, he may not fully recover; therefore, after initial resuscitation surgery is required without delay.
- The physical effects of the abscess. Although appearing to discharge outwards onto the skin, deeper tissues of the neck may be involved. The abscess may suddenly discharge into the airway, leading to an aspiration of abscess contents and subsequent aspiration pneumonia. Fistulation may form into the trachea or oesophagus, which can have unexpected effects with positive pressure ventilation. The mass effect of the abscess could obstruct the airway from within.

iv. After resuscitation, patient anaesthesia should start with inhalational induction with an agent such as sevoflurane. This is safer than an IV (rapid sequence) induction, as the airway may suddenly obstruct upon onset of paralysis if the abscess is large and compressing the trachea. The airway can be inspected when the patient is deeply asleep and then either intubated under deep inhalational anaesthesia or a muscle relaxant given when it is clear that the airway can be maintained. Endotracheal intubation should be performed as soon as possible to prevent contamination of the airway by abscess rupture. Surgery can then continue safely. Postoperative care could be complicated because of the presence of severe sepsis and ICU or high-dependency admission should be arranged.

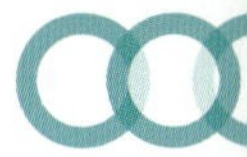

QUESTION 21

21 A CXR is taken (**21a**) of an 18-year-old front seat passenger in a car travelling at 45 mph (70 kph) that has collided with a tree. He was not wearing a seat belt and the airbag only partially inflated.

21a

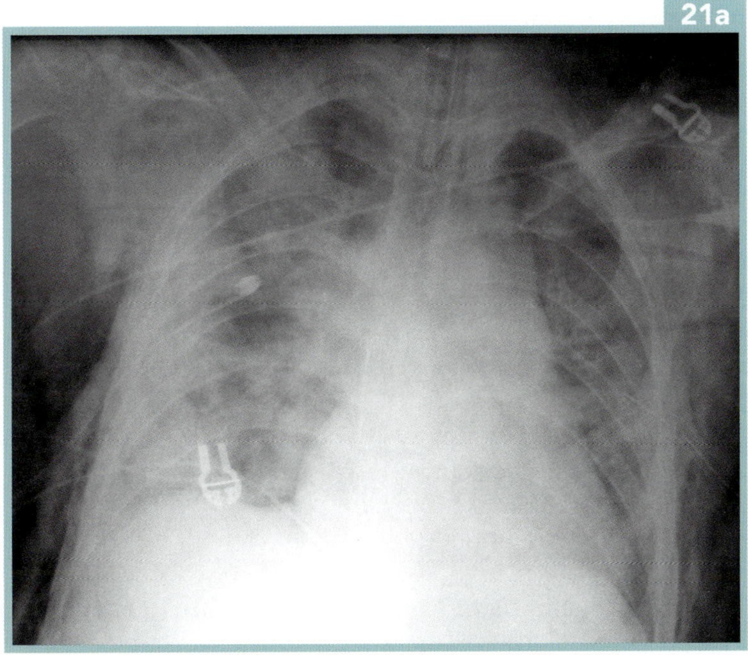

i. How would likely injuries be predicted?

ii. What are the immediate priorities when dealing with this patient?

iii. What does the radiograph show?

iv. What other investigation needs to be carried out to confirm or refute the potentially life-threatening provisional diagnosis?

Answer 21

21i. The mechanism of injury predicts likely pathology. Severe injuries (head, neck, thorax, abdomen, pelvis and limb) can be sustained by an unbelted front seat passenger who collides with the dashboard of the car at 40 mph (64 kph). Expulsion from the vehicle increases mortality by 300%.

ii. Airway, breathing and circulatory stabilisation should be established along ATLS guidelines as the X-rays are being taken. The CXR shows important signs for subsequent definitive management.

iii. A widened mediastinum (with abnormal contour), depression of the left mainstem bronchus and a small left-sided pleural cap (an area of opacity over the top of the lung parenchyma at the lung apex) all suggest a ruptured aorta. Other features on the CXR are:

- Hardware, multiple lines, ECG electrodes.
- Widespread subcutaneous emphysema suggesting pneumothorax.
- The left pleural drain is inadequate. Only a few centimetres of drain are inside the chest and a drain orifice appears to be at the skin. The drain needs to be re-sited deeper within the chest.
- A right-sided pleural drain is in place.
- Bilateral pulmonary contusions.

iv. Urgent aortic angiography and a cardiac/thoracic surgical opinion is required. Chest CT to diagnose aortic rupture is less invasive than angiography, but an angiogram should determine the precise site of the aortic tear. This patient's angiogram (**21b**) shows a typical tear (arrow) at the junction where the ductus arteriosis existed embryologically and inserts into the aorta alongside the superior aspect of the pulmonary artery. This is the weakest point along the aortic arch. Only the adventitial layers are preventing a massive bleed from this point of the rupture.

21b

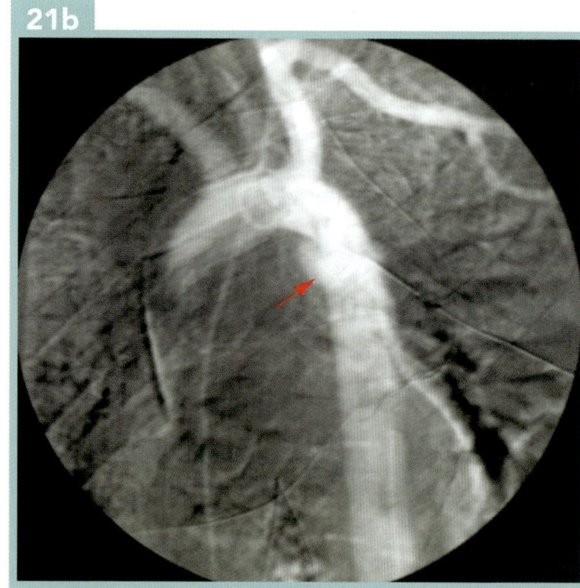

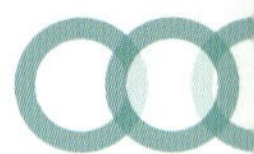

QUESTION 22

22 This lady (**22**) has presented to internal medicine with worsening of chronic shortness of breath. She reports that she has had 'heart trouble' for some time and has refused heart surgery due to anxiety. You have been asked to see her to sedate her for treatment of her breathlessness.

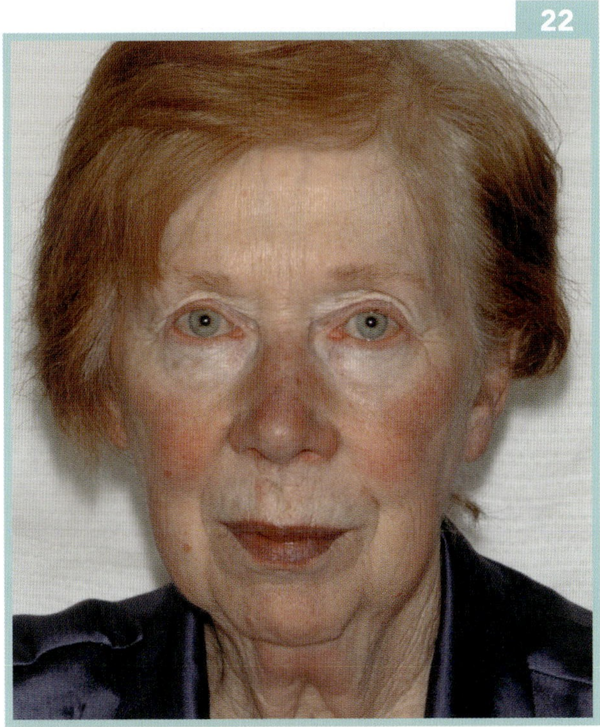

i. What kind of heart lesion does her facial appearance suggest, and why does this happen?

ii. What heart sounds would you expect to hear, and what other symptoms are associated with her 'heart problem'?

iii. What could cause her unexpected breathlessness?

iv. What treatment do you think requires sedation?

v. What surgical procedures has this patient refused?

vi. Had she presented with an acute abdomen, what principles should be employed to maximise her cardiovascular safety?

Answer 22

22i. The patient shows classical mitral facies due to severe advanced mitral stenosis. This 'malar flush' is thought to be associated with increased blood CO_2 levels due to pulmonary hypertension.

ii. Mitral stenosis is characterised by a loud opening snap with a mid-diastolic rumbling murmur loudest at the apex of the heart without radiation. Symptoms include blood-tinged frothy sputum and the symptoms of right heart failure because of persistent pulmonary hypertension (e.g. peripheral oedema including ankle swelling and hepatomegaly). Significant hepatic engorgement will lead to liver dysfunction in extreme cases.

iii. A sudden drop in cardiac output (in this case, the onset of AF) has caused her breathlessness. Other causes of decompensation are due to the increased cardiac demands of pregnancy, infection or metabolic disease (e.g. thyroid dysfunction). Atrial contraction contributes 40% of left ventricular filling in mitral stenosis (compared with 15–20% normally). When AF occurs, sudden cardiac decompensation can occur due to loss of the atrial kick.

iv. Electrical cardioversion of her new onset AF, the cause of her breathlessness.

v. Likely to be either a mitral valvotomy or open heart surgery for mitral valve replacement.

vi. Estimates of mitral valve area by transthoracic ECHO reliably indicate the severity of mitral disease. A normal adult mitral valve's cross-sectional area ranges from 4 to 6 cm^2. Stenosis is graded as mild (1.5–2.5 cm^2), moderate (1.1–1.5 cm^2) or severe ($\leq$1 cm^2). When anaesthetising someone with mitral stenosis, several features are important to maintain cardiac output:

- Heart rate is the primary consideration and should be maintained within the normal range. Bradycardia markedly reduces cardiac output because the stroke volume is limited by the stenotic valve. Tachycardia is even more detrimental to cardiac output as there is insufficient time for left ventricular diastolic filling due to the stenotic valve.
- Pulmonary oedema can develop suddenly if AF occurs or worsens with a rapid ventricular response. This must be treated aggressively (e.g. with cardioversion and/or an amiodarone bolus dose). Fluid balance should be carefully managed by giving enough to maintain left ventricular preload/stroke volume but not so much as to cause pulmonary oedema. Digoxin may control the ventricular rate of atrial arrhythmias.
- Monitoring pulmonary artery pressures with TOE and treating factors that increase it (e.g. hypercarbia, hypoxia, nitrous oxide) is important. A CVP line is also helpful to detect signs of right ventricular failure and for administering drugs rapidly to the heart.

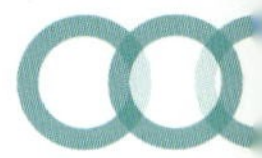

QUESTION 23

23 This 32-year-old man (**23**) is admitted after an incident. He is conscious. Respiratory rate is 24, pulse 110 and his BP is 95/50.

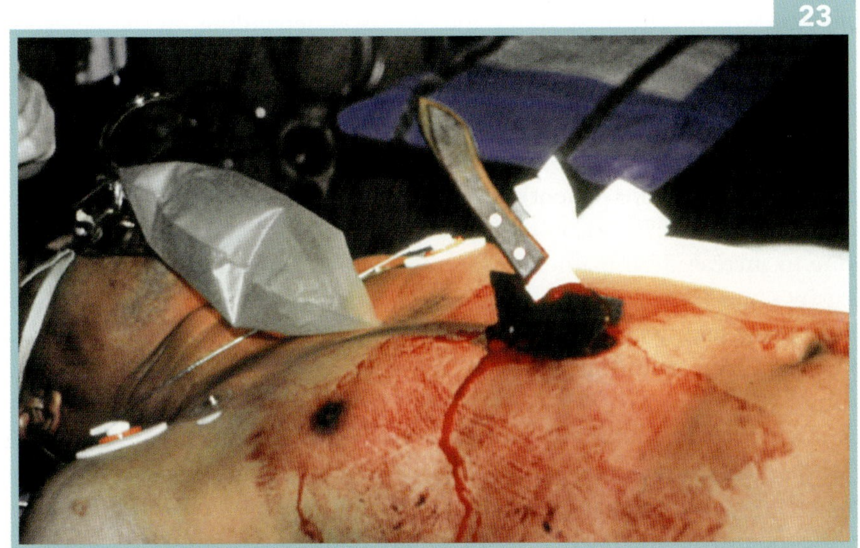

23

i. How would you categorise this patient's shock?

ii. Describe each category of shock and outline how you would treat each one.

iii. What six life-threatening thoracic injuries could this man have, which must be picked up in the primary survey prior to anaesthesia?

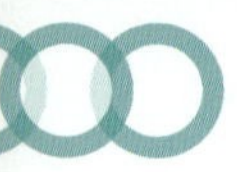

Answer 23

23i. He is stabbed in the chest and is correctly receiving high-flow oxygen through a trauma mask. He is conscious (implying a systolic BP >50 mmHg). He is in class 3 haemorrhagic shock as defined by the American College of Surgeons ATLS guidelines, which categorise shock into 4 classes depending on the percentage of blood volume lost by an adult patient.

ii.
- Class 1 (0–15%, 0–750 ml blood loss). Vital signs remain stable. Observe for potential further bleeding, especially if the source of bleeding is unclear. Make a surgeon aware of the patient's presence and rule out other injuries.
- Class 2 (15–30%, 750–1,500 ml blood loss). Characteristically, diastolic BP rises (due to increased sympathetic tone causing vasoconstriction), pulse pressure narrows and tachycardia occurs. This stage may not occur in elderly patients or in those taking certain medications (e.g. beta-blockers). Patients are usually anxious. Urine output is reduced. This is a potentially serious blood loss and a fluid challenge of 1,000–2,000 ml of Hartmann's solution should be given through two large bore (16 gauge) IV catheters. A surgical opinion is essential as further blood loss is likely and surgical or radiological/angiographic intervention may be required to stem bleeding. The patient must be observed for further evidence of haemorrhage, as he may only transiently respond to fluids.
- Class 3 (30–40% 1,500–2,000 ml blood loss). Systolic BP drops and tachycardia is marked. Air hunger with a raised respiratory rate is expected. Immediate administration of up to 2,000 ml of warmed Hartmann's given in 250 ml boluses is warranted to attempt restoration of systolic BP to approximately 90 mmHg until surgical control of bleeding is achieved. This should be followed by O-negative blood if BP remains unstable. Urgent surgical intervention is required to stop bleeding. Higher systolic BPs will exacerbate haemorrhage and administered fluids will dilute coagulation factors. Care must be taken to give enough, but not excessive, IV fluid until surgical control is reached. Thereafter, normal vital signs are desirable.
- Class 4 (40%, >2,000 ml blood loss). This is immediately life threatening. A patient needs surgical control of bleeding within minutes. Temporary restoration of volume should be attempted but this should not delay the start of surgery. Resuscitation and surgery should occur simultaneously.

iii. Airway obstruction; tension pneumothorax; large haemothorax, large open pneumothorax; flail segment; cardiac tamponade. All of the above could be present in this patient except flail segment (exclusively due to blunt trauma). In addition to intrathoracic damage, the abdominal cavity can extend up to the nipples, thus this injury is highly likely to have affected abdominal structures (e.g. liver, stomach, pancreas, spleen and bowel).

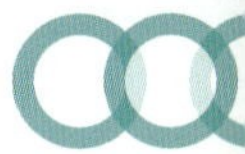

QUESTION 24

24 A 22-year-old male student has been admitted for elective excision of impacted molars under GA. At the preoperative assessment he states that on occasions he feels his heart pounding in his chest and he has mild breathlessness when this happens. His ECG is shown (**24**).

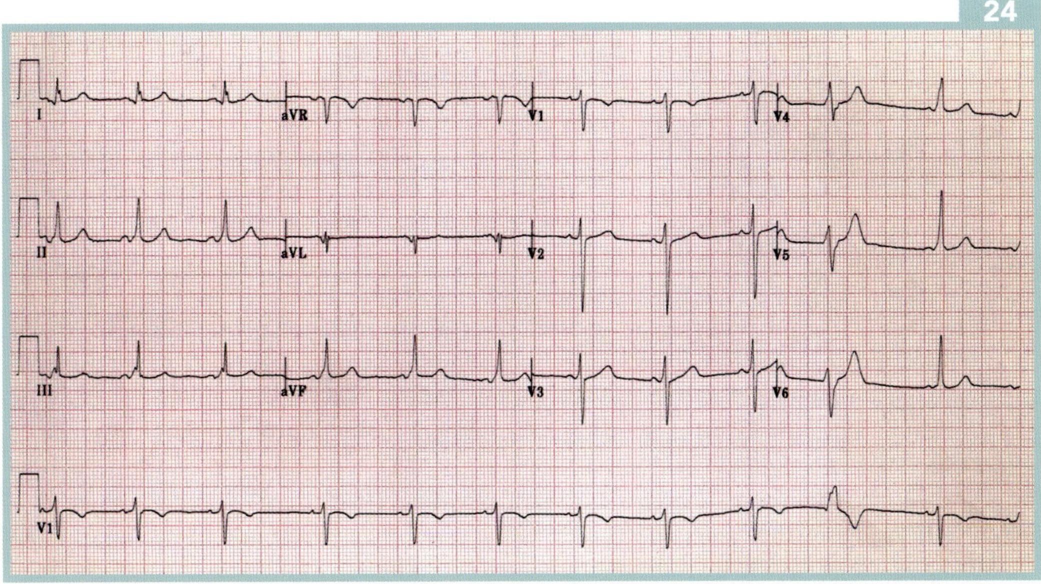

i. What does the ECG show?

ii. Should surgery proceed without any further action?

iii. If emergency surgery was required, how would anaesthetic management be modified to minimise risk, and how would the arrhythmia be managed?

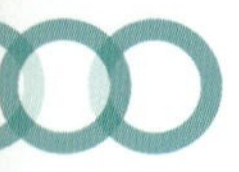

Answer 24

24i. Features of Wolf–Parkinson–White (WPW) syndrome. WPW is caused by an accessory pathway (the Bundle of Kent) which, when activated, causes a fast re-entrant tachycardia between the atria and the ventricles (i.e. a paroxysmal supraventricular tachycardia). Paroxysmal atrial flutter/fibrillation (PAF) is the commonest presentation of WPW but exceptionally, syncope and even death may result if the tachycardia is so rapid that ventricular filling fails. The ECG signs are a short PR interval and delta-shaped R waves that can be seen in leads II, III and aVF as well as V4–6.

ii. No. The operation is not an emergency and should be postponed until a cardiology opinion is obtained. Symptomatic WPW is best treated with radiofrequency cardio-ablation therapy and this should be done prior to elective surgery. Pharmacological treatment is also possible with Singh–Vaughan Williams Class Ia, Ic or III drugs.

iii. For emergency procedures, the condition has to be tolerated. Sympathetic stimulation makes acute paroxysmal atrial tachycardia more likely, so sympathomimetic drugs or excessive patient anxiety should be avoided. Antiarrhythmic medication should be continued. Adequate doses of an IV induction agent, supplemented with opioids or with a bolus of IV lidocaine, prior to direct laryngoscopy prevents excessive laryngeal sympathetic nervous system stimulation and the associated risk of tachyarrhythmias. Ketamine should be avoided. Amiodarone or procainamide are recommended for the treatment of PAF in patients with WPW. Both drugs increase the refractory period of the accessory pathways. Other antiarrhythmics, such as adenosine, verapamil, beta-blockers and digoxin, should not be used as they may increase the ventricular response during the dysrhythmia by suppressing the normal AV conduction pathways and accelerating conduction in the accessory AV pathway. If a tachyarrhythmia becomes life threatening during the perioperative period, emergency electrical cardioversion should be available.

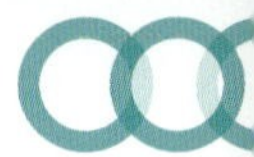

QUESTION 25

25 The vital signs chart for a 62-year-old man scheduled for laparoscopic cholecystectomy are shown (**25**). He was seen at a preoperative assessment unit 2 weeks ago. His BP at the clinic was 160/100, so he was told to present to the hospital the day before surgery for BP assessment. He started taking bendroflumethiazide (2.5mg orally) 2 months ago but has failed to attend for BP checks since. He has had morning headaches for the last 2 weeks.

i. Define hypertension.

ii. Comment on the BP readings on the chart.

iii. Would you proceed with operation on the next day? Justify your answer.

iv. What recommendations would you make with regard to his immediate BP management?

25

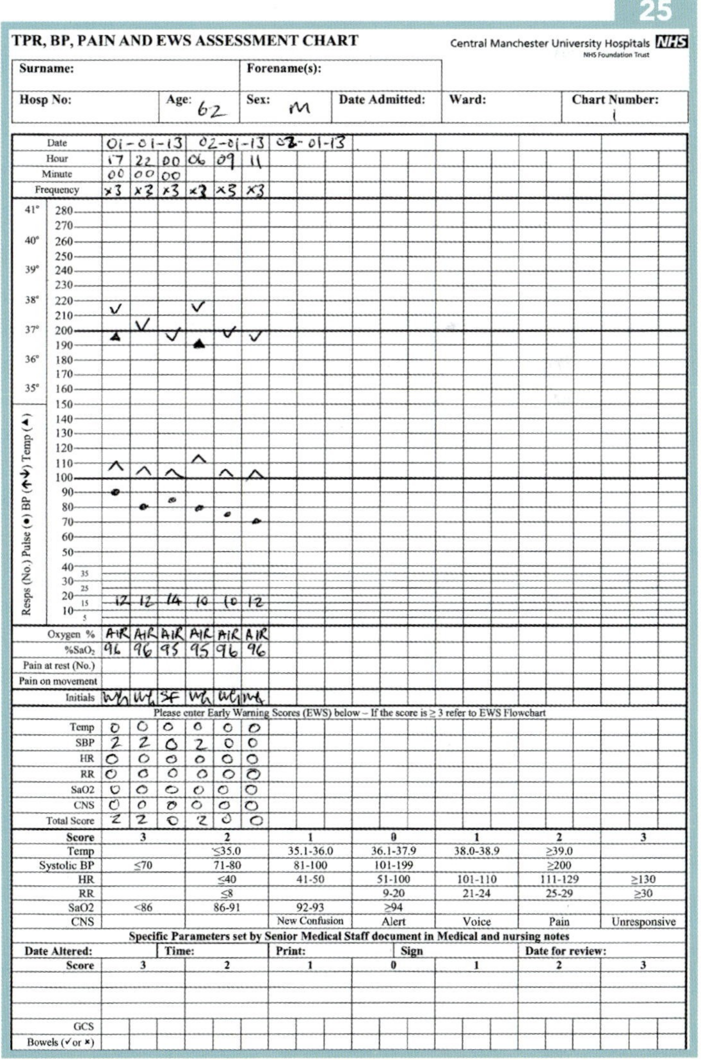

TPR, BP, PAIN AND EWS ASSESSMENT CHART Central Manchester University Hospitals NHS Foundation Trust NHS

Surname:		Forename(s):			
Hosp No:	Age: 62	Sex: M	Date Admitted:	Ward:	Chart Number: 1

Date	01-01-13			02-01-13			03-01-13
Hour	17	22	00	06	09	11	
Minute	00	00	00				
Frequency	×3	×3	×3	×3	×3	×3	

Oxygen %	AIR	AIR	AIR	AIR	AIR	AIR
%SaO_2	96	96	95	95	96	96
Pain at rest (No.)						
Pain on movement						
Initials	WH	WH	SF	WH	WG	MG

Please enter Early Warning Scores (EWS) below – If the score is ≥ 3 refer to EWS Flowchart

Temp	0	0	0	0	0	0
SBP	2	2	0	2	0	0
HR	0	0	0	0	0	0
RR	0	0	0	0	0	0
SaO2	0	0	0	0	0	0
CNS	0	0	0	0	0	0
Total Score	2	2	0	2	0	0

Score	3	2	1	0	1	2	3
Temp		≤35.0	35.1-36.0	36.1-37.9	38.0-38.9	≥39.0	
Systolic BP	≤70	71-80	81-100	101-199		≥200	
HR		≤40	41-50	51-100	101-110	111-129	≥130
RR		≤8		9-20	21-24	25-29	≥30
SaO2	<86	86-91	92-93	≥94			
CNS			New Confusion	Alert	Voice	Pain	Unresponsive

Specific Parameters set by Senior Medical Staff document in Medical and nursing notes

Date Altered:	Time:	Print:	Sign	Date for review:		
Score 3	2	1	0	1	2	3

GCS

Bowels (✓or ×)

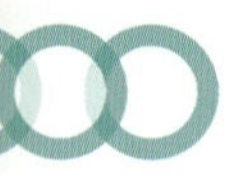

Answer 25

25i. Hypertension is defined by the UK National Institute of Clinical Excellence (NICE) 2011 Guidelines (categories in the USA are very similar, as described by the Center for Disease Control) in three stages:

- **Stage 1 hypertension.** Clinic BP is 140/90 mmHg or higher **and** subsequent ambulatory BP monitoring (ABPM) daytime average or home BP monitoring (HBPM) average BP is 135/85 mmHg or higher.
- **Stage 2 hypertension.** Clinic BP is 160/100 mmHg or higher **and** subsequent ABPM daytime average or HBPM average BP is 150/95 mmHg or higher.
- **Severe hypertension.** Clinic systolic BP is 180 mmHg or higher **or** clinic diastolic BP is 110 mmHg or higher.

ii. This chart shows severe hypertension as BP is between 210/110 and 195/105 for three consecutive readings, correctly done half an hour apart. Although with increased familiarity of the hospital surroundings and the procedure of having BP checked the hypertension may fall, this patient should continue to have half hourly BP checks for the rest of the day.

iii. With this level of hypertension, his surgery cannot go ahead until he is stabilised. He has severe hypertension complicated by symptoms (headache) and should remain in hospital and be seen by a hypertension specialist. Further investigations are needed to determine any end-organ damage (e.g. ECG, ECHO, FBC, urea, electrolytes, liver function tests, coagulation tests). If severe spikes of BP are seen, a 24-hour urine collection should be commenced and urinary vanillylmandelic acid and metanephrins measured to investigate for phaeochromocytoma. Plasma metanephrins, though sensitive to picking up phaeochromocytoma, are less specific than the urinary tests.

iv. With a diastolic BP <110 mmHg, postponing surgery is controversial. This man has hypertension above this and needs treatment. He is at risk of a hypertensive crisis. Without symptoms, such as headache or visual disturbances or end-organ changes (e.g. renal insufficiency or left ventricular hypertrophy with strain), surgery could be considered up to and including an arbitrary diastolic BP of 110 mmHg, which was suggested by a small but well quoted study, and subsequent meta-analysis of studies in perioperative risk in hypertensive patients corroborated this guidance. This patient should have additional antihypertensive medication started (either calcium channel blockers or beta-blockers, but not both).

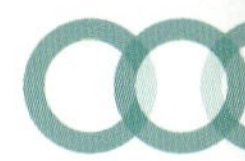

QUESTION 26

26 The molecule structure of a muscle relaxant drug is shown (**26a**).

26a

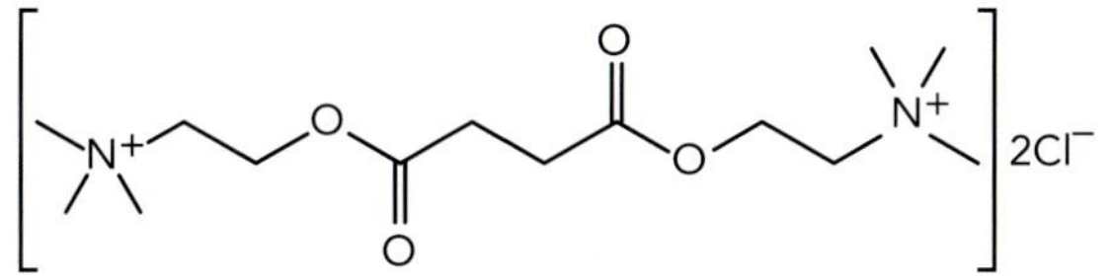

i. What is the drug?

ii. How does this drug work?

iii. Why is it short acting? Explain why, rarely, in some individuals it can last for a long time.

iv. Can this drug be used within 24 hours of a 30% body surface area burn?

v. What risks are associated with this drug in the burned patient?

vi. After a burn, is the patient more or less sensitive to non-depolarising muscle relaxants? Why?

Answer 26

26i. Suxamethonium (succinylcholine), which consists of two molecules of acetylcholine (ACh) joined by an ester link (shown as the red circle in **26b** and **c**). This structure (**26b**) gives rise to its neuromuscular blocking properties.

ii. ACh binds to the neuromuscular junction discharging the neuromuscular end plate causing muscle stimulation. Rapid metabolism occurs by acetylcholinesterase (in the synaptic cleft), breaking ACh down into inactive choline and acetate. Suxamethonium mimics ACh by depolarising the muscle membrane but then prevents repolarisation of the muscle membrane, thus 'blocking' the neuromuscular junction.

iii. Suxamethonium has an ester link (**26c**) (i.e. two carbon molecules joined by an oxygen molecule) (red circle in **26b**). This link is vulnerable to hydrolysis by plasma pseudocholinesterase, a ubiquitous enzyme in the blood. The breakdown of suxamethonium is therefore rapid in patients with normal levels of plasma cholinesterase. In rare cases, patients may have a deficiency of plasma cholinesterase, thus prolonging the action of suxamethonium. These conditions are: severe malnutrition or liver disease; drugs (e.g. anticholinesterases, chlorpromazine, echothioptate eye drops); genetically atypical plasma cholinesterases unable to metabolise the drug.

iv. Yes. The immediate risks of suxamethonium used in burned patients relate to a potentially difficult intubation.

v. Suxamethonium administered to facilitate intubation after a major burn can induce dangerous hyperkalaemia, but this effect takes several days to develop. The drug can be used within 24–72 hours of the injury. Beyond 72 hours and particularly between 9 and 60 days post burn, cardiac arrest from hyperkalaemia is likely. This occurs due to a proliferation of extrajunctional ACh receptors in and around the burned tissue, which when stimulated by suxamethonium cause a sudden large efflux of potassium ions into the bloodstream. Similar neuromuscular junction abnormalities and effects exist in patients with muscular dystrophies or paraplegia.

vi. Following a major burn, patients are relatively resistant to non-depolarising muscle relaxants because of an increase in the number of ACh receptors as described above. The response to muscle relaxants is abnormal for several months, and can persist as long as there are still large areas uncovered by the skin graft.

26b

$CH_3C(=O)OCH_2CH_2{}^{+}N(CH_3)_3$

26c

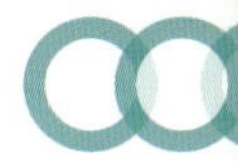

QUESTION 27

27i. How might these blood-stained swabs ('laparotomy sponges' and '4 by 4s') (**27**) be helpful in estimating intraoperative blood loss?

ii. List at least five static and/or dynamic methods of estimating blood loss.

27

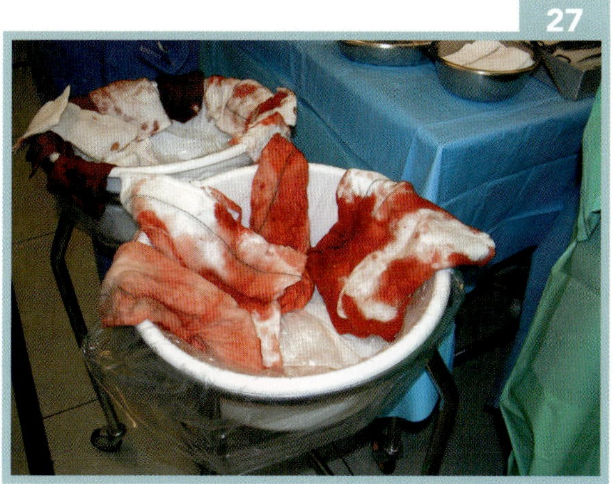

QUESTION 28

28 The base of a human skull is shown (**28**). The three arrows indicate a different foramen in the skull.

i. What are the three different foramina indicated by each coloured arrow called?

ii. Name the common structure that has branches that pass through each foramen and name each branch.

iii. Why is this anatomy important for an anaesthesiologist to understand?

iv. What practical procedure necessitates the passage of a needle through the foramen marked with the red arrow?

28

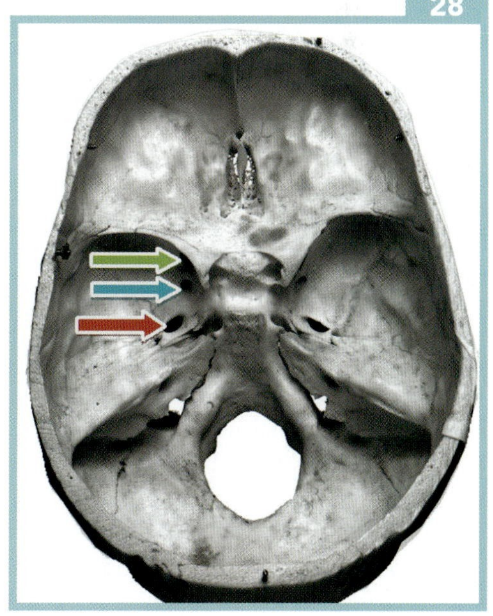

Answer 27

27i. Bloody swabs are weighed and blood loss estimated assuming that 1 ml of blood weighs 1 g. This is approximate, since the average specific gravity of RBCs is 1.0293 and of plasma 1.0270. Swabs should be weighed as soon as possible after removal from the field to minimise evaporative loss. This method is simple and widely used, but it generally underestimates blood loss by about 25%, representing unmeasured loss onto drapes, gowns, floor, etc. Volumetric means of measurement of loss (e.g. into suction containers) may also be recorded, but alone they have been found to have a very large error margin.

ii.
- CVP monitoring is believed to indicate a qualitative assessment of blood loss, since a decrease in central pressure indicates a deficit between circulating blood volume and volume of vascular bed. However, recent studies are questioning this assumption.
- In the trauma patient, estimation may be guided by site of injury; for example, a closed femoral fracture with moderate thigh swelling might be associated with up to 2 litres of blood loss. Changing cardiovascular parameters and skin and vital organ perfusion can give a rough indication of the extent of blood loss.
- Historically, colourimetric methods have been described whereby blood-stained swabs, gowns, etc, are washed in a known volume of solution. The haemoglobin concentration of this solution is then determined colourimetrically. This method has been shown to be no more accurate than the gravimetric method (weighing swabs).
- Dynamic variables such as pulse pressure variation due to controlled respiration have been shown to provide a more accurate reflection of the blood volume (preload) status of a patient.
- Advanced mathematical analysis of the peripheral arterial pulse wave form (e.g. Vigileo and FloTrac, Edwards LifeSciences™) has also been shown to indicate the status of the peripheral vascular resistance, which is also a dynamic indicator of the effective blood volume.

Answer 28

28i. Green arrow = superior orbital fissure; blue arrow = foramen rotundum; red arrow = foramen ovale.

ii. The trigeminal nerve, which has three branches: ophthalmic, maxillary and mandibular. Each branch passes through the respective foramen as listed above.

iii. The anatomy of the foramen ovale must be known in order to use regional anaesthesia for the treatment of intractable trigeminal neuralgia pain.

iv. The entire trigeminal nerve can be blocked by injecting local anaesthetic through the foramen ovale under radiological control.

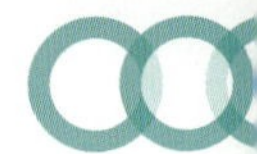

QUESTION 29

29i. Define chronic post-surgical pain.

ii. Describe how chronic post-surgical pain may occur and the risk factors for it.

iii. What is the incidence of chronic post-surgical pain in common operative procedures?

iv. How can this pain be prevented?

QUESTION 30

30 A 59-year-old man has ischaemic cardiomyopathy and worsening cardiac function. He is scheduled for insertion of a left ventricular assist device as a bridge to cardiac transplantation. On initiation of assist pumping and separation from cardiopulmonary bypass (CPB), the patient's oxygen saturation drops precipitously.

i. What are possible causes of this problem?

ii. A TOE probe is in place and shows this image (**30**). What is the diagnosis?

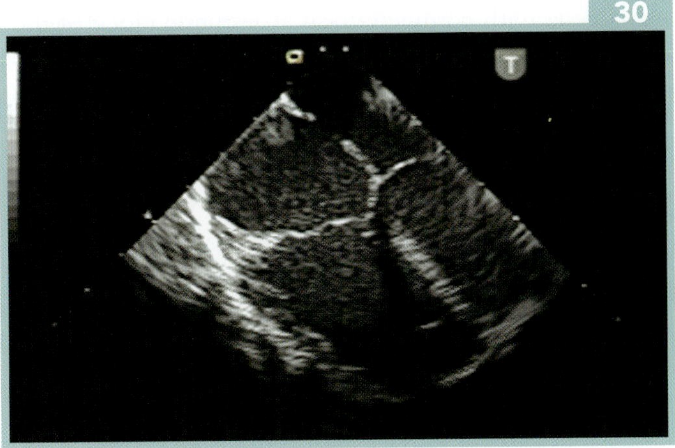

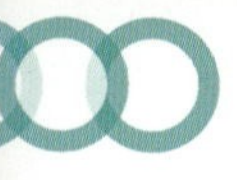

Answer 29

29i. Although relatively common, there is no universally acknowledged definition of chronic post-surgical pain. Most clinicians define it as pain developing after a surgical procedure; of at least 2 months duration; when other causes (e.g. malignancy/infection) have been excluded; or when pain from a pre-existing condition has been excluded.

ii. A peripheral nerve injury can lead to increased sodium channel expression causing increased sensitivity in pain fibres. These sensitised primary afferent nerves discharge spontaneously to increase glutamate release from nerve endings, which then act on glutamate receptors to trigger pain impulses, reduce pain thresholds and increase the effects of peripheral stimuli. A number of factors are thought to influence the development of the condition: pre-existing pain; genetic variability (single nucleotide polymorphisms coding for the catechomethyl-transferase enzyme are associated with the development of chronic pain conditions); and psychosocial factors such as severe fear of surgery or a history of depression/anxiety.

iii. Variable, depending on the surgery that has been carried out. Post-thoracotomy has the highest incidence (up to 50%), closely followed by vasectomy under GA. Breast surgery has a reported incidence of 30–35% and chronic postoperative pain levels with herniorrhaphy and lower uterine segment caesarean section scar pain ranging from 5 to 20%.

iv. The only proven method of preventing neuropathic pain from elective surgery is pre-emptive analgesia with complete local anaesthetic block of the affected nerves. This must be instigated prior to the first trauma and maintained for some hours postoperatively.

Answer 30

30i. Causes include failure to ventilate the patient as CPB is terminated, inadequate inspired oxygen concentration, pulmonary oedema, pulmonary embolus, patent foramen ovale (PFO) and atrial septal defect (ASD).

ii. The image is a four-chamber view, which reveals an ASD approximately 1 cm in size. Left ventricular assist devices fill by draining blood from either the left ventricular apex or left atrium. The presence of an ASD (or PFO) allows systemic venous blood to enter the assist device while bypassing the lungs. This results in a right-to-left shunt. Severe hypoxemia usually results. Closure of the ASD is necessary to remedy this problem.

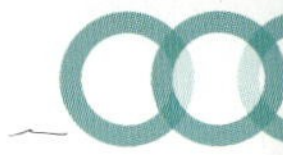

QUESTION 31

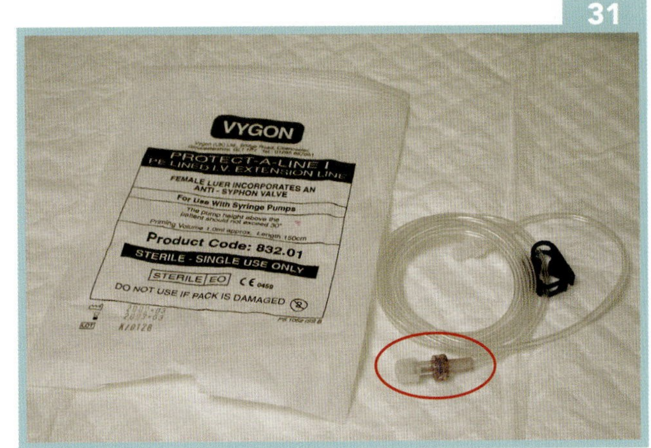

31

31i. What feature is highlighted in this patient-controlled analgesia (PCA) giving set (**31**, circle)?

ii. Why is it important?

iii. What problems are commonly associated with the use of PCA machines?

QUESTION 32

32 A 52-year-old man with emphysema is scheduled for release of a Dupuytren's contracture in his right hand under regional blockade. He has developed a 'frozen shoulder' and is unable to abduct the arm adequately to perform an axillary block. An alternative block is decided and a cross-sectional view of the arm at the site for this block is shown (**32**).

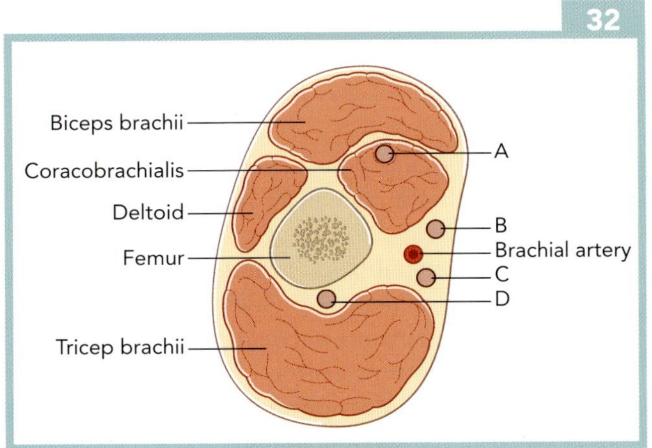

32

i. What is the name of this alternative regional block?

ii. Name each of the nerves labelled.

iii. Which of these nerves is commonly missed with the axillary block?

iv. Describe the movements you would anticipate on stimulation of each of these nerves.

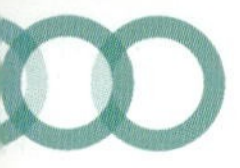

Answer 31

31i. An anti-siphon valve, or anti-flowback valve.

ii. If a syringe pump with standard giving set is placed above the level of the patient's right heart, a siphoning effect can develop, leading to potential rapid emptying of the syringe contents into the patient's intravenous line. Fatalities have resulted from this.

iii.
- Patients may not understand how to use the machine because of difficulty pressing the button (e.g. elderly patients, patients with learning difficulties).
- Patients may be physically unable to use the machine (e.g. arthritis affecting hand joints).
- Trained staff must be available to programme the device and monitor patient safety.
- Without a background infusion, patients might awaken in pain after a period without administering a PCA bolus.
- As a high-tech system, PCA is subject to potentially fatal errors. Human errors can occur in making up syringe contents or in programming the machine. As with all machinery, technical errors could, but rarely, occur.
- Adequate numbers of the machines must be available.

Answer 32

32i. A mid-humeral block.

ii. A = musculocutaneous nerve; B = median nerve; C = ulnar nerve, D = radial nerve.

iii. The musculocutaneous nerve. It emerges from the brachial plexus above the usual puncture site for an axillary nerve.

iv. The mid-humeral block is performed at the level of the insertion of deltoid muscle. Each nerve can be identified individually with a nerve stimulator:
- Musculocutaneous nerve: flexion of the elbow, supination of the forearm.
- Median nerve: pronation of the forearm, flexion of the lateral three fingers, flexion and adduction of the thumb; flexion and abduction of the wrist radially.
- Ulnar nerve: flexion and abduction of the wrist in an ulnar direction, flexion of the medial two fingers.
- Radial nerve: extension of the elbow, extension and abduction of the wrist radially, extension of the fingers.

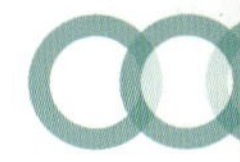

QUESTION 33

33 A plethoric 48-year-old man with severe ischaemia of his right foot scheduled for below knee amputation is shown (**33**). He smokes 40 cigarettes per day and suffers occasional tight chest pain that he has never reported. His haemoglobin (Hb) level is 190 g/l (19 g/dl).

i. What is the most likely diagnosis?

ii. Why does plethora occur?

iii. Why is it important to note his plethora, and how would you investigate it?

iv. What other diagnoses would you consider?

v. How should he be prepared for surgery?

33

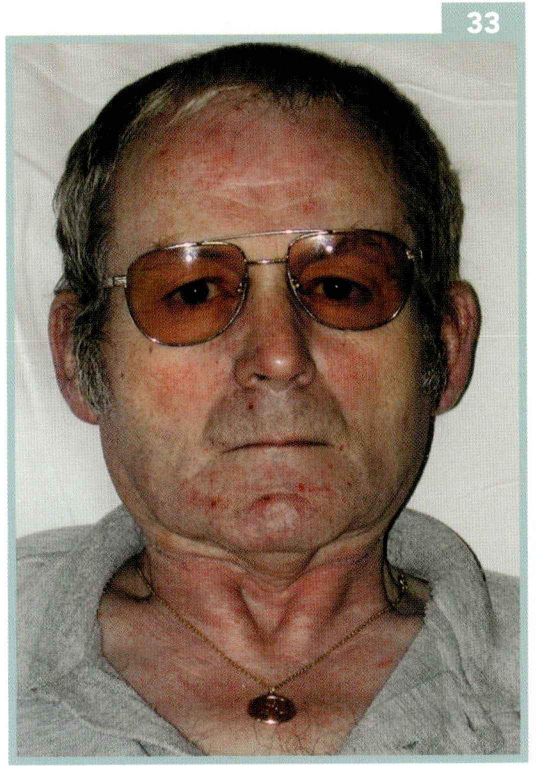

Answer 33

33i. This man has peripheral vascular disease, ischaemic heart disease, is a heavy smoker and is very polycythaemic. Smoking does not normally increase Hb levels above normal, so investigation is needed. The patient has polycythaemia rubra vera (PRV). Thrombotic events can occur including cerebrovascular accidents, transient ischaemic attacks, retinal vein thrombosis, central retinal artery occlusions, myocardial infarctions, angina, pulmonary embolism, hepatic and portal vein thrombosis, deep vein thrombosis and peripheral arterial occlusion. PRV may present with GI or other bleeding, vasomotor disturbances (headache, dizziness, acral dysaesthesia [i.e. pain or altered sensation of the palms and/or soles of the feet]), visual symptoms and, rarely, limb microvasculature occlusion leading to neurovascular pain named erythromelalgia.

ii. Renal hypoxaemia stimulates erythropoietin production by an oxygen sensor in peritubular interstitial cells. Renal hypoxaemia can occur secondary to high carbon monoxide levels (in smokers), living at high altitude or chronic lung/heart disease. Renal vascular disease or polycystic kidney can cause renal ischaemia with similar effects.

iii. Investigation of the polycythaemic patient includes: FBC (CBC) (to verify haematocrit: >54% in men or >50% in women is diagnostic); urea and electrolytes to assess renal function; red cell mass calculation (>125% of normal in pathological polycythaemia); CXR and arterial blood gases (to evaluate respiratory function and to exclude chronic hypoxia); abdominal ultrasound (for polycystic kidney disease); bone marrow aspiration (to examine red cell and other progenitors of blood components); erythropoietin levels (diagnostic of PRV if low with polycythaemia); blood viscosity (increased haematocrit promotes platelet/endothelium interaction causing thrombosis; therapeutic haematocrit and platelet count reduction decreases, but does not abolish, the risk of thrombosis).

iv. 'Apparent erythrocytosis' (high haematocrit without increased RBC mass) is associated with dehydration, use of diuretics, smoking and hypertension. Acquired secondary erythrocytosis can occur with either 'appropriate erythropoietin production' (from tissue hypoxia) or 'oxygen-independent erythropoietin production' (by tumours).

v. His cardiac symptoms must be investigated. PRV treatment involves phlebotomy (up to 500 ml daily) for haematocrit values <45% in men and <42% in women. Once haematocrit is controlled, surgery can proceed. In patients at high risk of thrombosis (age >60 or with previous thrombosis), chemotherapy with hydroxyurea can supplement phlebotomy. Low-dose aspirin (75 mg daily) is effective for alleviating vasomotor symptoms and its antithrombotic properties. Deep venous thromboprophylaxis should be used. The use of other anticoagulants remains controversial because of the increased risk of GI bleeding.

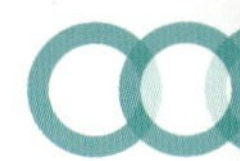

QUESTION 34

34i. What is represented in **34**?

ii. Explain the features marked (a) to (d).

iii. What are the potential pitfalls of meta-analysis?

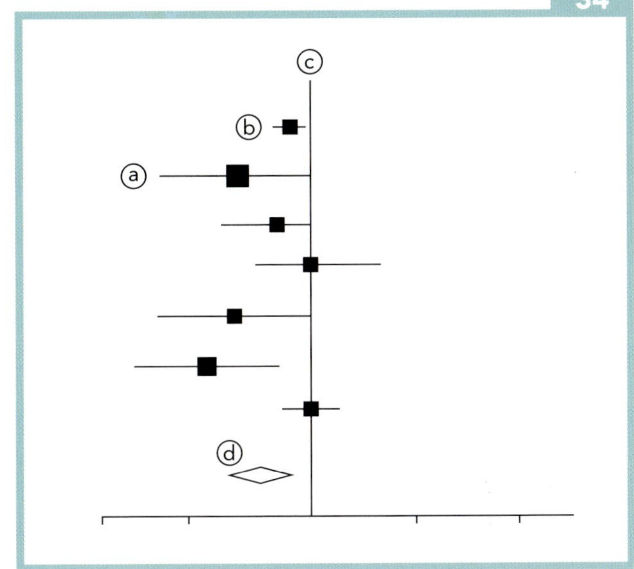

QUESTION 35

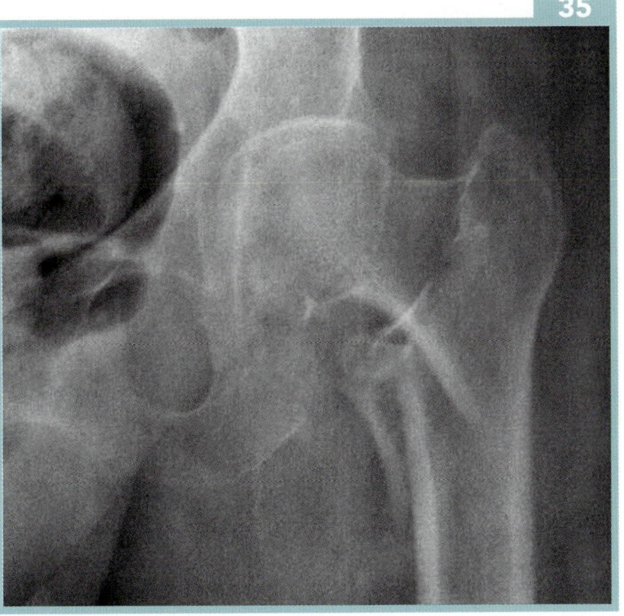

35 An obese 68-year-old woman with severe, steroid-dependent COPD is booked for a dynamic hip fixation of the left neck of the femur as an emergency (**35**). In addition to her normal steroids and nebulisers, the patient has received 40 mg enoxaparin (enoxaparin sodium) at 10 pm on the night before surgery as thromboprophylaxis. Spinal anaesthesia has been suggested for this patient because of her compromised respiratory function. What are the issues regarding neuraxial block in the presence of low molecular weight heparins (LMWHs)?

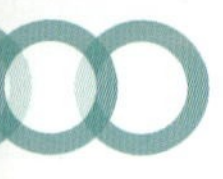

Answer 34

34i. This is a 'Forest Plot' or 'blobbogram', which is a diagrammatic representation of a meta-analysis of various randomised controlled clinical trials. Meta-analysis pools an estimate of the treatment effect by combining the odds ratios, or effect sizes, of all the studies. This example is a meta-analysis of seven randomised controlled trials of steroids given to mothers expected to give birth prematurely. Infant survival is compared in steroid and control groups.

ii. Horizontal lines represent 95% confidence intervals of individual studies analysed (a). The black square (b) on each line represents the study result expressed as an odds ratio (effect size). The size of the square, determined by numbers of subjects in the study, indicates the relative weighting of the individual study on the final, combined result. The vertical line (c) is the 'line of no effect' (often labelled as an odds ratio of 1 (i.e. where there is no difference in outcome between treatment and control groups). Odds ratios increase (move to the right) if the event is more likely and decrease (to the left) with increasing rarity. If a study demonstrates adverse outcome (i.e. neonatal death in this case), an odds ratio to the right of the line indicates that treatment had increased the risk of neonatal death. An odds ratio falling to the left of the line indicates that treatment reduced the risk of death. The diamond (d) represents the result of combining data from all the studies (the meta-analysis) with the centre of the diamond being the odds ratio of combined data. The width of the diamond represents the confidence intervals for this result.

iii. Meta-analysis can give misleading results. The most common problems are:

- Publication bias: positive studies are more likely to be published than negative studies, skewing the estimate of effectiveness of a treatment.
- Methodological weaknesses of individual trials, particularly smaller trials, weaken a meta-analysis.
- Heterogeneity of studies: subtle differences in study design, methods or patient population can cause pooled data to be inaccurate.

Answer 35

35 The use of neuraxial blockade in the presence of LMWHs is contentious owing to the increased incidence of epidural haematoma observed in North American patients (with possible subsequent paraplegia). Additional risk factors for epidural haematomas are being an elderly female, concomitantly taking other anticoagulants or antiplatelet drugs and using any kind of indwelling spinal/epidural catheter. Despite the much lower rate of epidural haematomas in Europe and the higher dose regimen of enoxaparin used in North America, both the European and American Societies of Regional Anaesthesia have recommended that neuraxial block should not be performed until at least 12 hours after the administration of a LMWH. Additionally, LMWHs should not be given for 2 hours after a neuraxial block or after withdrawal of an epidural catheter.

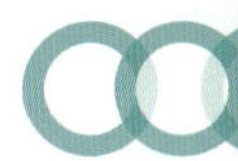

QUESTION 36

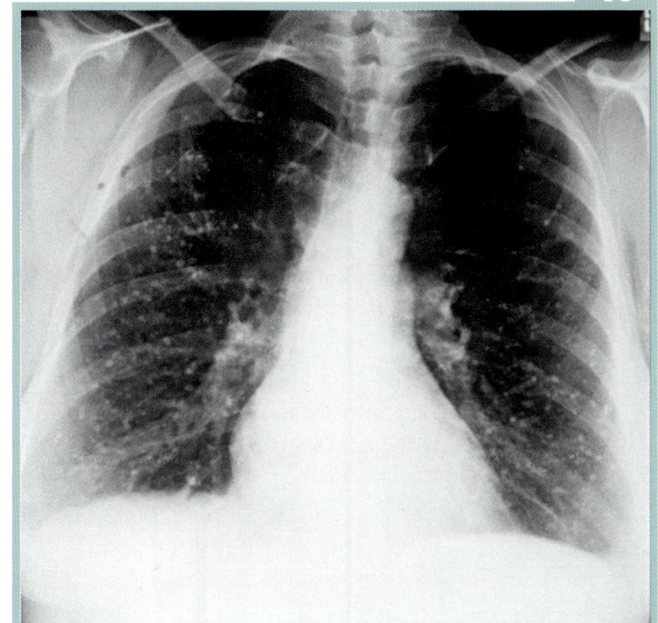

36 This CXR (**36**) is of a 46-year-old female patient from South Asia presenting for surgery to remove nasal polyps. She is otherwise healthy and denies weight loss, night sweats or shortness of breath, but was a hospital in-patient for one week with a "bad chest infection" 8 months ago.

i. What diseases are likely to cause such an appearance?

ii. How would you differentiate them?

iii. Does this radiographic appearance affect the conduct of GA?

QUESTION 37

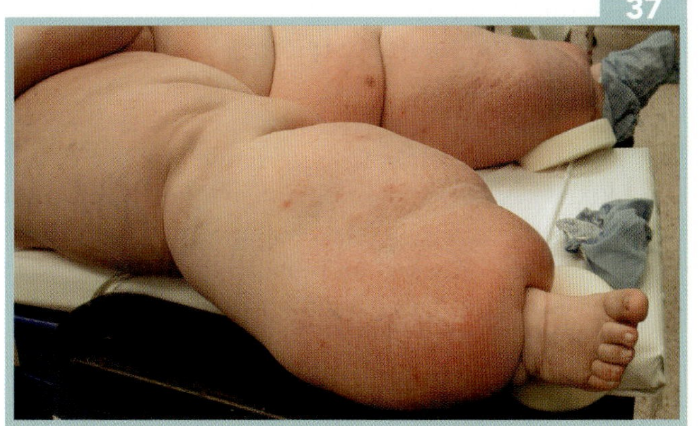

37 This patient (**37**) is taking warfarin.

i. She has no history of heart disease, so what is the warfarin most likely being prescribed for?

ii. Why is this lady particularly in need of warfarin, and what other risk factors should be considered?

iii. Describe your management of her coagulation both for routine surgery and for an emergency procedure (e.g. an axillary abscess).

Answer 36

36i. There are diffuse and uniformly distributed calcific densities throughout the lung fields and these are characteristic of an adult patient who has recovered from Varicella pneumonia (chicken pox). Miliary tuberculosis (TB) should also be considered, but the lesions are too large and the history does not fit with this diagnosis. These lesions are also characteristic of small pox (Variola), which has been eradicated by effective worldwide vaccination.

ii. The densities in the X-ray are larger (2–3 mm) than the typical 'millet' seed (1 mm) lesions seen with miliary TB.

iii. As the patient is healthy and denies any symptoms, serious pathology is unlikely. Pulmonary function tests should be ordered and correctly interpreted. The film should also be reported by a radiologist and discussed with a respiratory/ pulmonology expert, but anaesthesia can proceed unhindered.

Answer 37

37i. Thromboembolic disease. The patient had a venous thromboembolism 1 month ago.

ii. She is morbidly obese and this is a risk factor for thromboembolic disease. Other hypercoagulable conditions are pregnancy, malignancy (particularly bowel or pelvic), oral contraceptive medication, nephrotic syndrome and blood disorders such as Factor V Leiden and antithrombin III deficiency.

iii. For routine surgery warfarin should be stopped 4 days before surgery. Once the INR is under 2, an alternative perioperative prophylaxis should be started. Prior to surgery the INR should be under 1.5. In patients at high risk of thromboembolism, such as this patient, IV heparin should be started at 1,000 units/hour and adjusted to keep the activated partial thromboplastin time between 1.5 and 2.5 times normal. The infusion should be stopped no sooner than 6 hours before surgery and restarted 12 hours afterwards. This should be continued until warfarin is restarted and the INR is above 2. Additional methods of prophylaxis include compression stockings and intermittent pneumatic compression devices.

In emergency surgery there is not enough time for warfarin's effects to wear off and haematology advice should be sought. Fresh frozen plasma (10–15 ml/kg) and vitamin K (1–2 mg IM or slow IV) can be given to attempt to normalise the INR. If the patient had a thromboembolic event occurring more than 3 months ago, postoperative subcutaneous low molecular weight heparin may be sufficient. This should be continued for 24–48 hours post surgery and continued until warfarin is restarted and the INR is above 2.

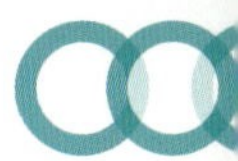

QUESTION 38

38i. Explain why on the graph below (**38**) the right-shifted curve 'delivers more oxygen' to the tissues. Merely saying that the right-shifted curve has a higher PO_2 at a given saturation (e.g. horizontal line 1) is not sufficient explanation.

ii. List four factors that will shift the curve to the right. Three of these factors are products of metabolism.

iii. Why would it be advantageous (useful) for these factors to shift the curve to the right?

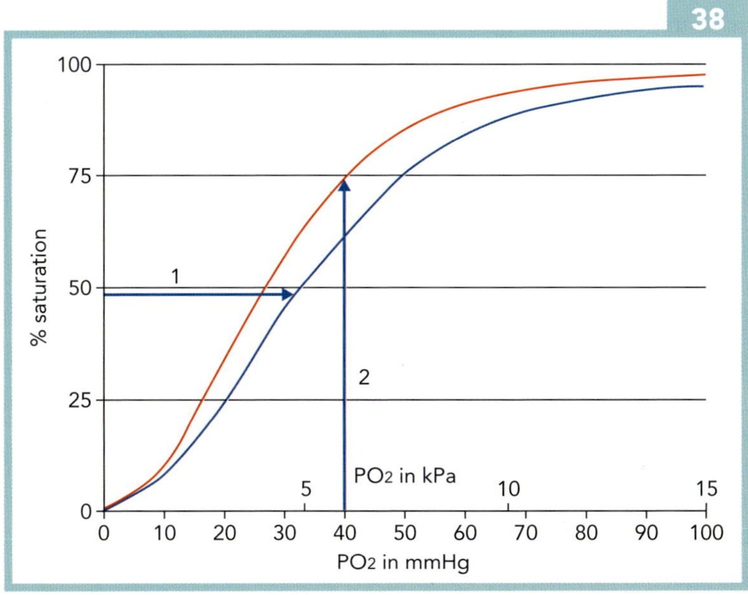

QUESTION 39

39i. Explain the shape (points A to E) of the normal capnograph trace shown (**39a**).

ii. How does the trace change in a patient with:

- Excessive dead space.
- Severe blood loss.

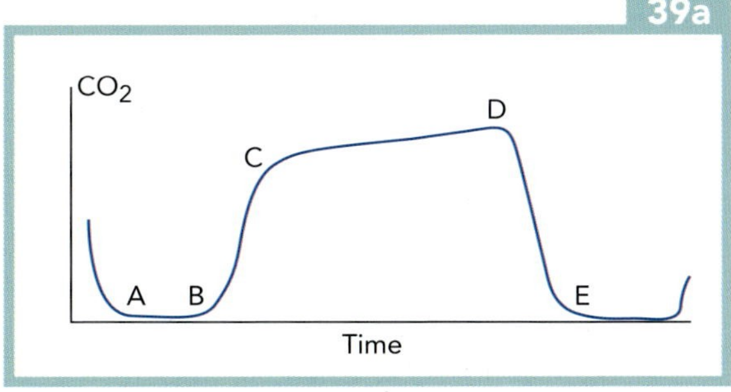

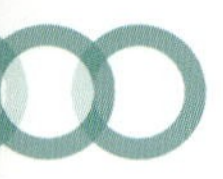

Answer 38

38i. At the arterial point, both the normal and right-shifted curves pick up virtually the same amount of oxygen (20 ml oxygen per 100 ml blood). However, at the venous point (e.g. vertical line 2 at PO_2 40 mmHg), the right-shifted curve is more desaturated (i.e. it gave up [delivered] more oxygen). In more detail, consider the y-axis, which displays oxygen content (on the right-sided y-axis): the normal curve would go from the arterial point with an oxygen content of 20 ml per 100 ml blood, to the venous point with 15 ml oxygen per 100 ml blood (i.e. delivering 5 ml oxygen per 100 ml blood). The right-shifted curve would go from an oxygen content of 20 to 12 ml oxygen per 100 ml blood (i.e. delivering 8 ml oxygen per 100 ml blood). At a venous PO_2 of 40 mmHg, the normal curve delivered 5 ml oxygen per 100 ml blood, while the right-shifted curve delivered 8 ml oxygen per 100 ml blood.

ii. Increases in H^+ (acidosis), CO_2, temperature and 2-3 di-phosphoglycerate.

iii. More oxygen would automatically be delivered to actively metabolizing tissues, without the energy expenditure of the body having to increase the cardiac output.

Answer 39

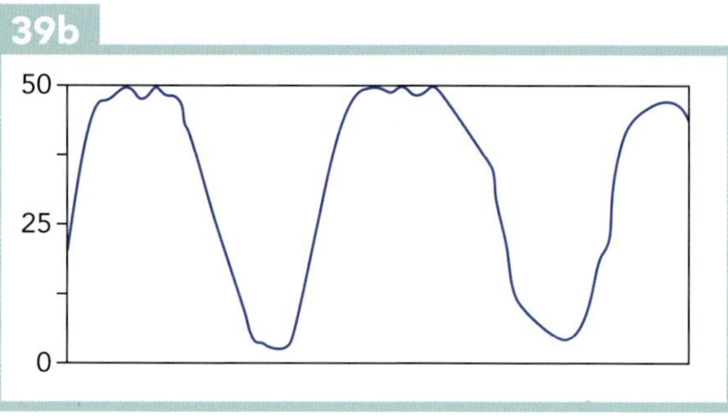

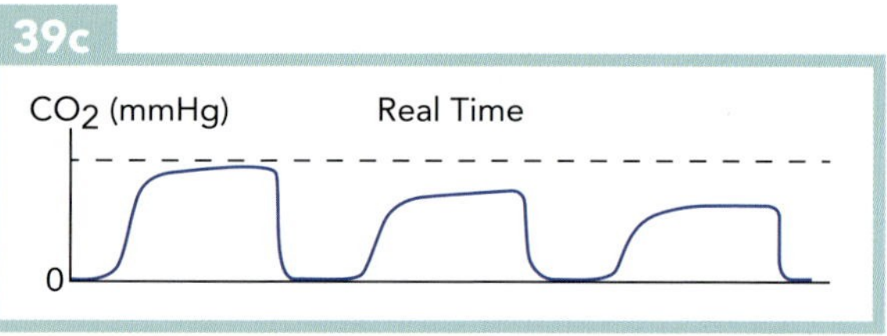

39i. A to B = initial expiration, anatomical dead space gas; B to C = mixed alveolar gas and alveolar dead space gas; C to D = alveolar 'plateau', horizontal in the 'ideal lung', slight slope (in real life the slope reflects ventilation/perfusion [V/Q] mismatching [see below]); D = end-tidal CO_2 level; D to E = inspiration.

ii.
- Dead space is shown when the CO_2 trace fails to return to zero (**39b**) at the end of each breath. Incomplete elimination of CO_2 is occurring and the patient could retain CO_2. This can be corrected by removal of any obvious equipment dead space in the breathing system or increasing the total fresh gas flow to the patient.
- As major blood loss is occurring, the CO_2 trace falls in amplitude (**39c**) because there is insufficient cardiac output to return CO_2 from the peripheral tissues to the lungs for exhalation. This indicates severe blood loss resulting in a decreased cardiac output. Hence, with a fixed minute ventilation (as on a ventilator), the capnograph may act as a 'cardiac output monitor'.

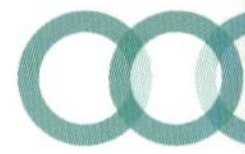

QUESTION 40

40 What is the relationship between arterial partial pressure of carbon dioxide (P_aCO_2) and end-tidal CO_2 ($ETCO_2$) in healthy lungs? What two factors determine this?

QUESTION 41

41 A normal flow trace on the monitor screen of an anaesthetic machine is shown (**41a**). Also shown (**41b**) is an abnormal flow trace from a different patient who has unexpected and unexplained hypotension. Your colleague suggests that it is possible to test quite quickly (in less than a minute or so) if the respiratory system is the cause of the hypotension.

i. Describe the abnormalities in the flow tracing in **41b**.

ii. Why does this type of abnormality lead to hypotension? What is this phenomenon called?

iii. What rapid test can be used on an anaesthetic machine to test if the ventilator pattern is the cause of the hypotension?

iv. How is this diagnosed with a typical ICU ventilator, and why is this important?

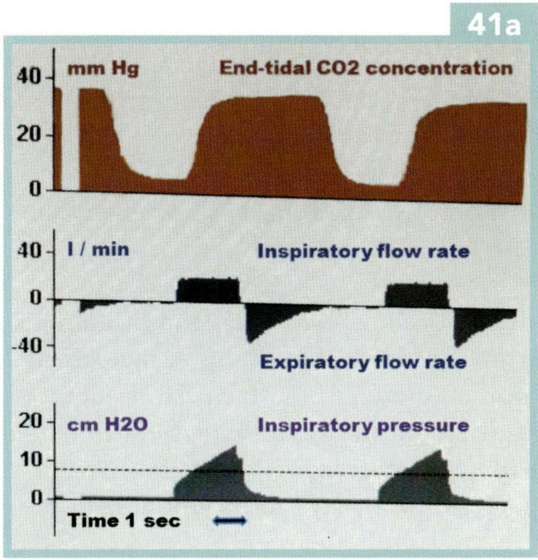

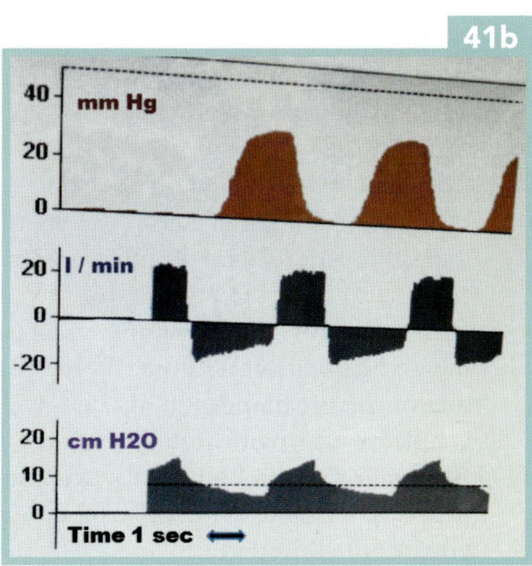

Answer 40

40 In the 'ideal lung' $PaCO_2$ and $ETCO_2$, ventilation and perfusion should match exactly with a ratio of 1. In reality V/Q mismatch (i.e. a spread of V/Q ratios) leads to alveolar dead space and a difference between $PaCO_2 - ETCO_2$. Two factors are important here:

- **Gravity causes variation in alveolar size.** At end-expiration, dependent alveoli and airways are 'squashed', while non-dependent alveoli/airways are relatively expanded. Thus they fill and empty asynchronously and the overall effect is V/Q <1. (Increase in West's lung zones 3 and 4.)
- **Gravity affects pulmonary perfusion.** Because the right heart circulation is a low pressure system, dependant regions are well perfused while non-dependent areas may be completely unperfused. Net effect: V/Q >1. (Increase in West's lung zone 1.)

Both factors occur in healthy adults. These effects are exacerbated by anaesthesia, age and smoking.

Answer 41

41i. The main (relevant to hypotension) abnormality is seen in the expiratory wave form. Exhalation is incomplete (the expiratory flow does not reach baseline or zero flow) by the time the next inspiration starts. Note also that the end expiratory pressure does not reach zero before the next breath.

ii. Incomplete exhalation leads to increasing volumes of air remaining in the lungs at end-exhalation, leading to an increased mean intrathoracic pressure and consequently decreased venous return with hypotension. This is called 'stepping' or 'auto-PEEP'.

iii. Disconnect the patient from the ventilator. Complete exhalation follows, with an increased venous return, and a rapid increase in the BP follows.

iv. ICU ventilators have a setting to intermittently occlude exhalation and measure the end expiration pressure. By measuring any build-up of pressure on the patient side of the breathing system, 'auto-PEEP' can be shown. If the I:E ratio on the ventilator is set with insufficient time for exhalation, auto-PEEP will result. Although this can be used therapeutically to 'recruit' alveoli in atalectatic lung, excessive PEEP, as with any excessive airway pressures, may cause barotrauma and possible pneumothorax.

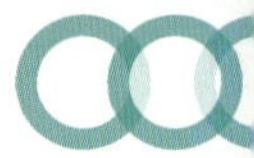

QUESTION 42

42 The adult advanced life support algorithm is shown (**42a**) with certain parts missing.

i. What three instructions are missing from the box marked 1?

ii. If the return of spontaneous circulation does not occur and the rhythm is not 'non-shockable', what does box 2 instruct one to do?

iii. What should box 3 say?

iv. What about box 4?

v. What do all the bullet points in the boxes headed Immediate post-cardiac arrest treatment, During CPR and Reversible causes indicate?

42a

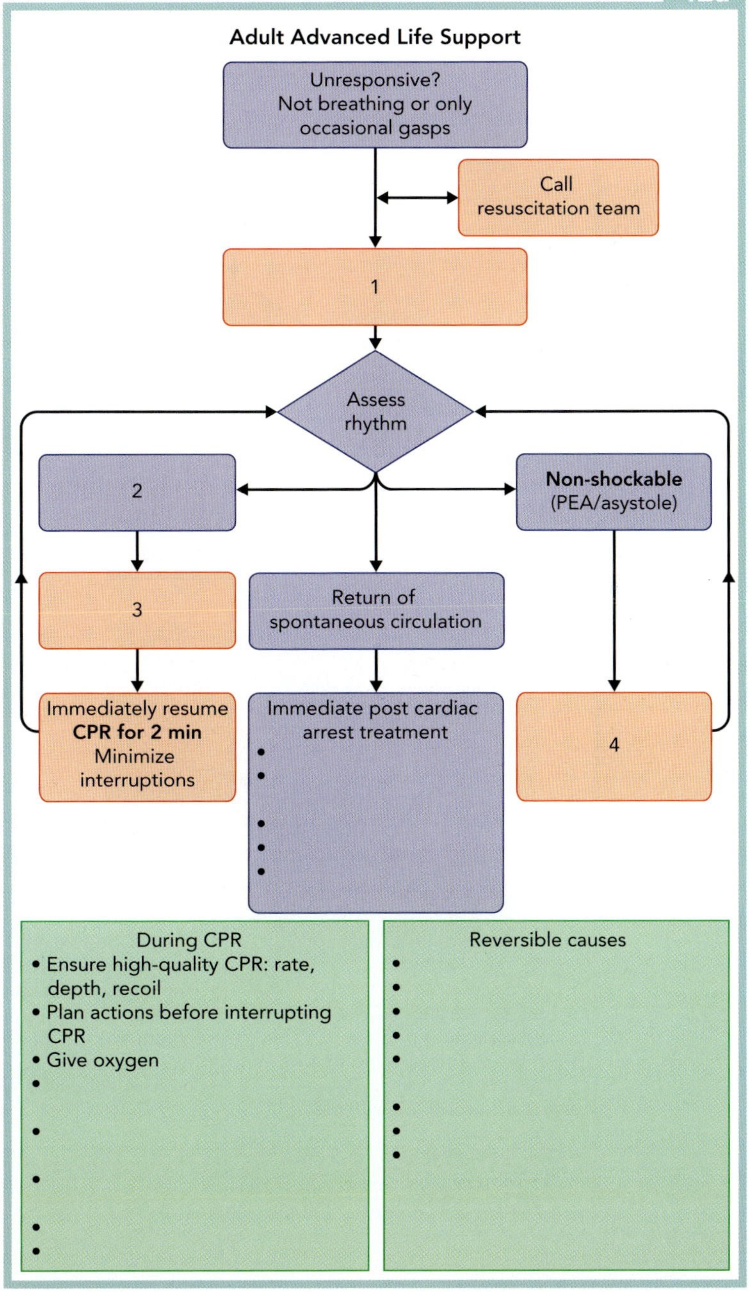

Adult Advanced Life Support

Unresponsive?
Not breathing or only occasional gasps

Call resuscitation team

1

Assess rhythm

2

Non-shockable
(PEA/asystole)

3

Return of spontaneous circulation

Immediately resume **CPR for 2 min**
Minimize interruptions

Immediate post cardiac arrest treatment
•
•
•
•
•

4

During CPR
- Ensure high-quality CPR: rate, depth, recoil
- Plan actions before interrupting CPR
- Give oxygen
-
-
-
-
-

Reversible causes
-
-
-
-
-
-
-
-

Answer 42

42 The complete adult advanced life support algorithm is shown (**42b**).

42b

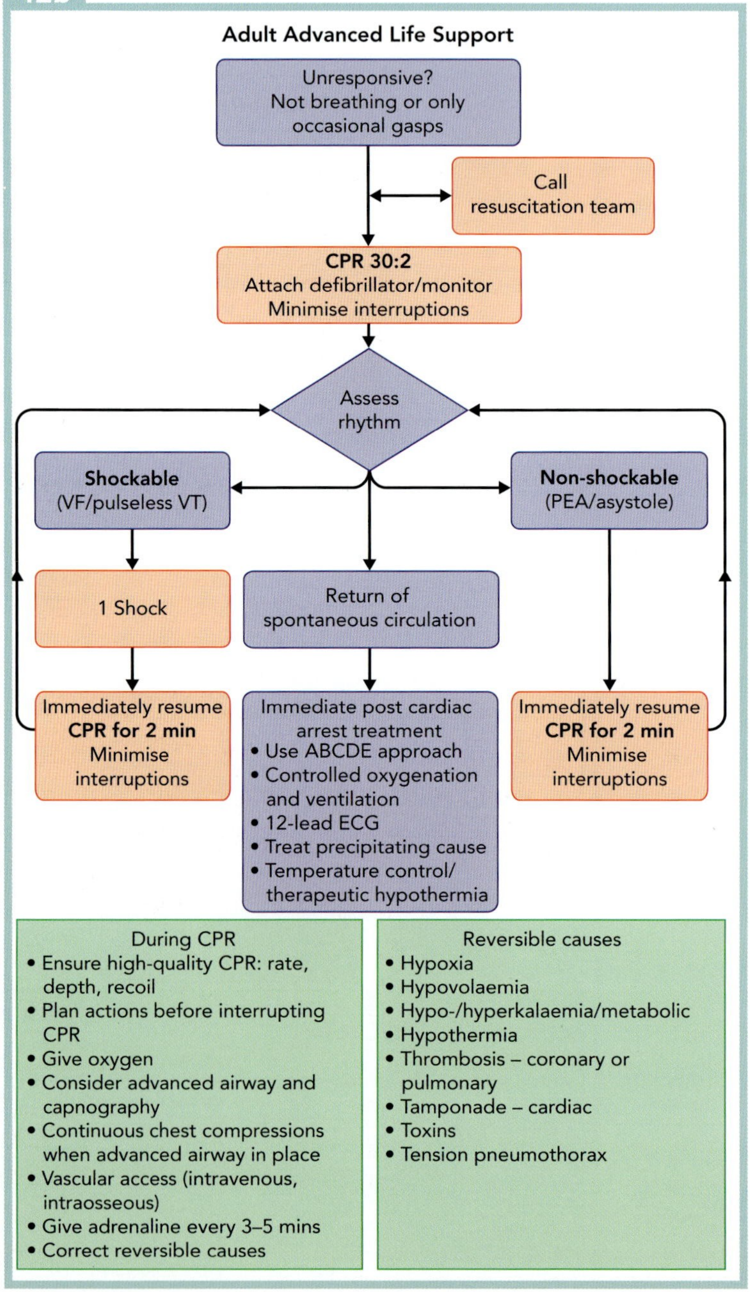

Adult Advanced Life Support

Unresponsive?
Not breathing or only occasional gasps

Call resuscitation team

CPR 30:2
Attach defibrillator/monitor
Minimise interruptions

Assess rhythm

Shockable
(VF/pulseless VT)

1 Shock

Immediately resume
CPR for 2 min
Minimise interruptions

Return of spontaneous circulation

Immediate post cardiac arrest treatment
- Use ABCDE approach
- Controlled oxygenation and ventilation
- 12-lead ECG
- Treat precipitating cause
- Temperature control/ therapeutic hypothermia

Non-shockable
(PEA/asystole)

Immediately resume
CPR for 2 min
Minimise interruptions

During CPR
- Ensure high-quality CPR: rate, depth, recoil
- Plan actions before interrupting CPR
- Give oxygen
- Consider advanced airway and capnography
- Continuous chest compressions when advanced airway in place
- Vascular access (intravenous, intraosseous)
- Give adrenaline every 3–5 mins
- Correct reversible causes

Reversible causes
- Hypoxia
- Hypovolaemia
- Hypo-/hyperkalaemia/metabolic
- Hypothermia
- Thrombosis – coronary or pulmonary
- Tamponade – cardiac
- Toxins
- Tension pneumothorax

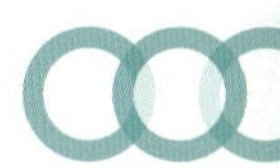

QUESTION 43

43

43 A 54-year-old man with stable angina, controlled by beta blockade and sublingual nitrate, presents for a day-case right cataract extraction and intraocular lens insertion. The axial length on the right eye is recorded at 27 mm. His cardiologist has told him it would be safer under LA. His ECG, U+E and physical examination are unremarkable.

i. What LA technique is most appropriate for this patient, and what other LA techniques are available? Justify your answer.

ii. Why is the axial length of 27 mm relevant?

iii. Explain how the technique in **43** is carried out and its advantages.

QUESTION 44

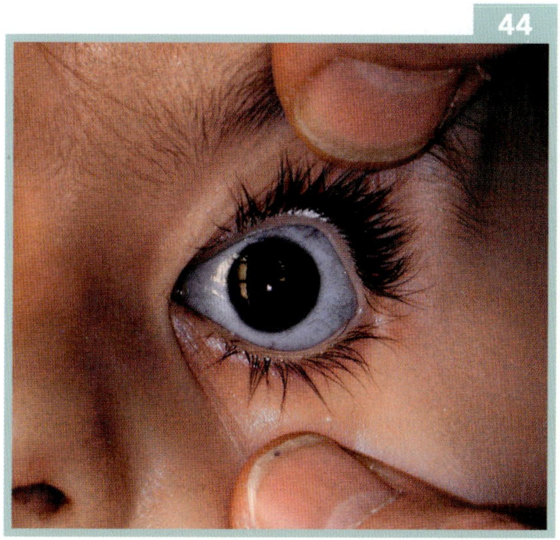

44

44 A child has long-standing skeletal problems. The characteristic blue sclera associated with this child's condition is shown (**44**).

i. What is this condition?

ii. What kind of surgery may be required?

Answer 43

43i. Subtenons LA technique, as shown in **43**. Other options are retrobulbar or peribulbar blocks (but both can cause retrobulbar haemorrhage), retinal vein or artery injection, ocular muscle paresis or globe perforation. Topical LA drops offer no akinesis so eye movement during surgery could cause serious complications.

ii. Retrobulbar and peribulbar blocks are more likely to perforate the globe if the axial length is >25 mm. Subtenons is safer with increased axial length due to a blunt needle being used and direct vision verifying the correct plane of infiltration.

iii. With a supine patient, topical LA drops anaesthetise the conjunctiva and then an eyelid speculum is inserted. The patient looks 'up and out' exposing the inferonasal quadrant. A small tent of conjunctiva is raised with fine non-toothed forceps approximately mid-way between the limbus of the eye and the visible edge of the inferonasal conjunctiva. A small incision is then made in the conjunctiva with ophthalmic scissors. Closed scissors are introduced through the aperture and a tunnel is fashioned to the bare sclera by blunt dissection through Tenon's capsule. A curved, blunt irrigating cannula is then inserted with a syringe. The syringe contains 4 ml each of 2% lidocaine and 0.25% bupivacaine to which 75–150 IU of hyaluronidase has been added. Hyaluronidase promotes diffusion of LA to peri- and retro-orbital tissues. Little resistance is found to injection. Slight eyeball proptosis is normal. Sensory nerve blockade and akinesia develop due to direct spread of LA onto the sclera, the Tenon's sheaths surrounding the insertion of the extraocular muscles and the retrobulbar cone on the extraocular muscles and motor nerves. Periorbital tissue can cause akinesia of the eyelids.

Answer 44

44i. Osteogenesis imperfecta (OI) (or 'brittle-bone disease'), an autosomal dominant generalised disorder of connective tissues. Fractures occur with minimal trauma. OI is characterised by combinations of short stature, blue sclerae, triangular facies, macrocephaly, hearing loss, defective dentition (translucent/opalescent teeth with increased susceptibility to caries), barrel chest, vertebral compression/scoliosis, progressive limb deformity and bowing due to recurrent fractures, joint laxity and varying degrees of growth retardation.

ii. Surgery is regularly required to repair fractures (commonly long bones). Selective orthopaedic procedures can improve the patient's ability to be independent. Physiotherapy (physical therapy) from early childhood can help to minimise fractures and maximise function. Some affected patients can walk with the use of a combination of bracing, surgery and physiotherapy to strengthen hip-girdle muscles and increase stamina. Intramedullary rods in the femurs may help if leg bowing is >40 degrees. The subsequent limb realignment provides some internal support for weight bearing, but does not decrease the rate of fractures.

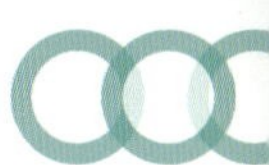

QUESTION 45

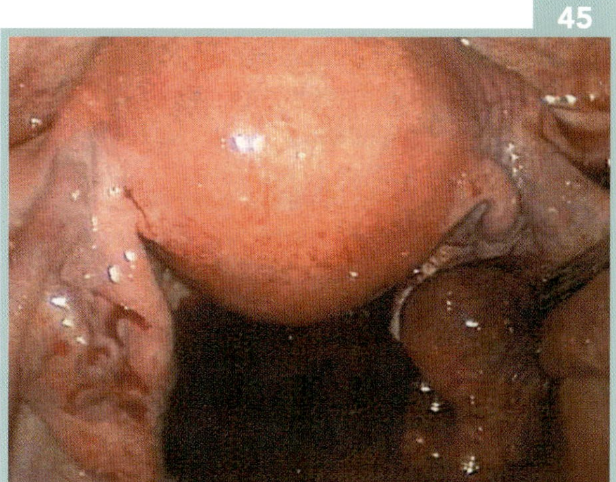

45

45 Shown is a laparoscopic view of the female reproductive organs with forceps alongside the right Fallopian tube (**45**). This 28-year-old woman presented with a history of right-sided stabbing-type pelvic pain, a small amount of vaginal bleeding and feeling faint.

i. What is the diagnosis?

ii. How is the diagnosis confirmed?

iii. What is the significance of 'feeling faint'?

iv. What operation is needed?

v. Describe the anaesthetic management of such a case.

QUESTION 46

46 A 54-year-old man is scheduled to undergo surgery because of the recent onset of angina. On physical examination a diastolic murmur is noted. This TOE is obtained preoperatively (**46**).

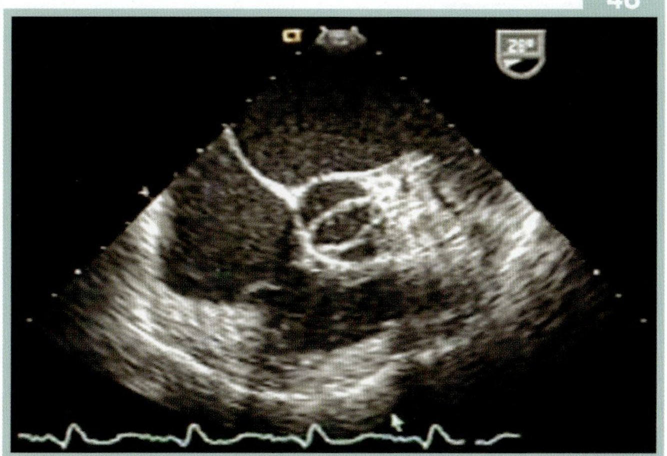

46

i. What is the diagnosis?

ii. What other diagnostic procedure needs to be performed?

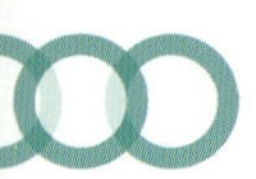

Answer 45

45i. Ectopic pregnancy. A fertilised ovum has implanted at a site outside the endometrium. Ectopic pregnancies are responsible for approximately 10% of maternal mortality.

ii. Laparoscopic direct vision surgery is recommended, although early pregnancy can be missed. Algorithms measuring serum progesterone, serial β-subunit of hCG measurement, pelvic ultrasonography and uterine curettage can also confirm the diagnosis.

iii. Significant blood loss may have occurred, resulting in shock.

iv. Laparoscopic salpingectomy is almost 100% curative, facilitates rapid recovery, preserves fertility and is low cost. Laparotomy only occurs when laparoscopy is too difficult, the surgeon is not laparoscopically trained or the patient is haemodynamically unstable.

v. Preoperative assessment (especially involving volaemic status) is mandatory. In stable patients blood is taken for FBC (CBC) and 'group and save' for a potential cross-match request. Shocked patients may need type-specific blood (available in 20 minutes) or, exceptionally, O-negative blood. A large bore (16 or 14 gauge) IV cannula should be inserted. Induction may suddenly drop BP because of concealed haemorrhage. Preoxygenation and a rapid sequence IV induction and a short-acting muscle relaxant (suxamethonium) is recommended. In shocked patients anaesthesia should occur in the operating room, fully draped, with the surgeon and team ready. Resuscitation should accept some hypotension until surgical control is achieved. Limited resuscitation to a BP of 90 mmHg systolic is now recognised to improve outcome in uncontrolled traumatic haemorrhage. When haemostasis is achieved, restoration of normal circulating volume and BP is the goal.

Answer 46

46i. The image shows that the aortic valve only has two leaflets (a congenitally bicuspid aortic valve). This patient has aortic valve insufficiency as the cause of his angina. Patients with a bicuspid aortic valve may develop aortic stenosis later in life.

ii. Coronary angiography should be performed to exclude coexisting coronary artery disease prior to aortic valve replacement.

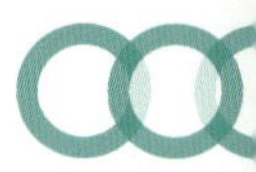

QUESTION 47

47 An ECG (top trace) and an arterial line with a normal arterial BP are shown (**47**). A series of three periods ('square waves') of high pressure are noted, with a rapid (precipitous) drop to normal (i.e. a pop-test or flush-test of the arterial line).

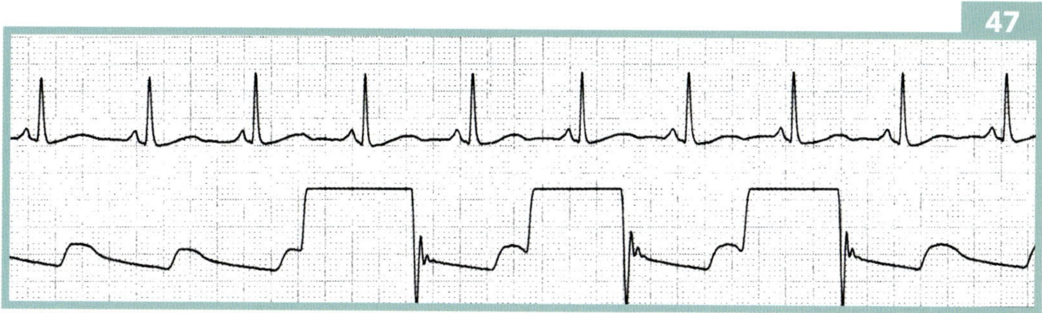

i. Describe the steps for performing a pop-test (flush-test).

ii. Describe the interpretation of this test as demonstrated by the graphic.

iii. Describe the concept of 'ringing' or 'oscillation' as related to underdamped arterial lines.

iv. What are the commonest reasons for under- and overdamping?

QUESTION 48

48 What is the formula for the oxygen (O_2) content equation of blood? Draw the oxygen dissociation curve for blood.

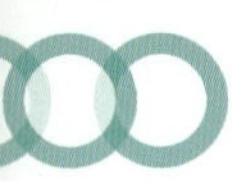

Answer 47

47i. A series of three 'pop-tests' or 'flush-tests' were performed. The flush valve was triggered (opened) and rapidly closed to cause a rapid decrease in the pressure in the arterial line.

ii. A normal test demonstrates 2–3 oscillation waves (back and forth pressure swings), as is shown in this test (i.e. indicates that damping is within acceptable limits).

iii. Ringing occurs in an underdamped arterial line and is diagnosed by multiple oscillating waves (typically up to five waves are seen.)

iv. Underdamping or 'ringing' occurs in cannulae that are too short or too stiff. More commonly, arterial lines are overdamped because of kinking of the line or a blood clot or air bubble in the line.

Answer 48

48 O_2 content = O_2 carried by Hb + O_2 dissolved in plasma

in more detail

O_2 content = (Hb concentration (g/dl) × % saturation × 1.34) + (P_aO_2 × 0.003)

1.34 = number of ml of O_2 carried per gram of Hb (the Hufner constant); 0.003 = the O_2 in ml physically dissolved in 100 ml of whole blood for each mmHg of O_2. The red, solid line on **48** shows oxygen saturation on the left y axis. The orange line (reading on the right-sided axis) shows the content of dissolved O_2. The blue line (reading on the right-sided y-axis) shows the O_2 content of Hb. The green line (reading on the right-sided y-axis) shows the total O_2 content of blood.

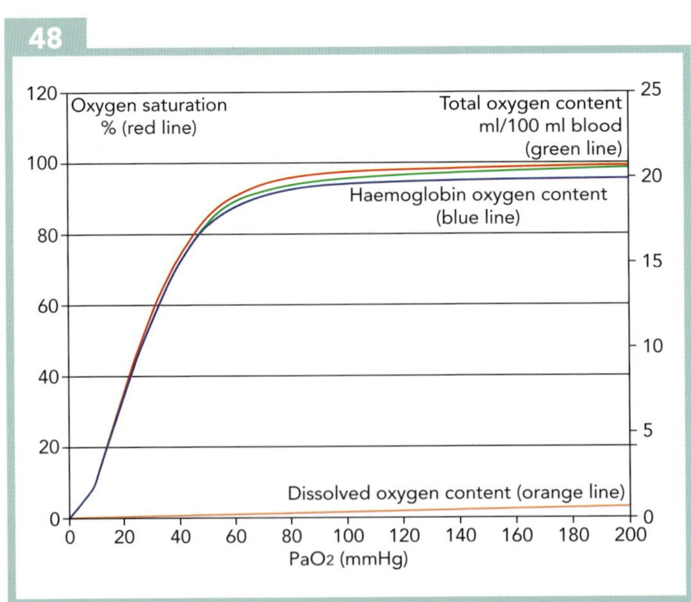

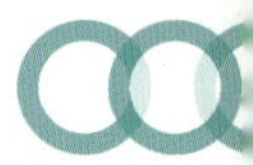

QUESTION 49

49i. Why is the formula for the oxygen content equation of blood important to the practice of anaesthesia?

ii. How is this altered when a patient has suffered significant smoke inhalation?

QUESTION 50

50i. A young healthy adult is in the recovery room after knee surgery and requires large doses of narcotics to control the pain. He seems to need increasing flows of oxygen to maintain a normal saturation. One of your colleagues makes the statement: "The patient's $PaCO_2$ is increased and that's why he needs extra oxygen". Do you agree? Explain your answer using the graph shown (**50**).

ii. A patient is in the emergency department after a motor vehicle accident. The patient has a small pneumothorax. One of your colleagues makes the statement: "This patient is on room air and the saturation is 98%, so the patient's alveolar minute ventilation is within normal limits". Do you agree? Explain your answer based on the graph shown (**50**).

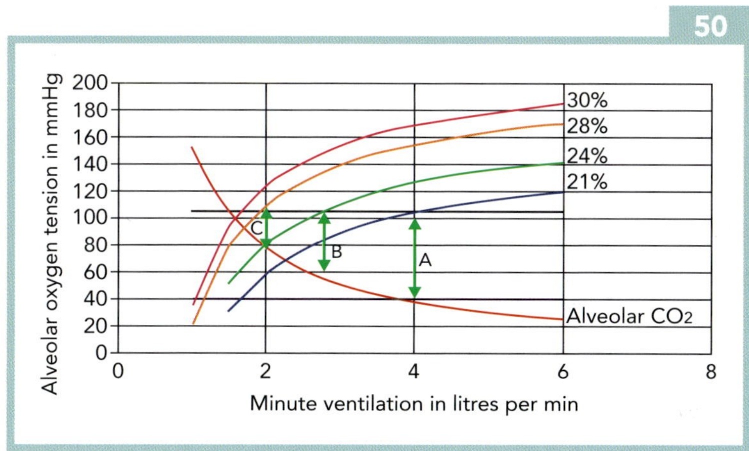

Answer 49

49i. The influence of Hb concentration and saturation is far greater on the carriage of O_2 than dissolved O_2. For safe anaesthesia, maintenance of adequate O_2 saturation and an Hb >7 g/dl (10 g/dl in ischaemic heart disease) allows adequate carriage of O_2 to the tissues. In cases of massive blood loss (>2 litres) it is important to order blood as soon as this blood loss is recognised to allow for maintenance of an adequate Hb level. This equation is also important for understanding 'goal directed therapy' where the 'goal' is adequate O_2 delivery (normally considered to be 600 ml/min/m^2 BSA). O_2 delivery is calculated by multiplying the above equation by the cardiac output. O_2 saturation should not be allowed to fall below 88% for any prolonged period. Because of the shape of the O_2 dissociation curve, saturation of <88% is associated with inadequate O_2 carriage in most patients.

ii. Smoke inhalation leads to high levels of blood carbon monoxide (CO). CO is 240 times more avidly bound to Hb than O_2, displaces O_2 from the Hb molecule and forms carboxyhaemoglobin. Carboxyhaemoglobin does not participate in O_2 carriage and the blood only carries O_2 in the dissolved form. Dissolved O_2 alone is inadequate for tissue gas exchange and leads to the cellular hypoxia seen in CO toxicity.

Answer 50

50i. Yes, your colleague is correct. During hypoventilation (such as following large doses of narcotics), the alveolar gas equation indicates that with decreased alveolar minute ventilation (while on room air – follow the 21% line to the left), the oxygen is not being replaced at a sufficient rate to maintain a normal alveolar P_AO_2 and CO_2 is displacing oxygen from the alveoli at this low ventilation. By increasing the FIO_2 (e.g. moving from A, to B to C on **50**), the amount of oxygen in the alveolar space is sufficient to maintain normal oxygenation, even with a decreased minute ventilation and an increasing CO_2 concentration.

ii. Based on the alveolar gas equation as shown in **50**, if the patient is on room air (21% line) and the P_AO_2, P_aO_2 and saturation are within normal limits, it is acceptable to make the statement that the alveolar minute ventilation is within normal limits. **Note:** On the 21% line it is clear that hypoventilation (moving to the left on the 21% line) leads to decreased saturation.

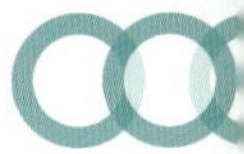

QUESTION 51

51 An 80-year-old man, admitted for an elective hernia repair, has fallen in the ward. He is now conscious, but slightly confused. His BP is 200/130, pulse 30. His ECG is shown (**51**).

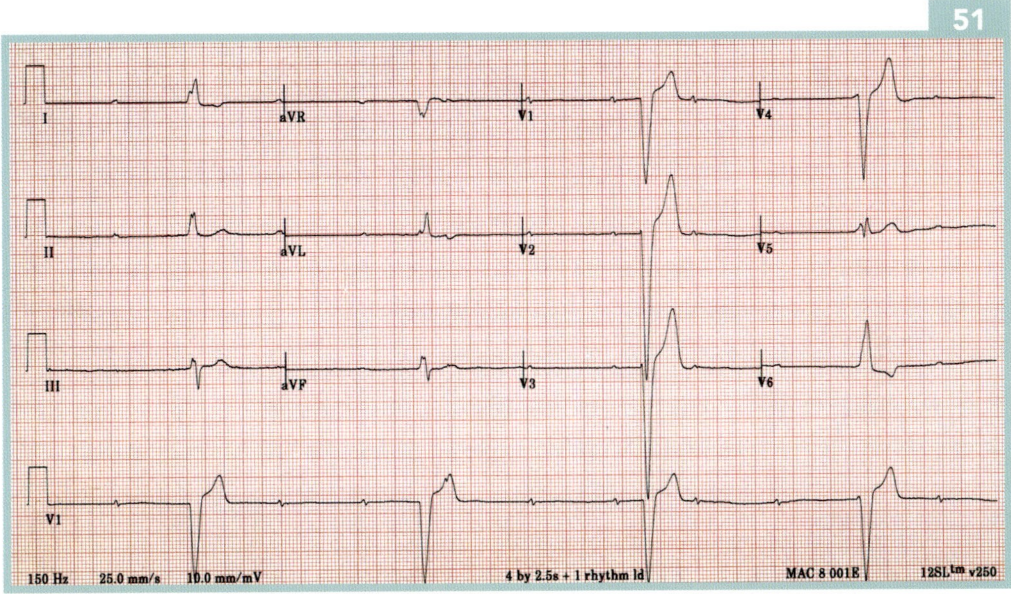

51

i. What has happened?

ii. Will IV atropine help?

iii. What treatment should this patient have?

QUESTION 52

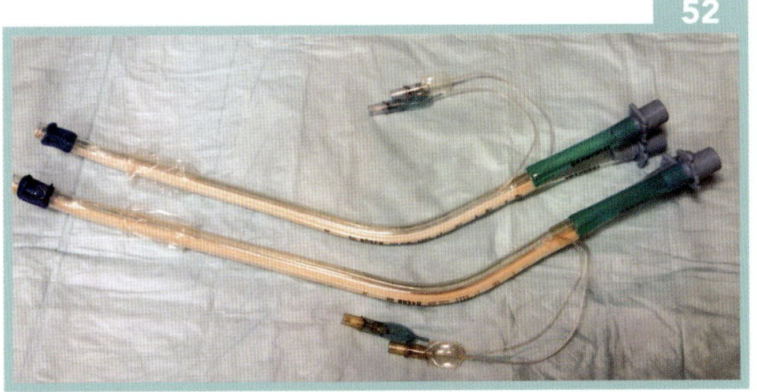

52

52i. What are the devices shown (**52**)?

ii. How would you recognise if they were left- or right-sided devices?

iii. With one-lung-ventilation (i.e. a +/- 50% shunt is created), the O_2 saturation often decreases, but CO_2 tensions do not change. Explain this phenomenon based on the differences in physiology between O_2 and CO_2.

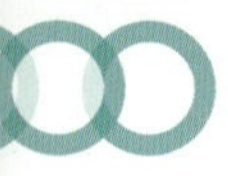

Answer 51

51i. The ECG shows 3rd degree (complete) AV block. The man is likely to have had a syncopal episode secondary to inadequate cardiac output due to a transient catastrophic reduction in heart rate. This is colloquially known as a 'Stokes–Adams attack'.

ii. He should receive high-flow oxygen and an IV line. Atropine (500 μg IV), repeated to a maximum of 3 mg, may be given but is unlikely to be effective, as atropine works via the sinoatrial node, which is blocked.

iii. Urgent transvenous pacing and transfer to a monitored bed is required. An acute coronary syndrome should be suspected and investigated with blood taken for FBC (CBC), U+E and serum troponin and a transthoracic echocardiogram performed. Any cardiac or other drug that slows AV conduction (e.g. topical preparations such as beta-blocker eye drops) should be stopped. The patient's hypertension is a baroreceptor reaction to the bradycardia and inadequate perfusion and may settle if his heart rate increases with treatment. If transvenous pacing is not readily available, an infusion of epinephrine (2–10 μg min^{-1}) may increase ventricular automaticity, although this can be hazardous in patients with a recent coronary event. Surgery should be postponed.

Answer 52

52i. Double lumen endotracheal tubes.

ii. Right-sided tubes have an adapted (shorter) bronchial cuff, sometimes with an opening in the cuff. This is to avoid obstruction of the right upper bronchus opening, which exits the right main bronchus within 1 inch (2.5 cm) from the carina.

iii. One-lung ventilation causes problems with oxygenation as red cells are limited in the amount of O_2 they can carry (20 ml O_2/100 ml blood at 100% saturation). The saturation of the red cells cause the O_2-haemoglobin dissociation curve to be flat above an arterial O_2 tension of +/-100–105 mmHg. When fully saturated blood from the ventilated lung mixes with blood from the non-ventilated ('shunted') lung, the mixture must contain less O_2 than 'full' saturation (i.e. the average of 20 ml O_2 and 15 ml O_2 (per 100 ml blood) from the ventilated and non-ventilated lungs, respectively, is 17.5 ml O_2 per 100 ml blood, which represents a saturation of 85%). **Note:** Dissolved O_2 (0.3 ml O_2 per 100 ml blood per 100 mmHg) does not usually contribute significantly to the blood O_2 content. CO_2, however, has a dissociation curve that is almost linear in the physiological range. Doubling the ventilation removes twice as much CO_2. When the blood from the ventilated lung (with below normal CO_2 content) mixes with blood from the non-ventilated lung (with venous levels of CO_2 content), the resulting CO_2 content is close to normal.

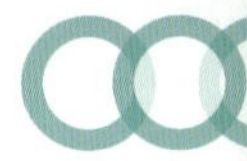

QUESTION 53

53 This man (**53**) was riding a motorbike, without a helmet, in a field. He hit a fence at about 32 kph (20 mph).

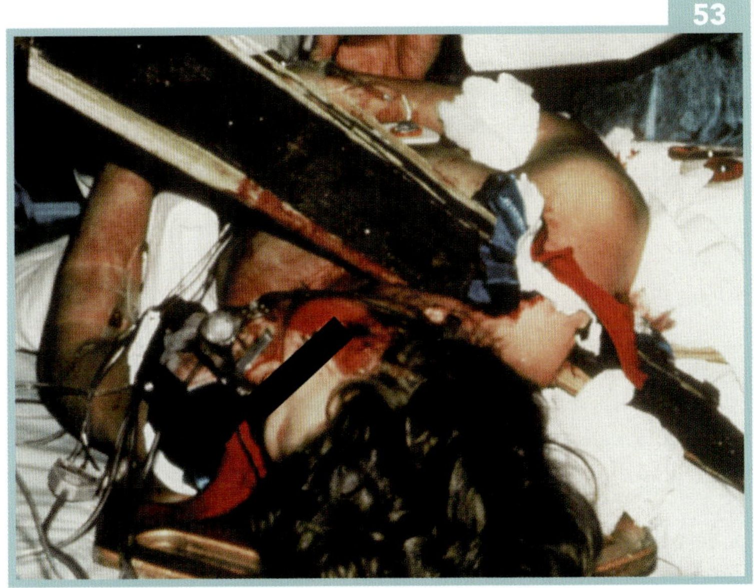

53

i. Prioritise the immediate management of this patient into five steps.

ii. How would you predict his injuries?

iii. What six life-threatening thoracic conditions must be considered?

iv. Comment on any management deficiencies seen in **37** that you could correct.

v. What other anaesthetic management should take place?

vi. What is damage control surgery?

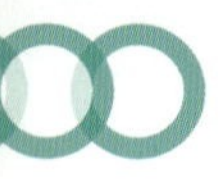

Answer 53

53i. **A**irway with cervical spine control and high-flow O_2 administration; **B**reathing with adequate ventilation; **C**irculation and haemorrhage control; **D**isability (neurological assessment); **E**xposure and complete **E**xamination.

ii. Establish the mechanism of injury (MOI). Consider major head trauma (no helmet); cervical spine injury; major chest/abdominal trauma. How he came to hit the fence could predict the nature of the injuries. Forty kph (25 mph) is sufficient to cause major head and spinal injuries. Ruptured aorta, ruptured spleen and fractured liver are possible.

iii. Airway obstruction, tension pneumothorax, open pneumothorax, massive haemothorax, flail chest with pulmonary contusion, cardiac tamponade.

iv. The O_2 mask is inadequate; a trauma mask with reservoir bag (delivering 85% oxygen) is required. Cervical spine stabilisation with in-line immobilisation by hand or a cervical collar is required. This is especially important due to this patient's MOI. In-line immobilisation is essential before intubation.

v. Bilateral chest drains, to prevent tension pneumothorax, are required before anaesthesia. Pneumothorax is likely and is exacerbated by positive pressure ventilation. Fluid replacement via two large-bore IV cannulae, commenced before surgery, prevents cardiovascular decompensation. The right arm cannot be used due to the location of the injury. BP should be restored to approximately 90 mmHg systolic using crystalloid IV fluids and blood until surgical control is obtained. Higher BPs encourage greater blood loss and coagulopathy by haemodilution. Ruptured spleen and other intra-abdominal injury should not be overlooked and leg/femoral veins should not be used for fluid resuscitation. Early intubation can help once the trauma team is assembled. Bleeding may need to be controlled by surgery before detailed assessment of all the injuries.

vi. 'Damage limitation surgery' (DLS) uses minimal surgical intervention to control bleeding, prevent contamination of a wound and prevent further injury. After DLS further resuscitation over some hours in critical care can correct hypothermia, coagulopathy and metabolic acidosis. Necessary definitive surgery can then be performed when the patient is rewarmed and stable.

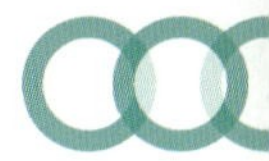

QUESTION 54

54 The reduction in plasma concentration of remifentanil that occurs after a 70 kg (150 lb), 170 cm (68 in) tall, 40-year-old man was given 1 μg kg^{-1} of remifentanil as a slow bolus injection is shown (**54a**). The pharmacokinetic model (for the same patient) that was used to simulate this and to calculate the plasma concentrations mathematically is also shown (**54b**).

i. How would you pharmacologically describe the fall of plasma remifentanil concentration in **54a**?

ii. What type of pharmacokinetic model is shown in **54b**?

iii. How do the compartments in this model relate to the different body tissues of this man?

iv. Why is this particular model useful for calculating the observed change in plasma concentration for remifentanil?

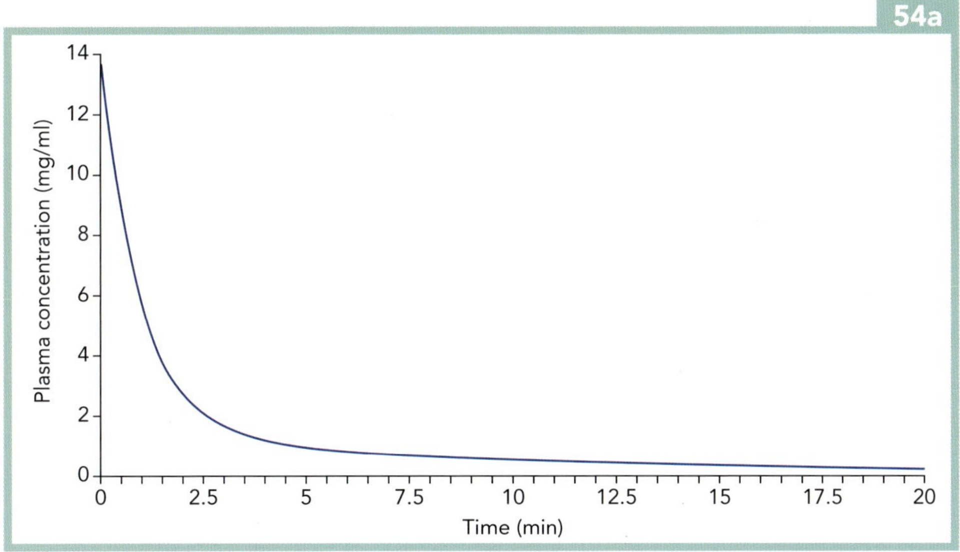

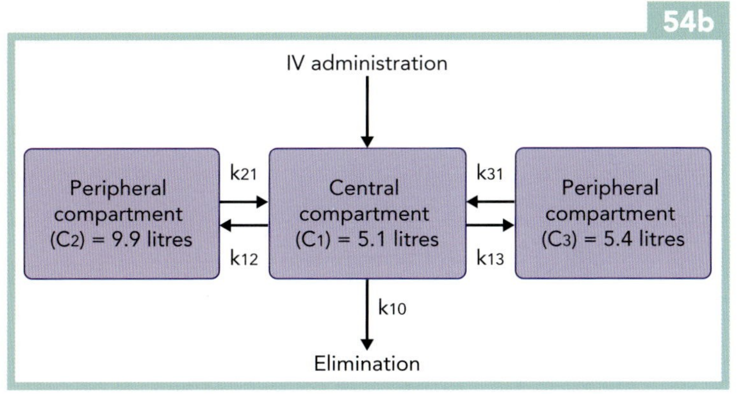

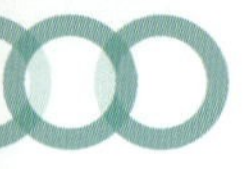

Answer 54

54i. This is an exponential graph of drug decay; in fact a tri-exponential function (see **54c**). The three solid lines show that the rate of decline in plasma concentration can be separated into three components.

ii. A three-compartment pharmacokinetic model: a central compartment (C_1) and two peripheral compartments (C_2 and C_3). Drug is delivered into (IV) and eliminated from the central compartment. Rate constants k_{12}, k_{21}, k_{13} and k_{31} determine the transfer of drug between the central and peripheral compartments. The elimination rate constant is k_{10}. Pharmacokinetic models attempt to describe the relationship between dose and blood concentration with respect to time.

iii. Compartments are a mathematical tool used to model how plasma concentration changes with respect to time. They do not, however, describe the concentration in any particular tissues and as such are not 'organ orientated'. In particular, the pharmacokinetic compartments do not relate to any particular organs. The traditionally quoted pharmacokinetic half-lives, such as $t\frac{1}{2}\alpha$ (redistribution half-life) and $t\frac{1}{2}\beta$ (elimination half-life), are used to describe mathematically the observed fall in plasma concentration. They are useful to pharmacologists in developing pharmacokinetic models, but when considered in isolation, none of these individual half-lives describe what is likely to happen to the plasma concentration when an infusion of anaesthetic drug is turned off. Complex logarithmic formulae (using these half-lives) are required to predict this.

iv. Mathematical analysis of the graph of concentration against time, for most anaesthetic drugs, reveals that they are tri-exponential drugs, which are best described by a three-compartment model. This can be useful in predicting when an IV agent will wear off.

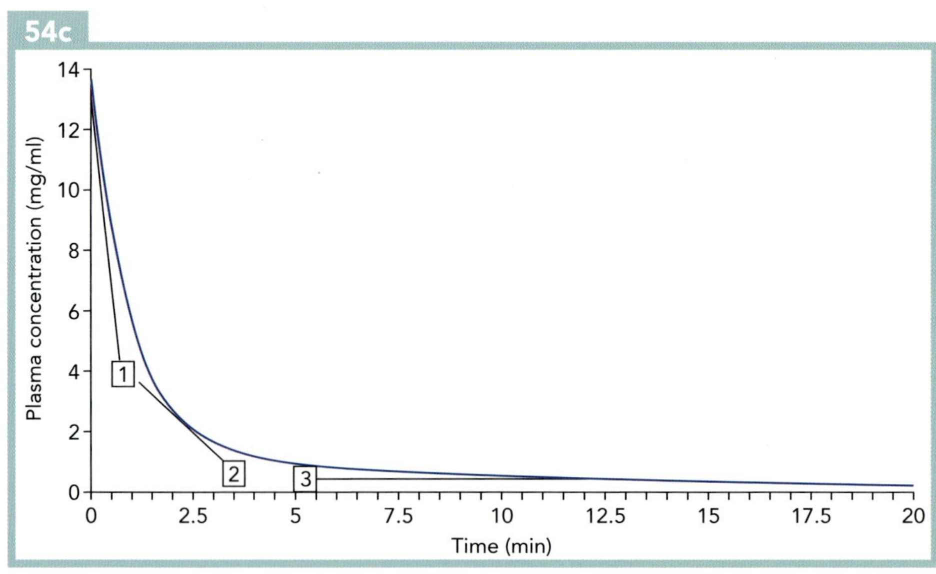

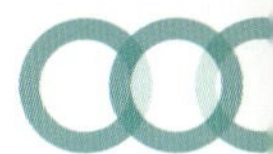

QUESTION 55

55 A device (**55a**) and the waveform it generates (**55b**) are shown. (Images courtesy Deltex Medical)

i. What is this device, and why is it useful?

ii. What does the green line show, and what is its relevance to patient care?

iii. What is the red arrow showing, and what is its relevance to patient care?

55a

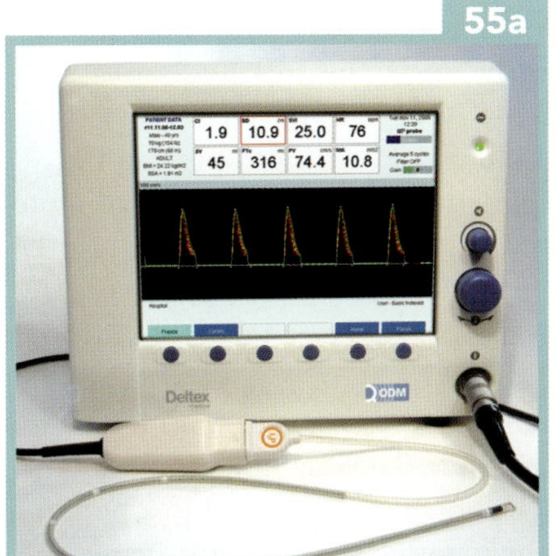

55b

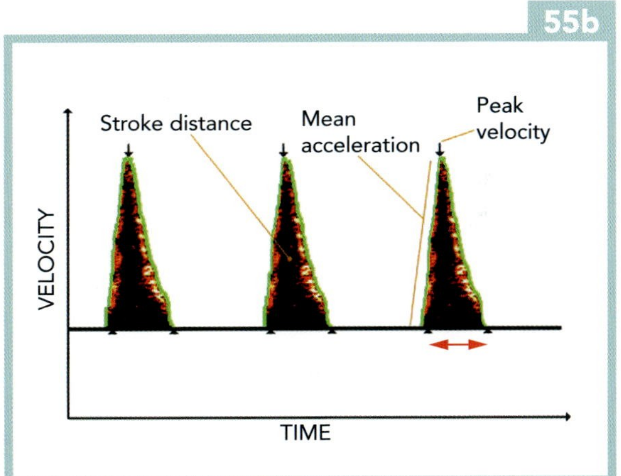

QUESTION 56

56 A 3-year-old boy weighing 14 kg (31 lb) presents for dental extractions and restoration under GA at a community hospital. He is extremely anxious and combative. The patient's natural father had a documented fulminant malignant hyperthermia (MH) crisis following GA for trauma. The father 'almost died' and spent 1 month in intensive care.

i. What is this patient's risk of MH susceptibility? Does the type of surgery affect risk?

ii. Would you recommend a muscle biopsy prior to the proposed procedure, during the dental procedure or not at all?

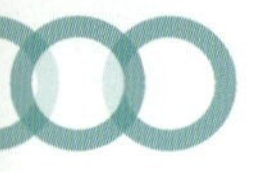

Answer 55

55i. An oesophageal Doppler probe. The device is used to aid perioperative fluid management by measuring blood flow (and therefore cardiac output) in the descending aorta. When optimally positioned, the waveform can be used to estimate cardiac output and intravascular filling and enable fluid or inotropic manipulations to be undertaken by the anaesthesiologist to optimise cardiac output to tissues. It has been found to be particularly useful in colorectal surgery when patients often are intravascularly deplete despite seemingly adequate fluid loading.

ii. It shows the velocity time envelope used to make calculations of cardiac output and stroke volume. Three main readings are used to do this: the peak of the green line, which is the peak velocity (PV) of blood in the aorta; the area under the green line curve is the stroke distance (SD); and the flow time, corrected for heart rate (FTc). Intraoperatively (and in ICU), fluid boluses and/or inotropes can be given and by measuring their effect, fluid management can be optimised, leading to enhanced tissue perfusion and improved perioperative outcome.

In addition to showing the waveform, the monitor displays numeric values of cardiac output, stroke volume, FTc, heart rate, PV and SD.

iii. The white arrow at the base of the waveform is known as the 'flow time' and depends on heart rate, left ventricular filling and afterload. The flow time corrected to a heart rate of 60 bpm (FTc) is inversely correlated with the systemic vascular resistance.

Answer 56

56i. There are three aspects of increased risk in this child:

- Genetics. Transmission of the genes for MH susceptibility is autosomal dominant. Therefore, there is a 50% risk that this child is also affected.
- Surgery. In a worldwide epidemiologic review of MH case reports, several types of surgery were shown to have an increased association with MH. The observed occurrence of MH during dental surgery was 56 times greater than expected.
- Patient. Not only is the incidence of MH increased in males, the fatality rate is also disproportionately increased. The most frequent age range in MH case reports is 3–5 years.

ii. It is not recommended that this child should undergo a muscle biopsy. This patient should receive a non-triggering anaesthetic agent and extended postoperative monitoring. Muscle testing is only performed at 40 centres in the world. The muscle sample must be obtained on-site. An age less than 4 years old and weight less than 20 kg (44 lb) are contraindications to muscle biopsy.

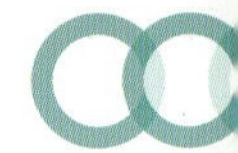

QUESTION 57

57 This child (**57a, b**) presented at 1 week of age because the parents noted difficulty with breathing and sucking.

i. What is wrong with this child, and how does the condition develop embryologically?

ii. What do the arrows in **57a** and **57b** show?

iii. What is the significance of the chest wall appearance (**57c**)?

iv. What are the implications for anaesthesia?

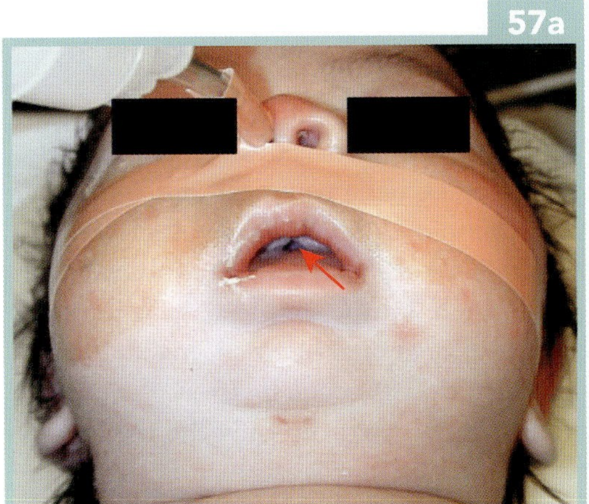

57a

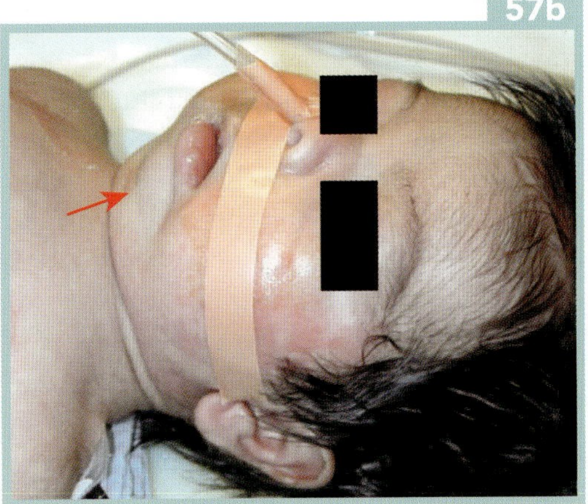

57b

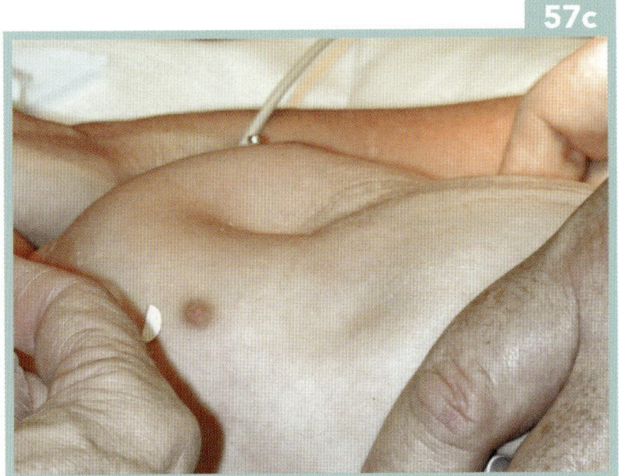

57c

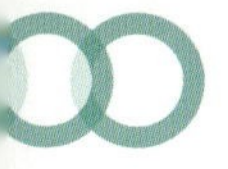

Answer 57

57i. The child has Pierre Robin syndrome, which results from a first embryonic branchial arch malformation causing micrognathia, glossoptosis and cleft palate.

ii. The arrow in **57a** shows a cleft palate between the teeth. There is also a symmetrically receded micrognathia (**57b**, arrow), which is confirmed by the radiograph (**57d**).

iii. The chest wall is receded because the child has difficulty in the inspiratory phase of respiration. This can be evident at birth but may not be severe for the first week. Periodic cyanotic attacks, laboured breathing and recession of the sternum and ribs (apparent when the child is supine) are common. The baby may be permanently mentally retarded secondary to periods of asphyxia.

iv. Immediate airway maintenance is critical. Keeping the baby prone with its head suspended by a pulley in a stockinette cap may be sufficient, but in severe cases the tongue tip may be sutured temporarily to the lower lip or anterior mandible. Tracheostomy is rarely required. Implications for anaesthesia centre on difficult airway management because of mandibular recession and the cleft palate. Airway maintenance must be constantly evaluated as the ET tube may kink and obstruct. Soft palate repair may cause airway swelling and the ET tube should remain for 48 hours post surgery to prevent airway obstruction. Congenital heart anomalies (e.g. ventricular or atrial septal defect, patent ductus arteriosus) occur in 15–20% of cases of Pierre Robin syndrome. The palatal defect varies widely from only the uvula to two-thirds of the hard palate and is horseshoe shaped. The small mandible often achieves catch-up growth by 4–6 years of age, but is always somewhat abnormal.

57d

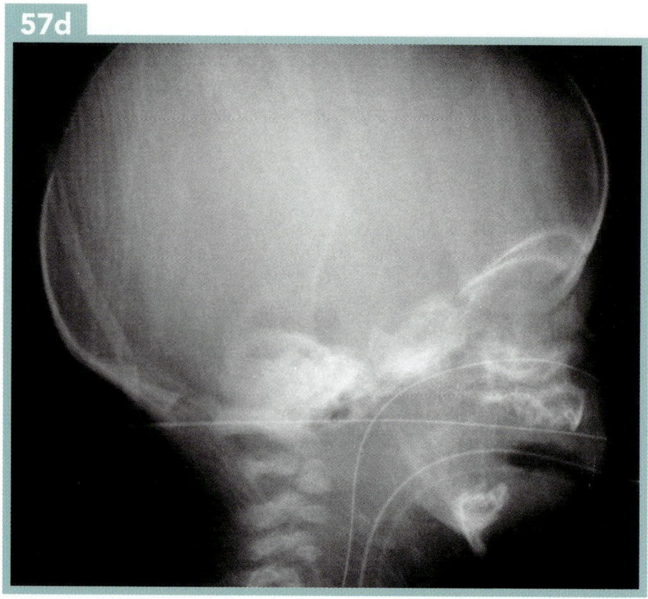

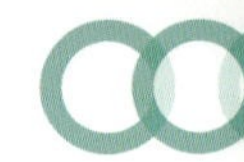

QUESTION 58

58 This 20-year-old woman was kicked by a horse (**58a**). She did not lose consciousness and was orientated prior to the induction of anaesthesia. She has no neck pain and an MRI of her cervical spine excluded a cervical spine injury.

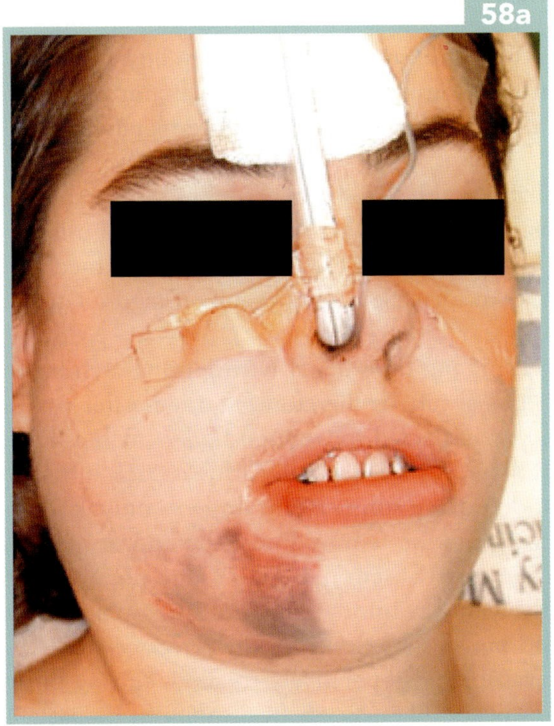
58a

i. What injury is likely? What investigations would assist diagnosis?

ii. Operative surgery on her jaw is planned. What anaesthetic problems may complicate induction?

iii. What anaesthetic techniques can be used for induction?

iv. What postoperative precautions need to be planned for?

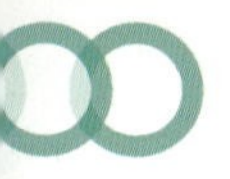

Answer 58

58i. A fractured mandible. She is unlikely to have a brain injury as she did not lose consciousness. Planned surgery is assisted by CT (**58b**) of the jaw. A 3-D CT image can also be constructed where facilities exist.

ii. Fractured mandible can cause a difficult airway due to loose teeth, oral bleeding, unstable fractures and a full stomach (due to swallowed blood). A fracture close to the articular joint may cause trismus, which may not relax on induction. A failed intubation drill should be thought through preoperatively.

iii. Awake nasal intubation with a fibreoptic scope is the safest option but may be difficult due to the patient's pain. Inhalational induction using a rapidly acting agent (e.g. sevoflurane) is an alternative. This should be performed on a tilting table with suction and facilities to turn the patient rapidly if regurgitation or vomiting occurs.

iv. Intermaxillary fixation and transdental wiring using arch bars will be carried out by the surgeons. A nasal tube is therefore required. After nasal tube placement, the mouth should be inspected for foreign bodies such as loose teeth and bone fragments and suctioned to clear blood. A throat pack in the oropharynx absorbs secretions and blood during surgery. The surgeon must know of the presence of the throat pack, as it must be removed near the end of surgery before jaw wiring starts. Antiemetics (e.g. ondansetron, 8 mg IV) are required as the jaws will be wired postoperatively and vomiting could lead to asphyxiation. Dexamethasone (6 mg IV) can also prevent vomiting and help reduce swelling. Wire cutters must be immediately available postoperatively to allow cutting of the wired jaws should airway obstruction occur. The nasotracheal tube can be partially withdrawn and used as a nasopharyngeal airway at the end of the case. Postoperative restlessness could be due to hypoxia in addition to pain, and the patient must be closely monitored until fully awake.

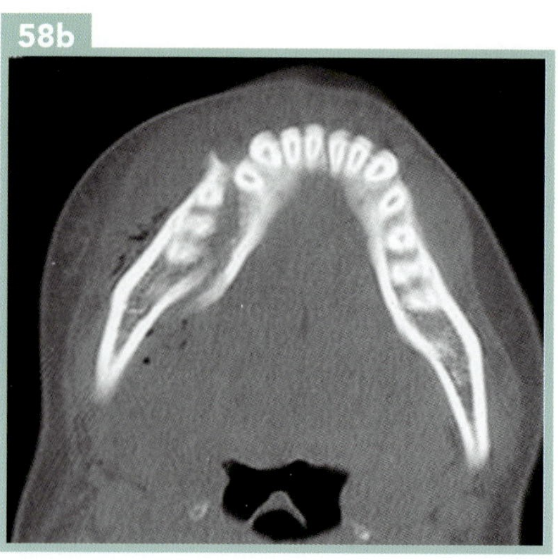
58b

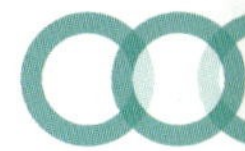

QUESTION 59

59 A 3-year-old child is brought to the hospital with a 2-day history of coughing. The child is not asthmatic, has not had any recent symptoms of an upper respiratory tract infection and does not have a fever.

i. Based on the X-rays (**59a, b**), what is this child's most likely diagnosis, and what operative intervention is necessary?

ii. What special anaesthetic considerations are important?

iii. How long should a child be fasted for prior to surgery?

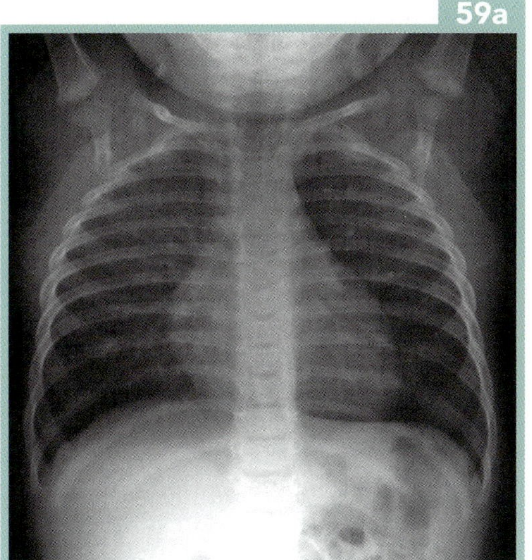
59a

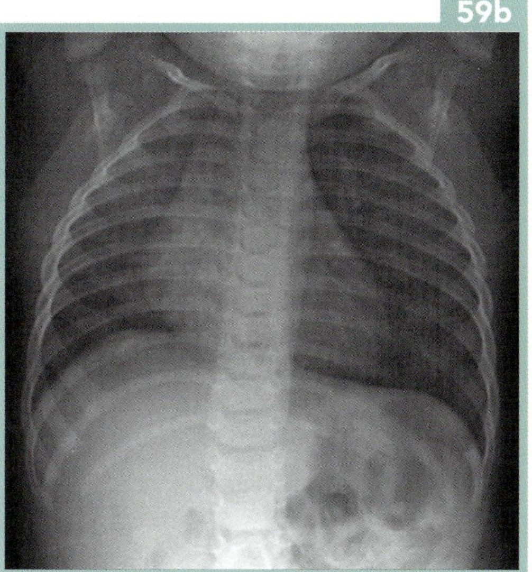
59b

QUESTION 60

60i. What are the risks for anaesthesia based on Child's classification (see case **219**)?

ii. How does severity of liver disease influence potential anaesthetic management?

Answer 59

59i. There is likely a foreign object in the right mainstem bronchus. Note the loss of normal vascular markings and hyperinflation of the right lung field (which does not decrease with exhalation). Such obstructions are usually non-radiopaque (in this case a carrot) and they create a 'ball valve' obstruction of the bronchus, allowing air to enter the right lung but not to escape. This child will require a general anaesthetic for rigid or flexible bronchoscopy and removal of the foreign object.

ii. An important consideration for this child is that positive pressure ventilation can aggravate the hyperinflation of the right lung, leading to compromise of venous return to the heart and/or a tension pneumothorax. Options for anaesthesia include mask induction with maintained spontaneous ventilation or total intravenous anaesthesia with spontaneous ventilation until the surgeon places the bronchoscope. However, if there is any risk of aspiration, or the child fails to maintain an adequate airway, the trachea should be intubated prior to presenting the airway to the surgeon.

iii. Children are considered fasted if they have had no clear fluids within 2 hours of surgery, no milk products (including breast milk) for 4 hours prior to operation and no solid foods for 6 hours prior to surgery.

Answer 60

60i. This classification has relevance to risk assessment for elective anaesthesia. Anaesthesia causing an abrupt acceleration of liver disease, resulting in fulminant hepatic failure, is the most serious outcome for the anaesthesiologist to consider. Child's C category indicates the risk of liver failure from major surgery and/or anaesthesia is >30%. Adverse outcome is only slightly increased for Child's A patients compared with matched controls without liver disease.

ii. Regardless of the severity of liver disease, the anaesthetic should be planned to have the least insult to the liver. Maintenance of liver blood flow and substrate delivery are major goals, as acceleration of liver disease is based on the multiple potential causes for reduced liver blood flow. Hypotension, vasoconstriction and cavity manipulation are the obvious causes. Direct anaesthetic drug effects are difficult to quantify, but drugs that require minimal hepatic metabolism are ideal. Some agents have intrinsic hepatic toxicity (i.e. halothane) and should be avoided. It is tempting to select regional anaesthesia but (1) central axis block could result in hypotension with adverses affects, (2) coagulation might also be abnormal, leading to increased risk of intrathecal or epidural bleed, and (3) poor liver synthetic function may result in low plasma cholinesterase levels, thus prolonging the plasma half-life of ester local anaesthetics.

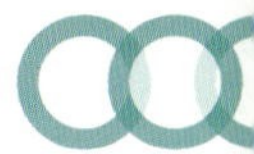

QUESTION 61

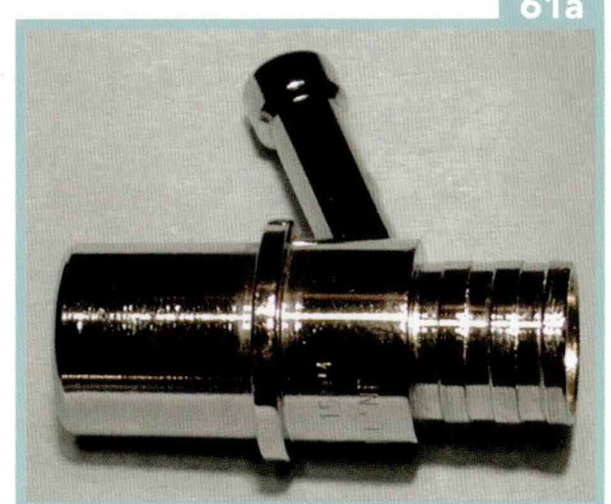
61a

61i. What is the archaic piece of equipment shown (**61a**)? (It has subsequently been replaced by a plastic disposable version, but the principles are the same.)

ii. Which Mapleson breathing system is it?

iii. Why have these metal reusable systems been replaced with plastic disposable versions?

iv. What is the minimum gas flow rate to prevent entrainment of room air for spontaneous breathing when this device is used exactly as shown? (**Note:** Such high-flow rates are not used in clinical practice as the wastage of fresh gas would be excessive and polluting.)

v. How is this piece of equipment modified by additional hardware such that it can be used in the operating room? Comment on how the gas flows are modified.

vi. What additional item is added to this device to enable controlled ('hand') ventilation?

QUESTION 62

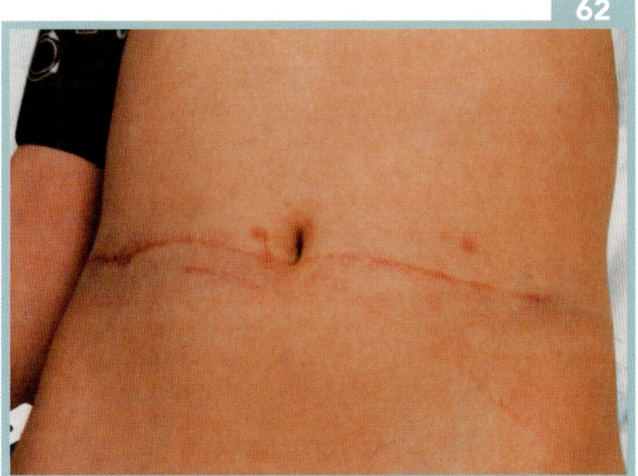
62

62 Shown (**62**) is the abdomen of a back seat passenger involved in a road traffic accident/motor vehicle accident.

i. What is this sign due to?

ii. What is the significance to the anaesthesiologist?

iii. Name five significant injuries that may have happened as indicated by this sign?

Answer 61

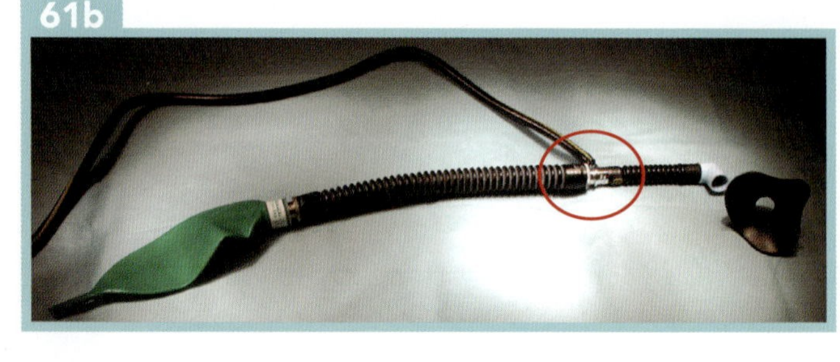

61b

61i. A classic 'Ayres T piece'.

ii. A Mapleson E breathing system.

iii. Plastic, single-use, disposable systems prevent contamination with viruses and/or prions and are cheaper to produce.

iv. A classic 'Ayres T piece' would have to have a gas flow of Pi (π) times minute ventilation (about 15–30 l/min for an adult) to prevent entrainment of room air (or gases from the expiratory limb). This is because there is no reservoir in the expiratory limb ('dead space'), therefore the fresh gas flow rate must exceed maximal (peak) tidal flow, approximately 15–30 litres per minute. This is neither economical nor practical.

v. The additional equipment to make an Ayres T piece practical is shown (**61b**). The long corrugated tubing introduces an expiratory limb 'dead space', which acts as a reservoir of fresh gas during the expiratory pause. This reduces the required minute volume from 30 l/min to twice minute volume (10–15 l/min (adult) or 100 ml/kg/minute for a child). This tubing is now disposable and plastic and the way all the component parts fit together is shown in **61b** (circled).

vi. A green reservoir bag. This is used in paediatric practice, is known as the 'Jackson Rees' modification and enables hand ventilation. An outlet at the distal end also allows venting of excess gases.

Answer 62

62i. The petechial stripe across this patient's abdomen has been caused by a rear seat belt in the car.

ii. This is a highly significant sign, as to generate this sign the vehicle can be assumed to be travelling at at least 64 kph (40 mph). At this speed significant deceleration injuries can occur.

iii. The mechanism of injury should alert suspicion of intra-abdominal haemorrhage from any organ, ruptured intra-abdominal viscus, ruptured spleen or liver, diaphragmatic rupture or any injury caused by rapid flexion deceleration of the thorax onto the thighs, such as head/neck/thoracic injury.

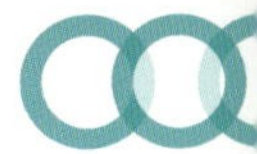

QUESTION 63

63i. What is illustrated in **63a**?

ii. What is indicated by the point marked A?

iii. What is indicated by the point marked B, and why is it important to understand why this is used?

iv. What does the blue line represent?

v. How do the curves of perfluorocarbon solutions, fetal blood and sickle cell blood differ from the normal curve illustrated by the red line?

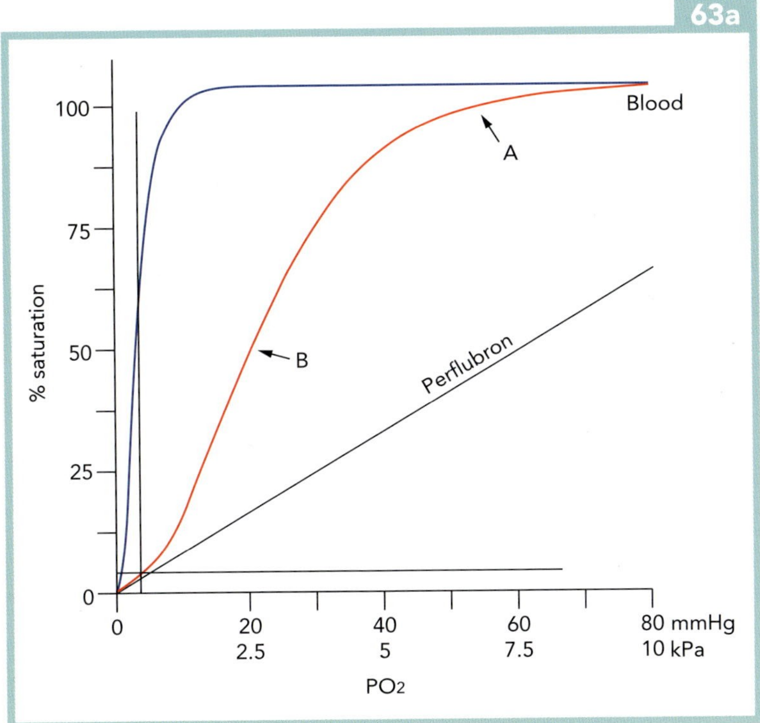

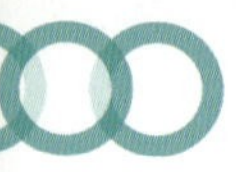

Answer 63

63i. The oxygen dissociation curve for normal adult haemoglobin (Hb).

ii. This point indicates an Hb O_2 saturation of 97%, above which good oxygenation of blood is guaranteed; this is the norm for an adult breathing room air at sea level.

iii. The P50 (normal value 3.73 kPa (28 mmHg)). This is the O_2 partial pressure in blood that leads to a Hb O_2 saturation of 50%. P50 is used to compare O_2 carriage in normal Hb with other types of Hb such as fetal Hb, abnormal variants of the Hb such as methaemoglobin, sickle cell anaemia, thalassaemia and other abnormal Hbs.

iv. CO has an affinity with Hb 240 times more than O_2. In CO poisoning the dissociation curve of carboxyhaemoglobin is very much shifted to the left (blue line on **63b**). Carboxyhaemoglobin is incapable of O_2 carriage, so high apparent 'saturations' actually reflect poor available O_2.

v. Perfluorocarbons do not have a sigmoid shaped dissociation curve, so oxygen carriage is linear (see **63b**). Perfluorocarbons need a high inspired O_2 concentration before clinically useful O_2 carriage can occur. Fetal Hb is designed to function at lower O_2 tensions than adults and therefore is to the left of the adult curve. The sickle cell Hb O_2 dissociation curve is to the right of the normal curve and loads O_2 less avidly than normal Hb. Sickle cell Hb is poorly soluble and crystallises, causing red cell deformation (sickling) with red cell fragility and thrombus formation.

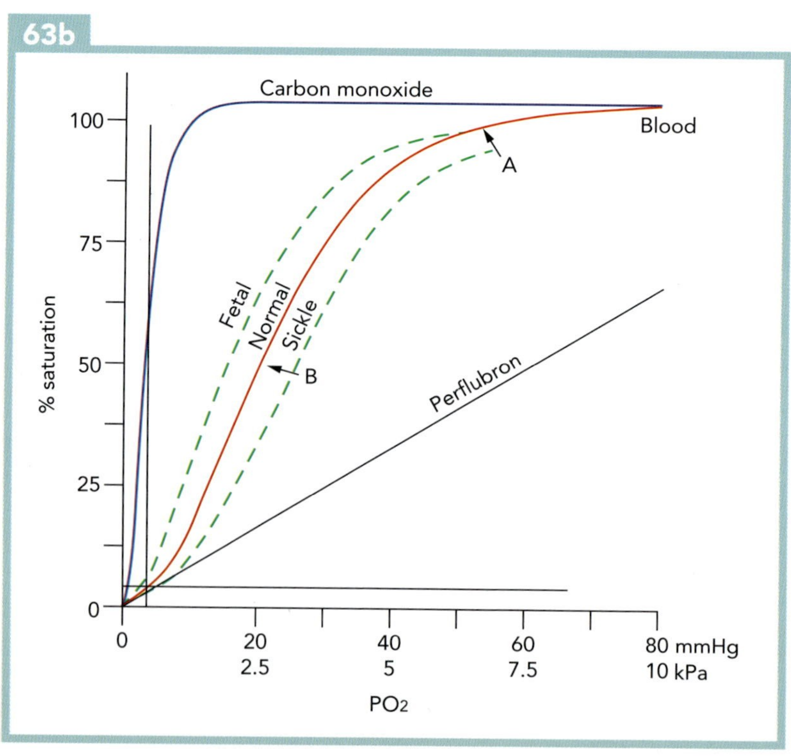

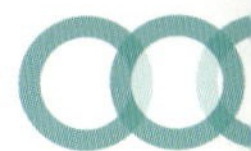

QUESTION 64

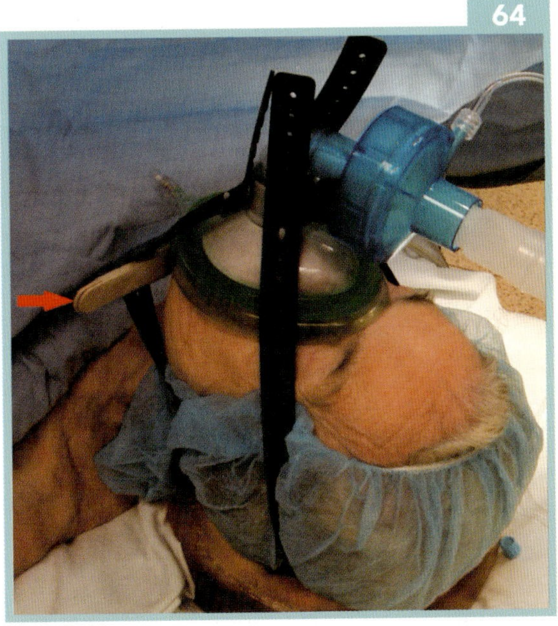

64 A patient is having difficult and prolonged lower limb surgery under a successful spinal anaesthetic block with a tourniquet inflated for almost 90 minutes. However, she is starting to experience anxiousness, restlessness and backache. The surgeon announces 30 minutes to completion of surgery. The patient had indicated that she had had prior 'bad experiences' with midazolam and propofol. Your colleague regularly and successfully uses mask anaesthesia with low concentrations of volatile agents for these cases of prolonged tourniquet use (**64**).

i. Mask anaesthesia could endanger the patient's eyes. Why?

ii. Mention two methods of preventing mechanical trauma to the eyes when using an anaesthetic mask.

iii. What would be an alternative way of maintaining the airway?

QUESTION 65

65i. What proportion of newborns require resuscitation?

ii. What factors contribute to making the neonate's first breath difficult?

iii. What three factors need to be assessed to determine the need for, and extent of, resuscitation? Give a description of the incremental steps implemented, dependent upon the assessment of the neonate.

iv. List the five elements of the APGAR score.

Answer 64

64i. If the mask 'cuff' presses on the eyes, periorbital tissue damage could result. Also, fat-soluble volatile agents could irritate the eyes directly or be absorbed into any oil-based eye ointments that may have been used.

ii. As indicated in **64**, a 'platform' (in this case, a tongue spatula) can change the direction of forces of the straps and prevent the mask from 'riding up' into the patient's eyes. Alternatively, the whole chin of the patient can be placed in the wide (lower) portion of the anaesthetic mask, preventing the mask from 'riding up' and also lifting the jaw upwards.

iii. A laryngeal mask airway could be used if the patient was anaesthetised deeply enough to allow its insertion.

Answer 65

65i. Approximately 6%.

ii. During the first breath, a negative pressure of >40 cm H_2O is needed to expand the lungs and overcome the viscosity of fluid-filled airways (100 ml). The opening of alveoli reduces pulmonary vascular resistance, decreases left atrial pressure and causes functional closure of the foramen ovale.

iii. Skin colour, heart rate (HR) and respiratory effort:
- Pink, HR >100 bpm, regular respiration: keep warm and dry.
- Pink, HR >100 bpm, irregular respiration: give O_2 and observe.
- Cyanosed or white, HR <100 bpm, irregular or absent respiration: advanced life support.

iv. See Table below.

	Score of 0	Score of 1	Score of 2	Acronym component
Skin colour/ complexion	Blue or pale all over	Blue at extremities: body pink (acrocyanosis)	No cyanosis; body and extremities pink	Appearance
Pulse rate	Absent	<100	≥100	Pulse
Reflex irritability	No response to stimulation	Grimace/feeble cry when stimulated	Cry or pull away when stimulated	Grimace
Muscle tone	None	Some flexion	Flexed arms, legs that resist extension	Activity
Breathing	Absent	Weak, irregular, gasping	Strong, lusty cry	Respiration

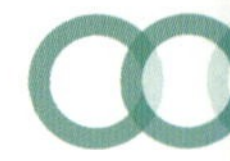

QUESTION 66

66 List the steps in the standardised resuscitation of the newborn.

QUESTION 67

67 An ECG taken on a patient with chronic renal failure who has presented with a ruptured aortic aneurysm (AA) is shown (**67**). The anaesthesiologist plans a rapid sequence anaesthetic induction with 3 minutes of preoxygenation followed by rapidly injected predetermined doses of thiopentone (thiopental) and suxamethonium (succinyl choline). Cricoid pressure is used to prevent aspiration of gastric contents. Comment on the plan to anaesthetise this patient with regard to:

67

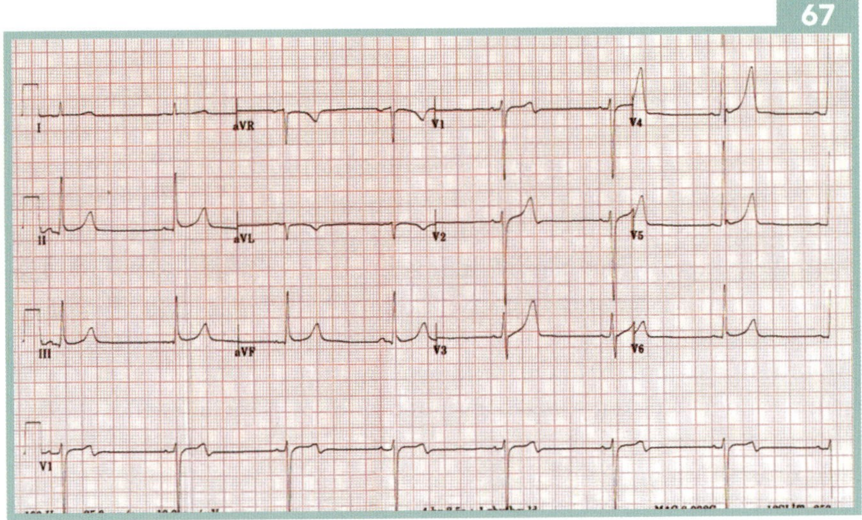

i. Optimal preoperative assessment and what you need to know.

ii. The choice of drugs for induction.

iii. General measures to care for this patient postoperatively.

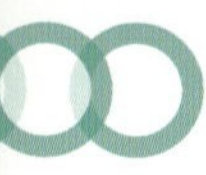

Answer 66

66 • Airway. Open and clear the airway, suction to mouth and nares.
• Breathing. Give 5 breaths, maintain 2 seconds inspiration with inflation pressure of 30 cm H_20. Ventilate at a rate of 30–40 breaths/minute.
• Circulation. Cardiac recovery is rapid when oxygenation is corrected. If the heart rate (HR) is <60 bpm or falling and below 100 bpm, start cardiac compressions. Compress the lower third of the sternum to a depth of 2–3 cm with two thumbs at 120 compressions/minute. If HR is >100 bpm, ventilate until spontaneous respiration returns. If HR does not recover, consider epinephrine (10 μg/ml IV, ideally via an umbilical venous catheter) or via the ET tube. Rarely, 4.2% sodium bicarbonate (1–2 mmol/kg) and/or a fluid bolus (10–20 ml/kg IV) of albumin or colloid may be needed. Administration of drugs should not interrupt chest compressions.

Answer 67

67i. The ECG shows 'tented' (coming to a point) peaked T waves, pathognomonic of hyperkalaemia. QRS complex duration is long at 112 ms (should be <110), further evidence of hyperkalaemia. Broad high T waves that do not 'tent' are probably due to ischaemia, particularly of the left anterior descending coronary artery. This ECG suggests that dangerously high serum potassium levels are present. (Serum potassium was 6.7 mmol/l.) Suxamethonium administration is contraindicated as potassium may rise by a further 0.5–1 mmol/l (i.e. to a level that can cause dangerous arrhythmias ± cardiac arrest). A suxamethonium-induced potassium surge is poorly understood but may relate to the acetylcholine receptor. Suxamethonium binds to this receptor and holds it open, allowing a potassium leak from the muscle endplate. Uraemia also exacerbates hyperkalaemia. An alternative muscle relaxant should be selected.

ii. This patient needs to be safely anaesthetised to prevent aspiration of gastric contents and allow rapid surgical control of the intra-abdominal haemorrhage. Dialysis should occur prior to surgery, but in this case this is not possible. Vecuronium (0.1 mg/kg) or rocuronium (0.6 mg/kg) are alternatives to suxamethonium and in the event of a failed intubation both can be reversed by the selective relaxant binding agent drug sugammadex (4 mg/kg) (not currently licenced in the USA). For continuing relaxation atracurium is useful, as it breaks down by Hoffmann degradation into inactive metabolites.

iii. Renal failure is highly likely due to the shock associated with AA rupture. The anaesthesiologist should maintain renal perfusion pressures where possible. Nephrotoxic drugs (e.g. NSAIDs, ACE inhibitors and aminoglycoside antibiotics) should be avoided and renally excreted drugs (e.g. certain antibiotics, digoxin, beta-blockers, diuretics and lithium) should be minimised.

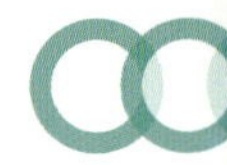

QUESTION 68

68 A patient presents to the emergency room with upper abdominal pain and long-standing COPD. He has air under the diaphragm on CXR and is not receiving any supplemental oxygen. His blood gas results are shown below:

pH	= 7.23 (H^+ = 60 nmol/l)
PO_2	= 8.0 kPa (60 mmHg)
PCO_2	= 7.5 kPa (55 mmHg)
HCO_3^-	= 18 mmol/l
Base excess	= -10

i. Interpret the blood gas results in terms of the clinical information that you have.

ii. What is the significance of the air under the diaphragm?

iii. Why has an anaesthesia consultation been asked for?

QUESTION 69

69 Shown are three oesophageal Doppler waveforms under three baseline circumstances and then an intervention has occurred in each case to change the waveforms into three different shapes (**69**). (Image courtesy Deltex Medical.)

i. What suboptimal conditions exist in each of the three baseline conditions a, b and c?

ii. What intervention has occurred in each case to improve the 'treated' waveform?

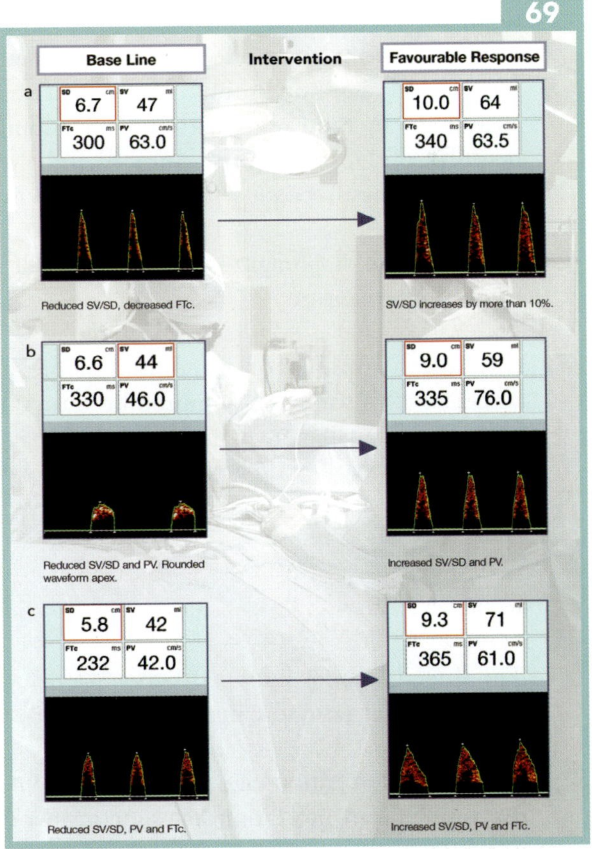

Answer 68

68i. Interpret blood gases thus. Check patient details, time of the sample and FIO_2. Look at PaO_2 (for hypoxaemia), pH/H^+ (for acidosis or alkalosis), $PaCO_2$ (to determine the respiratory component of the acidosis/alkalosis), bicarbonate or base excess (to determine any metabolic component). The anion gap should finally be calculated.

FIO_2 is 21% (room air). The patient is hypoxic, although a PO_2 of 8 kPa (60 mmHg) could be normal in severe COPD. Chronic retention of CO_2 is unlikely as bicarbonate rises in chronic CO_2 retention to compensate for chronic hypoventilation and bicarbonate is normal here. High-flow oxygen via a trauma mask should be commenced as the patient may be shocked from fluid depletion (nausea/vomiting/nil by mouth status) and possible blood loss. Increasing somnolence indicates CO_2 retention. Blood gases should be repeated 20–30 minutes after starting O_2 therapy to exclude retention and ventilatory support may be needed if CO_2 is retained. Oxygen use should be guided by O_2 saturations (94–98%, or 88–92% in CO_2 retention).

The marked acidosis compromises cardiac function and makes life-threatening arrhythmias and/or reduced cardiac contractility likely. The high CO_2 shows a respiratory acidosis; the low bicarbonate and negative base excess show a metabolic component too. Metabolic acidosis in an acute surgical patient is often due to shock or sepsis. Shock should always be considered and rapidly corrected prior to anaesthesia by fluid resuscitation. CVP monitoring, serial echocardiography and oesophageal Doppler during surgery all help to optimise perfusion. In summary, this patient has hypoxia with a metabolic and uncompensated respiratory acidosis.

ii. Air under the diaphragm is pathognomic of intestinal perforation and needs surgical intervention.

iii. Anaesthesia consultation is required before surgery. Postoperative ventilation in ICU after this surgery is required because the baseline gases show significant ventilatory impairment with a high CO_2 level. The abdominal wound will further inhibit respiration and clearing of respiratory tract secretions.

Answer 69

69i. The three baselines show: (a) hypovolaemia; (b) left ventricular inadequacy or failure; and (c) probable high afterload with vasoconstriction.

ii. The three interventions are: (a) administration of a 500 ml fluid bolus over 10 minutes; (b) commencement of inotropic support in a patient with a suspected myocardial infarction; and (c) administration of a vasodilator.

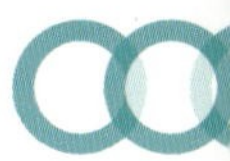

QUESTION 70

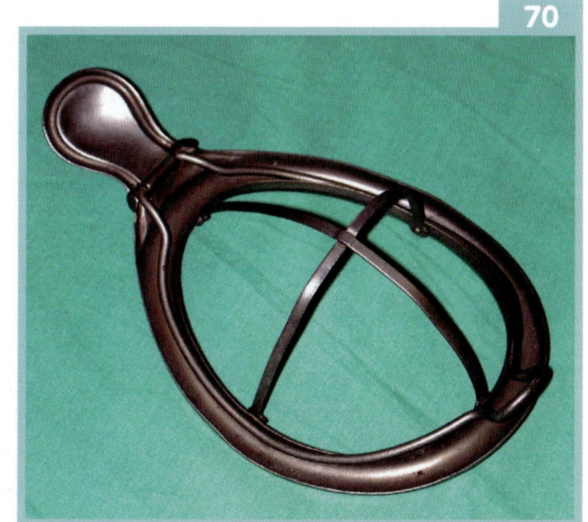

70i. What is the archaic piece of equipment shown (**70**), and how is it used?

ii. If ether was being used with this equipment, describe the stages of anaesthesia that would be gone through when anaesthetising patients from awake to deeply unconscious.

iii. Why does a modern day anaesthetist/anaesthesiologist need to know this information?

QUESTION 71

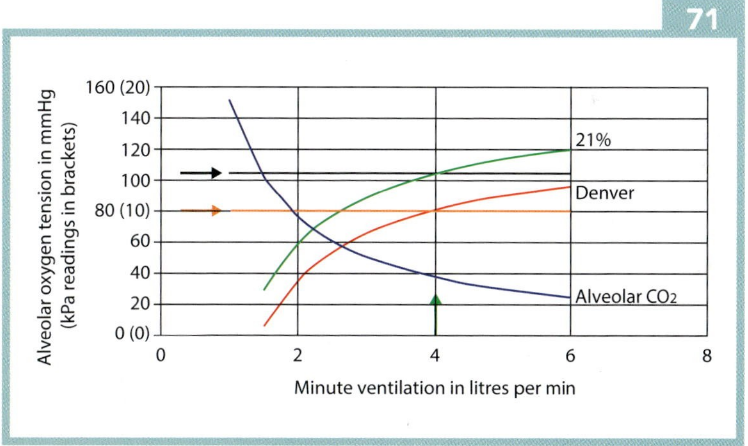

71 A graphic representation of the alveolar gas equation is shown (**71**). The effects of increasing the alveolar minute ventilation on the PCO_2 and PO_2 are also demonstrated. Note that without compensation (by hyperventilation) the alveolar oxygen tension (and the P_aO_2) will be around 80 mmHg (10.5 kPa) (green arrow intersection with the Denver line).

i. Using the graphic, explain why hyperventilation from 4 l/min to 6 l/m in Denver, Colorado, corrects alveolar O_2 tension from 80 mmHg to 100 mHg.

ii. Does atmospheric pressure and/or hyperventilation change the contribution of water vapour in decreasing the alveolar PO_2?

Answer 70

70i. A Schimmelbusch mask. A piece of gauze is laid over the mask and clipped between the edges of the rim of the device. Anaesthetic liquid is then dripped onto the gauze. It is the classical 'open' circuit and is dangerous for the patient in that volatile liquid can come into contact with the skin. Scavenging of vapour is not possible, therefore the operator will inhale anaesthetic vapour as well as the patient.

ii. Ether anaesthesia is incredibly safe. Cardiovascular depression occurs well after cessation of breathing, so unless the patient is ventilated with ether, cardiovascular depression is unlikely. Ether anaesthesia causes the patient to pass through various stages of anaesthesia as described by Guedel (see below). Anaesthesiologists using ether tried to maintain a state of surgical anaesthesia. Optimally this would consist of no eyeball movement, regular and deep breathing and moderate sized pupils.

Stage	Physical condition	Description
1	Analgesia	Beginning of induction to loss of consciousness
2	Excitement or uninhibited	Loss of consciousness to onset of automatic response breathing. There may be struggling, breath-holding, vomiting, coughing, swallowing
3	Surgical anaesthesia	Onset of automatic respiration to respiratory paralysis
4	Overdosage	From onset of diaphragmatic paralysis to death

iii. Current inhalational anaesthetic agents mimic the stages of anaesthesia seen by ether, but because of the lesser lipid solubility of modern agents, the stages are passed through more quickly. Even with modern monitoring there is no current accurate and infallible monitor of anaesthetic depth. Signs such as lacrimation, pupil size, pulse, BP, depth and rate of respiration (in spontaneously breathing patients) are still useful adjuncts by which to judge depth of anaesthesia.

Answer 71

71i. When breathing room air in Denver, Colorado (atmospheric pressure 640 mmHg (85 kPa), the PO_2 is 125 mmHg (16.6 kPa), which leads to an alveolar PO_2 of 80 mmHg (10.6 kPa) and the subject being relatively hypoxic. This hypoxia stimulates minute ventilation, decreases the alveolar CO_2 partial pressure and supplies additional oxygen to the alveolar space, so improving both the alveolar and arterial PaO_2.

ii. The saturated vapour pressure (SVP) at 37°C is 47 mmHg (6.2 kPa). The only factor that affects SVP is temperature. Neither the altered atmospheric pressure nor the hyperventilation affects the SVP of water vapour.

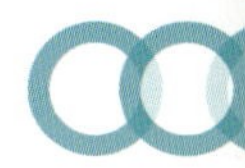

QUESTION 72

72 This patient (**72a**) is about to undergo carotid surgery under regional anaesthesia using a deep cervical plexus block.

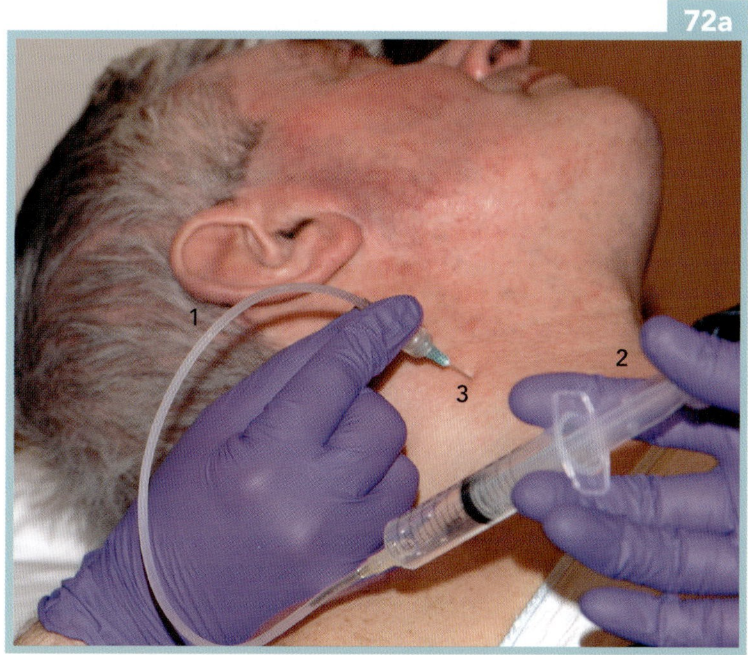

i. Is this block alone sufficient for this surgery?

ii. What are the landmarks indicated by points 1, 2 and 3?

iii. Which cervical dermatomes are blocked for this procedure to be successful?

iv. Outline the anatomy of the procedure and how it is performed.

v. Is regional anaesthesia preferable for this surgery?

vi. What complications can occur using this regional block?

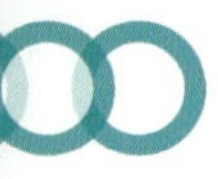

Answer 72

72i. Yes, but a combination of deep and superficial cervical plexus blocks works best.

ii. The block should be performed at C3 (point 3). The mastoid process (point 1) is used to identify the position of the first cervical vertebra (**72b**). The cricoid cartilage and the C6 transverse process (Chassaignac's tubercle) are at point 2. Using these two landmarks, the cervical processes are palpated manually. Point 3 is identified approximately 1 cm posterior to the posterior border of the sternocleidomastoid muscle.

iii. Dermatomes C2, C3 and C4.

iv. The supine patient turns his head to the opposite side from surgery. Under strict sterile technique, intradermal infiltration with local anaesthetic is performed and a 2.5 cm 25 gauge needle is introduced at right angles to the skin aiming in a slightly caudal direction (to avoid intrathecal injection). After location of the C3 vertebra (or if the patient reports paraesthesia in the distribution of the cervical plexus) 20 ml of local anaesthetic (usually 0.375% levo-bupivacaine) is injected. An assistant injects the solution as it is important to keep the needle as still as possible while the injection is taking place. Additional infiltration of the angle of the jaw also prevents the pain of the surgeon's retractor on the angle of the jaw during the procedure. The surgeon may supplement the block by a small amount of local anaesthetic on the carotid sheath.

v. A large trial of GA versus LA for carotid endarterectomy demonstrated no difference in the complication rate for either technique.

vi. Include: vertebral artery injection producing immediate loss of consciousness or seizure; subarachnoid injection; epidural injection; phrenic nerve palsy, which can lead to serious embarrassment of respiratory function in a patient with advanced lung disease. Less severe complications include local haematoma, transient Horner's syndrome, transient laryngeal nerve palsy and stellate ganglion block.

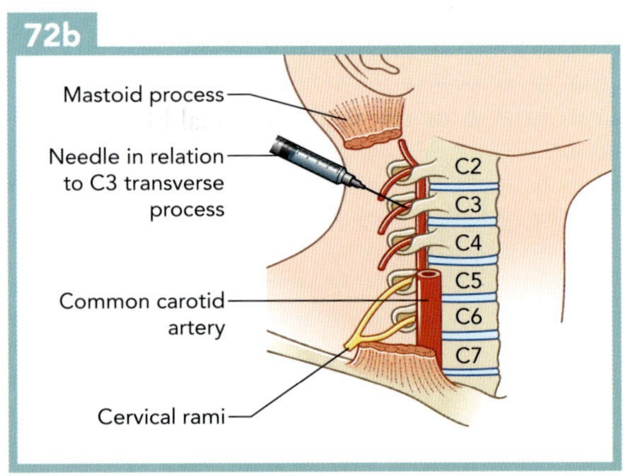

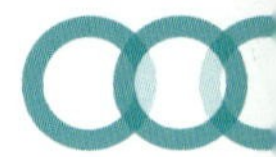

QUESTION 73

73i. What does this CT scan demonstrate (**73a**)? Describe its features.

ii. Describe a likely presentation of a patient as in **73a**.

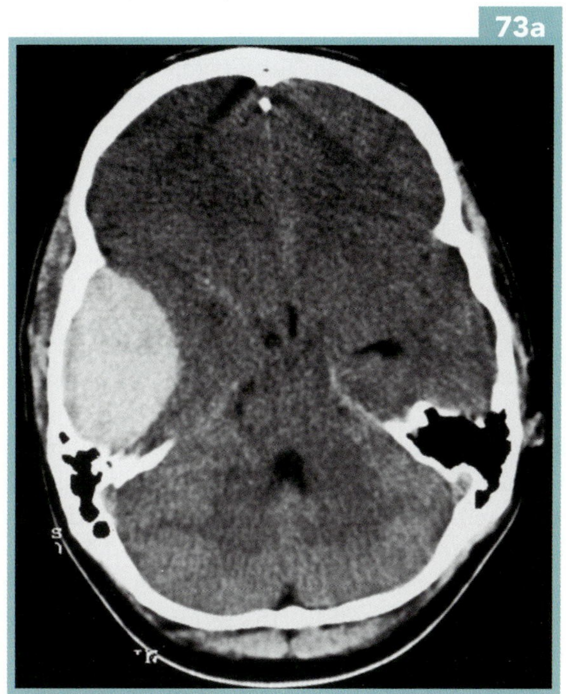
73a

QUESTION 74

74i. Define chronic kidney disease (CKD) in terms of glomerular filtration rate (GFR).

ii. List the causes.

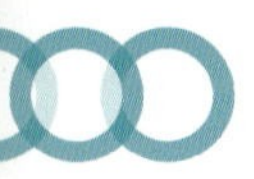

Answer 73

73i. An acute extradural haematoma (EDH) with accumulated blood between the dura mater and the skull. The classical lentiform (lens-like) appearance is shown.

ii. EDH is usually caused by head injury affecting the middle meningeal artery as it crosses the temporal bone. Rapid development of focal signs (e.g. contralateral unilateral weakness or visual loss) results from ipsilateral compression of crossed pyramidal pathways or the posterior cerebral artery, respectively. A lucid interval (temporary recovery of consciousness) may be described. Raised ICP with decreased conscious level and ipsilateral fixed dilated pupil subsequently occurs, leading to death if untreated.

Answer 74

74i. CKD is a permanent (usually progressive) reduction in renal function defined by stages according to GFR:

- **Stage 1.** Slightly diminished function; kidney damage with normal or relatively high GFR (≥90 ml/min/1.73 m^2). Kidney damage is defined as renal pathological abnormality or markers of renal damage (e.g. blood or urine tests or imaging studies).
- **Stage 2.** Mild reduction in GFR (60–89 ml/min/1.73 m^2) with kidney damage.
- **Stage 3.** Moderate reduction in GFR (30–59 ml/min/1.73 m^2).
- **Stage 4.** Severe reduction in GFR (15–29 ml/min/1.73 m^2). Preparation for renal replacement therapy (RRT).
- **Stage 5.** Established kidney failure (GFR <15 ml/min/1.73 m^2) (needs permanent RRT), or end-stage renal disease (ESRD). Patients may remain asymptomatic down to a GFR of 50 ml/min/1.73 m^2.

ii. Causes of CKD (from European Dialysis and Transplant Registry) are listed below:

	% of total
Glomerulonephritis	24.1
Pyelonephritis (stones, obstruction, reflux nephropathy)	16.6
Uncertain aetiology	14.4
Diabetes (non-insulin and insulin dependent)	13.1
Renal vascular disease (including hypertension)	9.8
Polycystic kidney disease	8.2
Multisystem disease (e.g. SLE)	4.8
Analgesia nephropathy	2.6
Amyloidosis	1.6
Renal vasculitis	0.7
Hypoplastic kidneys	0.5
Nephrotoxicity (e.g. cisplatinum, ACE inhibitors, aminoglycoside antibiotics)	0.2
Other	3.4

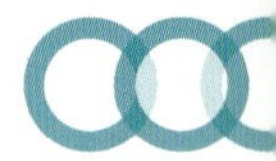

QUESTION 75

75i. What does this CT scan demonstrate (**75**)? Describe these features.

ii. Describe a likely presentation of a patient as in **75**.

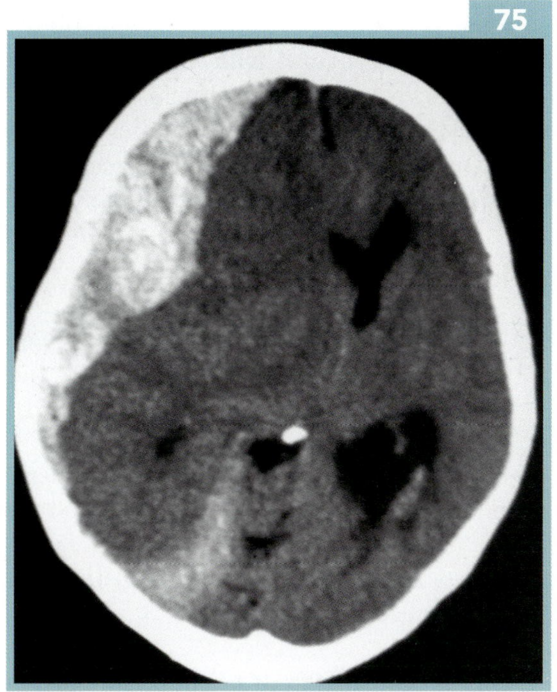

QUESTION 76

76 Describe how the degree of chronic kidney disease can be estimated from preoperative serum electrolytes.

Answer 75

75i. An acute subdural haematoma (SDH). Bleeding from the bridging veins between the dura mater and the arachnoid mater 'hugs' the internal aspect of the cranium and forms a crescent shape.

ii. SDH is classified as acute, subacute or chronic depending on the speed of onset. Acute bleeds occur from obvious trauma with high speed acceleration/deceleration injuries. Acute SDHs mimic extradural haematomas but have a worse prognosis due to the severity of the trauma causing other injuries and/or cerebral contusion. Chronic SDHs present subtly with symptoms of headache, fluctuating drowsiness, confusion, falls or ataxia and may go unnoticed for some weeks, particularly in the elderly. They are associated with minor or no trauma, alcoholism, age over 50 and systemic anticoagulation.

Answer 76

76 An estimate of GFR is calculable by knowledge of the patient's age, gender, body weight and urea/creatinine applied to the Cockcroft–Gault formula:

GFR in ml/min = [(140 – age in years) × weight (kg)]/plasma creatinine (μmol/l) × 0.82 (subtract 15% for females)

Renal function can also be estimated from serum creatinine. This guidance applies to elderly patients with known renal impairment
Reduced GFR (50 ml/min/1.73m^2) = serum creatinine rarely above 140 mmol/l (1.58 mg/dl)
GFR of 30–50 ml/min/1.73m^2 (moderate CKD) = creatinine up to 170 mmol/l (1.92 mg/dl)
GFR of 15–29ml/min/1.73m^2 (severe CKD) = creatinine to rise to 350 mmol/l (3.95 mg/dl)
GFR of <10 ml/min/1.73m^2 causes creatinine to rise to above 700 mmol/l (7.9 mg/dl) and may be life threatening.

Note: Serum creatinine can vary enormously (i.e. a young 100 kg body-builder may have a normal creatinine of 150 μmol/l [1.7 mg/dl], whereas for an elderly lady the same creatinine would indicate significant renal impairment).

QUESTION 77

77 The results of the European Carotid Surgery Trial (ECST), where patients are being treated for 82% or greater carotid stenosis by either carotid endarterectomy (CEA) or non-operative conservative treatment (prohibition of smoking, treatment of raised BP and use of antiplatelet drugs), are shown (**77**).

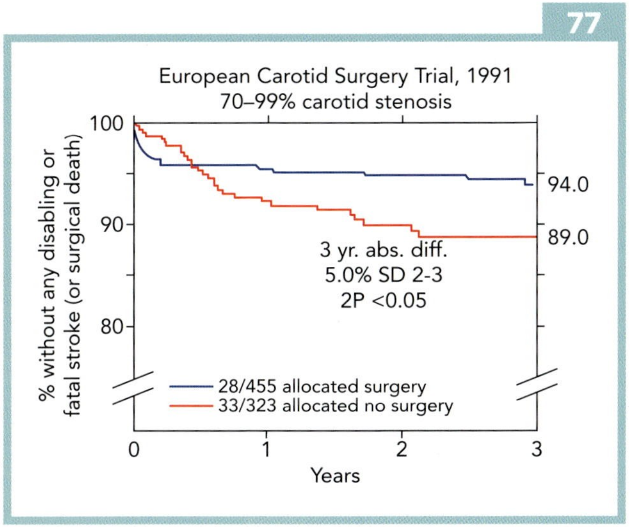

i. What is this kind of plot called?

ii. How is it carried out?

iii. What is a censored value?

iv. Is it worth performing CEA for patients of this type?

v. How should the graph be interpreted?

vi. Why does the graph fall by steps?

Answer 77

77i. A Kaplan Meier (K-M) survival curve, also a 'life table'.

ii. K-M plots record the survival time of subjects in two treatment groups against time. Survival time is the time from randomisation for the operative procedure (or start of conservative treatment) until time of death. Often used to predict time of death, this analysis can be applied to other situations (e.g. to detect the time when symptoms of a condition start). The end point is clear (death), but the start time of observation must be clearly defined (usually time of diagnosis). In CEA, delay between diagnosis and operation is important, as deaths occur during this period. In the ESCT, time from diagnosis to operation had to be <1 year.

iii. Censored values are 'lost' values because the period of observation was longer than the event being observed and patients withdrew for any other reason (e.g. non-consent).

iv. Yes. The lines cross early, showing the effect of immediate postoperative mortality. After the operative period, the lines cross again so at 1 year CEA patients are surviving at a much higher rate. Surgery is justified in patients with >82% stenosis.

v. In K-M plots, the probability of surviving a given length of time is calculated by considering time in many small intervals. The probability of surviving 2 days after CEA can be considered to be the probability of surviving 1 day multiplied by the probability of surviving the second day given that the patient survived the first day. This second probability is the 'conditional probability'. If $p100$ is the probability of surviving to the 100th day, conditional on having already survived the first 99 days, then the overall probability of surviving 100 days after a CEA is given by $p1 \times p2 \times p3 \ldots p99 \times p100$. The probability is 1 on days when nobody dies, so calculations are simplified by the fact that it is only necessary to calculate the probabilities for days when at least one person dies.

vi. The survival curve steps down as patients die. Censored values (e.g. due to patient withdrawal) are conventionally indicated with a tick.

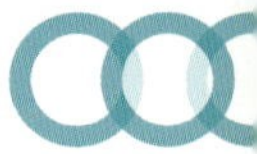

QUESTION 78

78i. Does the lateral cervical spine film shown in **78a** show any inadequacy or abnormality?

ii. Two CT images of a single vertebra of the same patient are shown in **78b**. Which vertebra is shown, and are there any abnormalities?

iii. What lessons should be learned from these two radiological investigations?

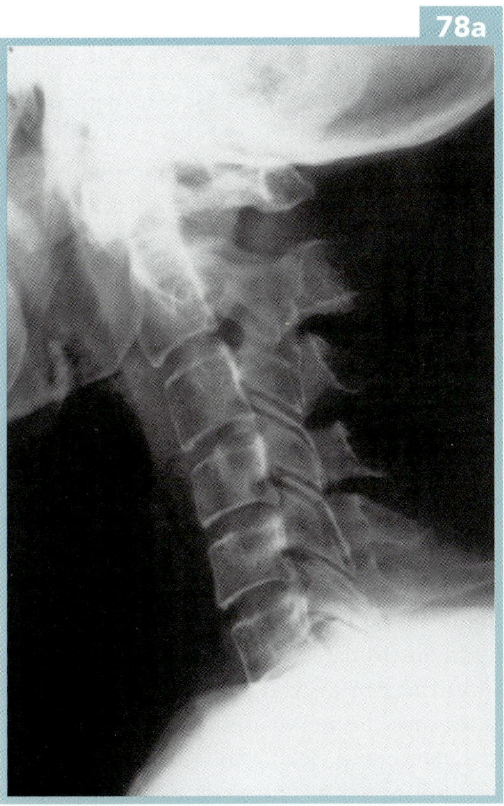
78a

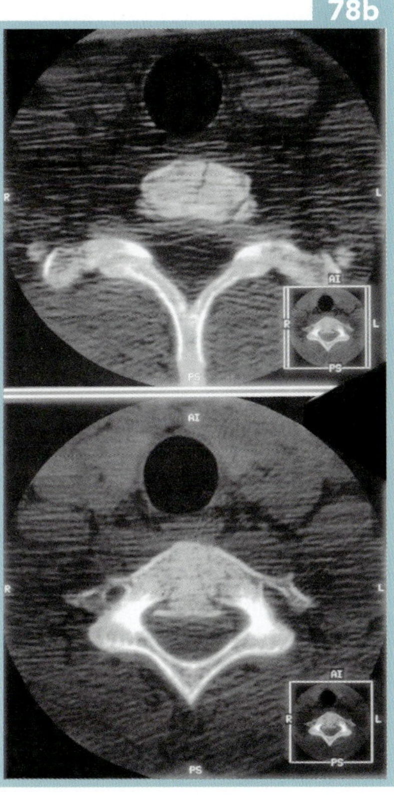

78b

QUESTION 79

79i. What procedure is being shown (**79**)?

ii. How is accurate needle placement ensured?

iii. Comment on the 'transarterial' technique.

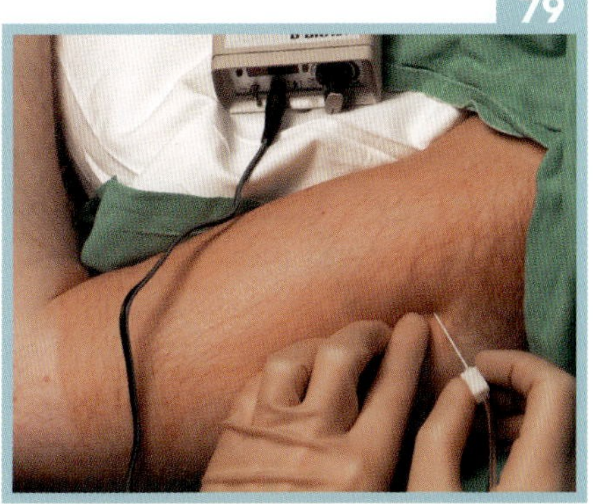
79

Answer 78

78i. The film is inadequate; the C7/T1 junction cannot be seen. The film shows loss of normal lordosis with abnormal straightening of the cervical spine, a sign of possible spinal damage. No other abnormality is visible on the X-ray.

ii. The CT scan of the same patient shows the fractured body of C7 with retropulsion of bone fragments into the spinal canal. There was no cord injury.

iii. Cervical spine injury should be assumed in all unconscious trauma patients. A lateral cervical spine film must show vertebral bodies C1 to C7. If these vertebral bodies are not shown, a 'swimmers view' could be requested but in major trauma cases, CT of the lower neck can be combined with thoracoabdominal CT to reveal the required structures. Inadequate cervical spine X-rays must never be accepted. With unsatisfactory X- ray views and no CT, the cervical spine must remain immobilised until suitable radiological or physical examination ensures that there is no cervical injury.

Answer 79

79i. The axillary approach to blocking the brachial plexus.

ii. Formerly, 'soft' end-points were used to confirm accurate placement of the needle, such as feeling a 'click' on entering the sheath or paraesthesia in the distribution of any of the cords of the brachial plexus. These methods can be inaccurate and subjective. Using a current generator and an insulated needle (as shown) to detect paraesthesia or contractions/twitching in the hand is the minimum method now expected. The use of ultrasound helps localise the nerve, minimises tissue damage and allows the relationship between the nerve and needle to be directly visualised and subsequent distension of the sheath on injection of the local anaesthetic.

Confirmation of successful placement can be made by adequacy of anaesthesia or imaging of radiopaque contrast within the plexus sheath. With successful placement it is possible to feel a 'sausage' of local anaesthetic within the sheath. The axillary approach, although excellent for forearm and hand surgery, may not anaesthetise the musculocutaneous nerve, resulting in tourniquet discomfort, and missing of the eminence of the hand may result.

iii. The brachial plexus in the axilla is known to run alongside the brachial artery, so arterial puncture and blood flow is actively sought and then local anaesthetic deposited both deep and superficial to the artery. This simple but hazardous technique has been superceded by the use of ultrasound.

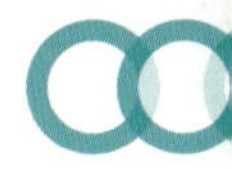

QUESTION 80

80i. Why might this patient (**80a**) present an airway problem?

ii. List the factors that may contribute to a difficult airway.

iii. Draw a diagram of the Mallampati system for preoperative prediction of a difficult airway.

iv. Describe how it can be used to predict ease of intubation at laryngoscopy?

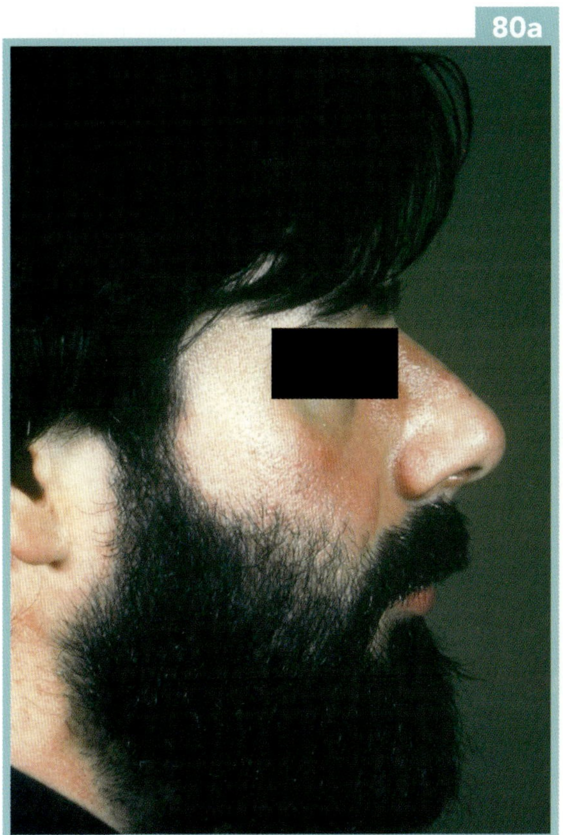

80a

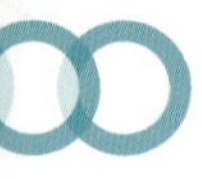

Answer 80

80i. In this case marked micrognathia is concealed by the beard (**80b**). Application of a facemask and intubation are challenging and the larynx may not be visible at laryngoscopy.

ii. Receding mandible; obesity; reduced atlanto-occipital joint movement (e.g. rheumatoid arthritis, past spinal surgery or neck trauma, Down's syndrome); prominent incisor teeth; high arched palate (e.g. Marfan's syndrome).

iii. Preoperative airway assessment follows the Mallampati classification. An open mouth and oropharyngeal view (**80c**) is classified as follows:

- Class 1. Faucial pillars, soft palate and uvula visualised.
- Class 2. Faucial pillars and soft palate visualised but uvula is masked by tongue.
- Class 3. Only the soft palate can be seen.
- Class 4. No soft palate can be seen.

80b

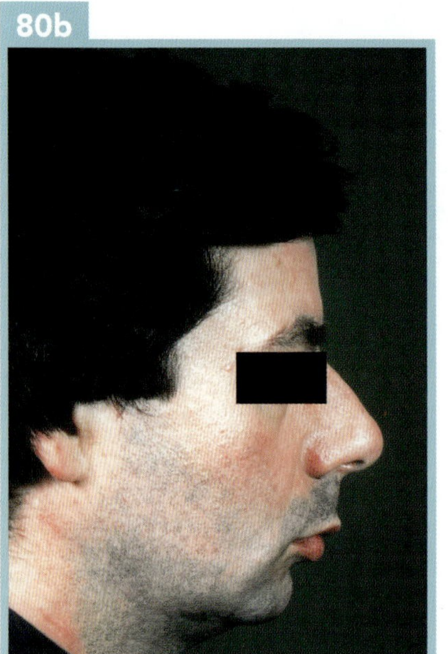

iv. 80% of Class 1 patients and 65% of Class 2 are easily intubatable. Classes 3 and 4 predict very difficult intubation. Ease of intubation should be routinely checked at the preoperative visit by Mallampati assessment. This patient was Mallampati Class 3 and fibreoptic intubation was required.

80c

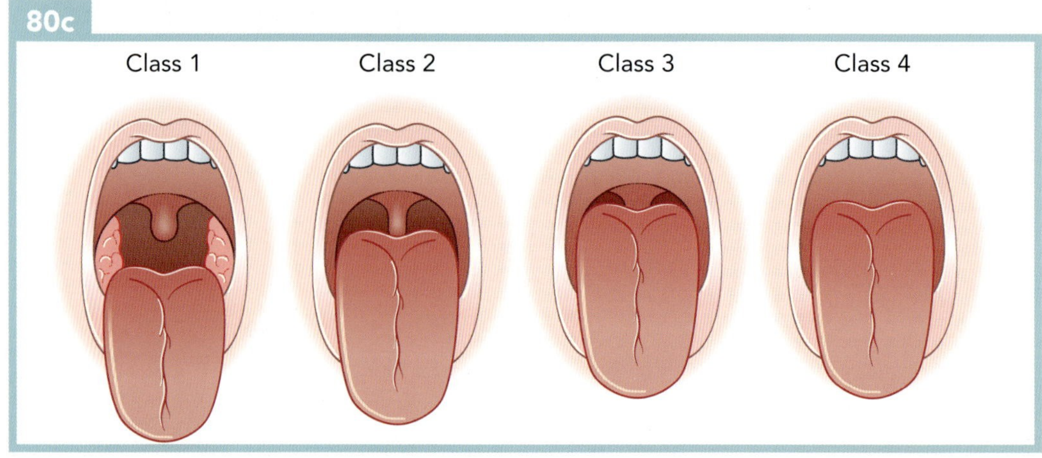

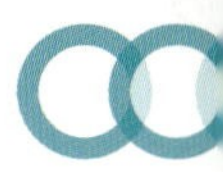

QUESTION 81

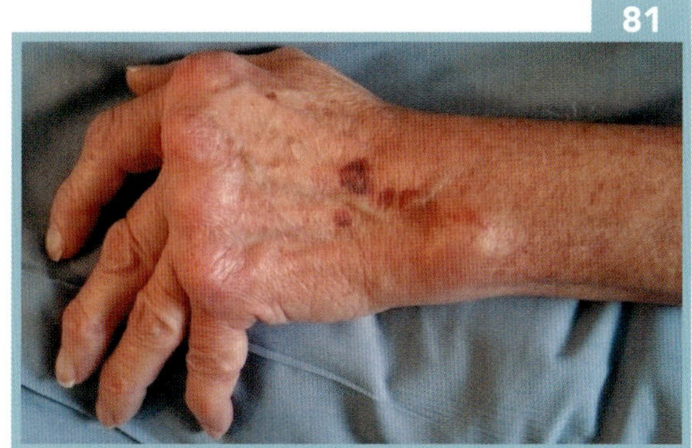
81

81i. What is the likely pathology affecting this female patient's hand (**81**)?

ii. Describe the key abnormal features illustrated.

iii. What preoperative investigations would help determine the extent of the disease.

QUESTION 82

82 Three tracings of relevance are shown (**82**): impedance pneumogram signal indicating chest movement; pneumotachogram indicating flow through the nose and/or mouth; and saturation (SpO_2). What type of apnoea is indicated by this tracing (i.e. does this patient show central or obstructive apnoea)? Explain your answer.

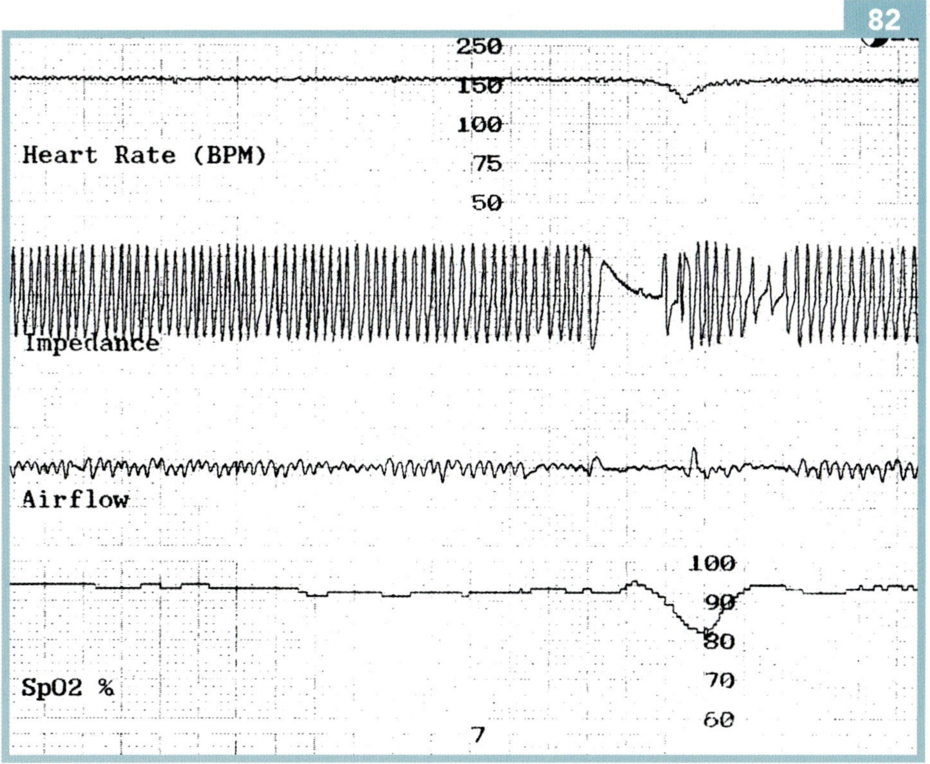

82

Answer 81

81i. Rheumatoid arthritis.

ii. The joints show swelling, deformity, changes in the overlying skin (e.g. erythema, microinfarcts) and abnormalities of surrounding structures (muscle wasting). Swellings around rheumatoid joints are of three types: hard/bony; joint effusions; synovial thickening.

iii. FBC (CBC), U+E, C-reactive protein and ESR are required. In patients with suspected respiratory compromise, blood gases are useful as rheumatoid lung may affect gas exchange. Anaemia is common but preoperative transfusion is rarely indicated even if Hb has fallen to 70 g/l (7 g/dl). The patient may have adapted to this Hb level but when haemorrhage is likely, cross-matched units should be ordered as relatively little blood loss may render such a patient critically anaemic.

Chest and cervical spine (c-spine) X-rays are important. CXR may reveal rheumatoid lung disease with pulmonary effusion, parenchymal or pleural rheumatoid nodules and signs of restrictive lung disease (e.g. kyphosis or bony collapse of the spine). C-spine films may show atlantoaxial subluxation (>3 mm from the anterior arch of the atlas to the odontoid process). Manipulation of the head may cause odontoid compression of the cervical cord, medulla or vertebral arteries, producing pyramidal signs, tetraplegia or even death. Preoperative neurological complications should be noted and care taken to avoid worsening them (e.g. peripheral nerve compression [carpal tunnel syndrome] and cervical root compression). Preoperative ECG is mandatory. Cardiological problems with pericardial thickening or effusion, pericarditis/myocarditis (associated with atypical chest pain or dysrhythmia), coronary arteritis, cardiac valve fibrosis, rheumatoid nodules in the conducting system with aortic regurgitation are all possible. If cardiopulmonary exercise testing is not possible, a cardiologist can perform a 'dobutamine stress test' to determine cardiological reserve. Patients receive a graded increasing dobutamine dose by infusion. Cardiovascular parameters associated with myocardial ischaemia can be documented and steps taken to prevent these from developing under anaesthesia.

Answer 82

82 The lack of chest movement (impedance pneumogram becoming 'flat') indicates that the apnoea is not obstructive, and therefore probably of central origin.

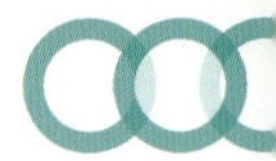

QUESTION 83

83 A male patient slipped on ice and fell heavily 48 hours ago and has broken ribs. He complains of a severe sharp pain in his left chest, worsened by inhalation, and had an obvious pneumothorax on CXR on admission, which is now being treated with a chest drain. He is pyrexial (39°C [102.2°F]) and has severe pain on coughing. He is neither coughing effectively nor expectorating secretions and is in danger of developing pneumonia.

i. What practical procedure is being carried out (**83a**), and why?

ii. Describe the procedure. **Note:** Modern practice would demand a sterile field with drapes applied to the patients back. The drapes have been omitted for anatomical clarity.

iii. Draw the anatomy of structures that must be known in order to safely perform this procedure.

iv. What are the risks of this procedure?

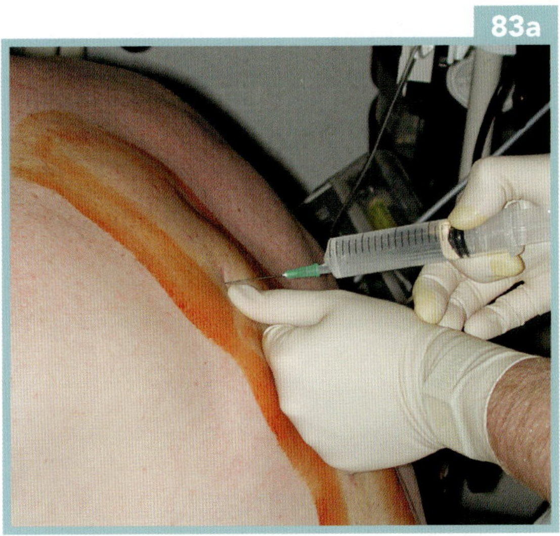
83a

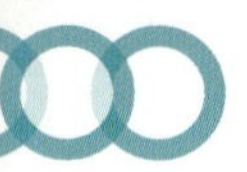

Answer 83

83i. An intercostal nerve block; provides excellent short-term analgesia to enable expectoration.

ii. With full aseptic technique, the lower edge of the affected rib has a 21G needle inserted 20° cephalad to the skin at the posterior angle of the rib. Both posterior and anterior intercostal nerve divisions are blocked. The needle is then 'walked off' the inferior rib edge and inserted approximately 1 cm cephalad. The tip of the needle should now be close to the intercostal nerve. Needle aspiration now verifies that neither air (indicating pleural puncture) nor blood (indicating blood vessel puncture) is present. A standard dose of 3–6 ml of 0.5% bupivacaine (ideally levo bupivacaine with 1:200,000 adrenaline) is injected into the sub-intercostal region. This procedure is repeated at least two rib spaces above and below the painful area up to the maximum dose of local anaesthetic (2 mg/kg for bupivacaine). This can be repeated 4–6 hours later, up to 3 or 4 times.

iii. The anatomy is shown in **83b**. The yellow, red and blue structures are the intercostal nerve, artery and vein, respectfully.

iv. Pneumothorax by pleural puncture. Must be avoided if the patient requires GA or air transport. As the intercostal vein and artery lie close to the intercostal nerve, inadvertent puncture of the intercostal vessels or local anaesthetic toxicity (causing seizure or cardiac arrest) can occur because of rapid absorption of local anaesthetic by this vascular area. Needle shearing of the intercostal nerves can lead to long-term nerve damage, irritation or neuritis.

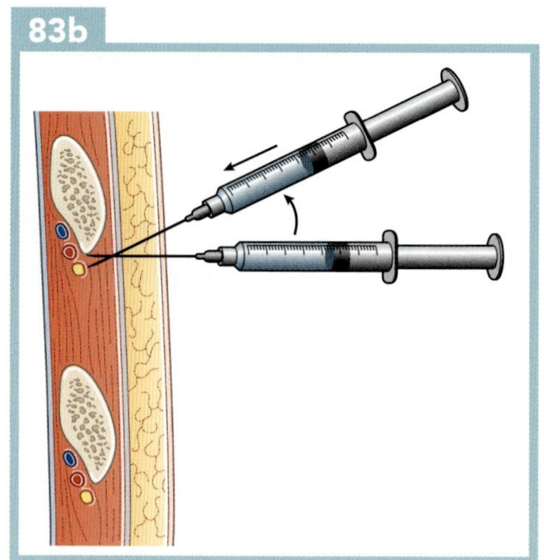

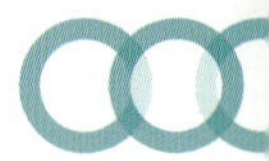

QUESTION 84

84i. Define what an inotrope is.

ii. Why is this different from a vasopressor?

iii. Catecholamines form the majority of inotropes administered by infusion for the treatment of circulatory inadequacy in critically ill patients. Describe how catecholamines exert their action.

iv. Comment specifically on dopamine's mode of action.

v. For each of the drugs listed, fill in the blanks in the Table below.

Drug	Adrenoreceptors stimulated	Actions (on heart rate [HR], stroke volume [SV], vascular tone)
Adrenaline		
Dobutamine		
Dopamine		
Dopexamine		
Noradrenaline		

QUESTION 85

85 A TOE image is shown (**85**).

i. What is this view called?

ii. Which structures are indicated by A, B and C?

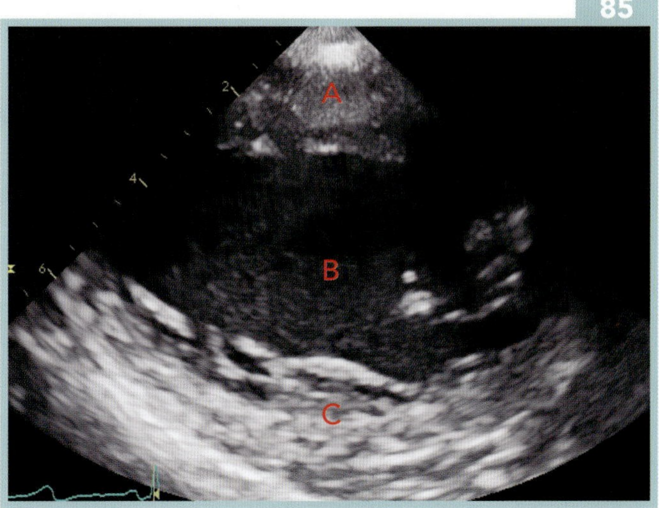

Answer 84

84i. An inotrope increases the force of cardiac contraction.

ii. A vasopressor causes constriction of vascular smooth muscle and elevates BP. Vasopressors and inotropes work via the autonomic nervous system and adrenoreceptors.

iii. Catecholamines work by binding to three major classes of adrenoreceptors: α-adrenergic, β-adrenergic and dopaminergic (DA) receptors. Adrenoreceptors constitute a complex group of glycoproteins that allow catecholamines to alter cellular function. Although as many as eight subtypes of adrenoreceptor exist, for practical purposes there are two types of each adrenoreceptor: α_1 and α_2, β_1 and β_2, and DA_1 and DA_2. The most important in understanding catecholamine actions are summarised as:

- 1: peripheral arteriolar vasoconstriction.
- 1: cardiac effects are increased heart rate and force of contraction.
- 2: bronchial smooth muscle dilation. Vasodilatation in skeletal muscle. Also some positive inotropic and chronotropic cardiac effects.
- D: increased renal blood flow at low dose, inotropic effects at medium dose.

iv. The dopamine receptor and subsequent effect is dose dependent:

- 1–2 mcg/kg/min: acts on DA receptors causing renal vasodilation and increasing urine output.
- 2–10 mcg/kg/min: also acts on β receptors and increases cardiac output.
- >10 mcg/kg/min: has effects on α_1 receptors, causing arterial vasoconstriction.

v.

Drug	Adrenoreceptors stimulated	Actions (on HR, stroke volume [SV], vascular tone)
Adrenaline	β1, β2, α	↑HR, ↑SV, vasoconstrictor (↑BP)
Dobutamine	β1, β2	↑HR, ↑SV, vasodilator (↓BP)
Dopamine	α, β1, β2, DA	Low dose: DA effects Intermediate dose: inotrope High dose: vasopressor
Dopexamine	β2, DA	↑HR, splanchnic vasodilator
Noradrenaline	α	Vasoconstrictor

Answer 85

85i. This view is called the transgastric, two-chamber view.

ii. A indicates the liver; B indicates the left ventricular cavity; C indicates the anterior wall of the left ventricle.

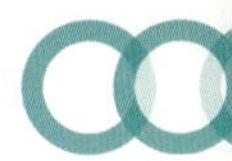

QUESTION 86

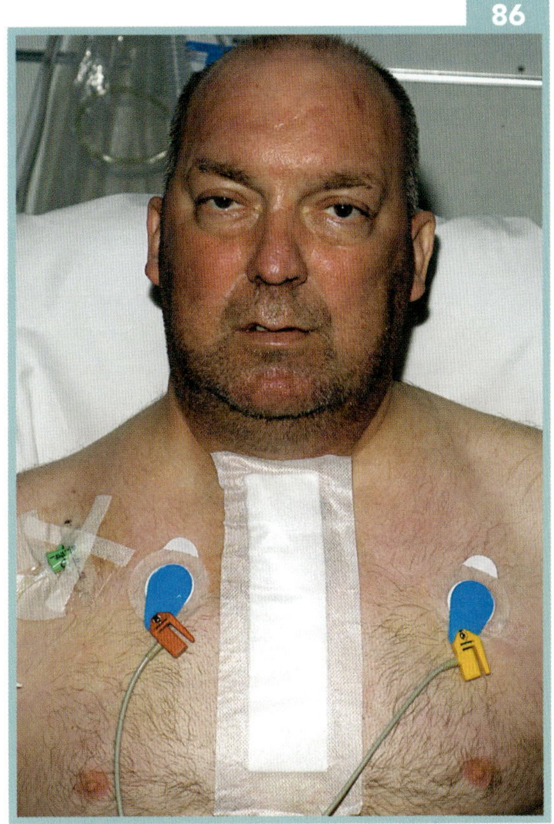

86 The man shown (**86**) presented with lethargy, double vision and difficulty chewing food that worsened with fatigue and in the latter half of the day.

i. What is a possible diagnosis?

ii. Why does this condition occur?

iii. The patient has had surgery via his anterior chest wall. What is this for?

iv. Why is anaesthesia challenging in these patients?

QUESTION 87

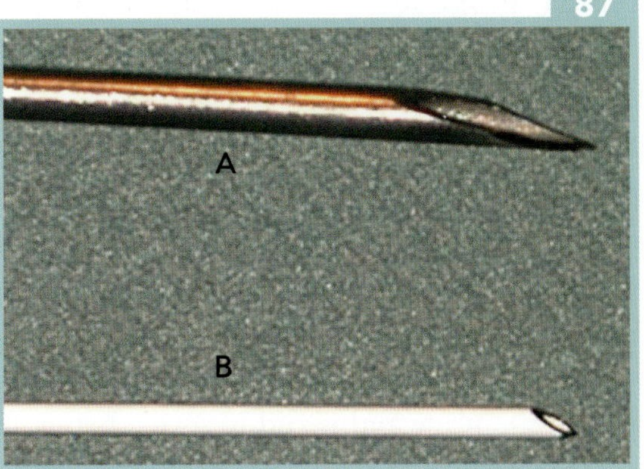

87i. What is meant by a single bevel needle in contrast with a double bevel needle? Which is the single bevel needle and which the double bevel needle in **87**?

ii. What are the advantages of each?

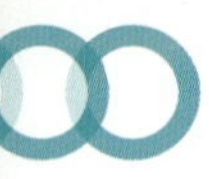

Answer 86

86i. Myasthenia gravis (MG). Muscle fatigability worsening through the day is characteristic of MG. Note the patient's drooping eyelids. Facial/bulbar myasthenic weakness leads to classical symptoms of double vision and chewing difficulties.

ii. Autoimmune antibodies block nicotinic acetylcholine receptors (AChRs) in the postsynaptic neuromuscular junction, causing muscle weakness.

iii. Thymectomy is recommended and within 2–5 years of surgery symptoms unpredictably may improve. Thymus produced helper T cells interact with B cells forming antibodies to attack the AChRs. Ten percent of patients with MG have a thymic tumour and 70% have hyperplastic changes indicating an active immune response.

iv. Muscle relaxants should be avoided but if essential, drugs that decay spontaneously by Hoffman degradation (atracurium/mivacurium) should be used. Neuromuscular transmission should be monitored by nerve stimulator.

Most anaesthetic problems relate to reversal of neuromuscular blockade with cholinesterase (ChE) inhibitors (e.g. neostigmine). Inadequate doses of inhibitor may mimic a myasthenic crisis with profound weakness; too much causes a cholinergic crisis with queasiness, loose stools, nausea, vomiting, abdominal cramps and diarrhoea. Increased bronchial and oral secretions with severe generalised weakness, swallowing problems and respiratory failure may be precipitated. ChE inhibitors should be avoided and postoperative ventilatory support is safer by allowing relaxants to wear off without reversing agents. Medical treatment of MG may be maintained, tapered or discontinued depending on the outcome of surgery.

Answer 87

87i. A single bevel needle has the tip cut in a single plane. The double bevel needle has two separate angles cut into the tip of the needle (easier to see in the upper part of the tip of the upper needle). Needle A is the double bevel needle.

ii. The double bevel needle is said to be 'sharper' and cuts through skin and tissues much more readily. The single bevel needle is perceived to be more blunt, requires more force to cut through tissues, demonstrates a better 'pop through' into a new tissue plane and is said to give a better 'feel' of the type of tissue being traversed. The single bevel needle is also less likely to damage ('cut into') a nerve. For the last two reasons, the single bevel needle is often preferred for regional anaesthesia.

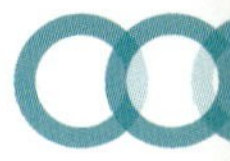

QUESTION 88

88 Platelets are an essential component of the clotting cascade and aggregate by stimulation of intraplatelet calcium (as shown in the centre of **88**). Various drugs (labelled on **88**) can inhibit this aggregation. What is:

- Drug A: a cyclo-oxygenase inhibitor with a long duration of action. A very commonly prescribed drug.
- Drug B: acts positively on adenylate cyclase and increases cyclic AMP.
- Drug C: acts on GP receptors on the platelet surface and is administered by IV infusion.
- Drug D: covalently binds to adenine diphosphate on the platelet wall. Used in a similar way to drug A, it is more expensive but associated with less GI haemorrhage.
- Drug E: used during percutaneous coronary intervention to prevent intracoronary coagulation during the procedure.

ADP = adenosine diphosphate; cAMP = cyclic adenosine monophosphate; GP = glycoprotein; PGG_2 = prostaglandin G_2; PAR = protease activated receptor; PGH_2 = prostaglandin H_2; PGI_2 = prostacyclin; TXA_2 = thromboxane A_2; vWF = von Willebrand factor.

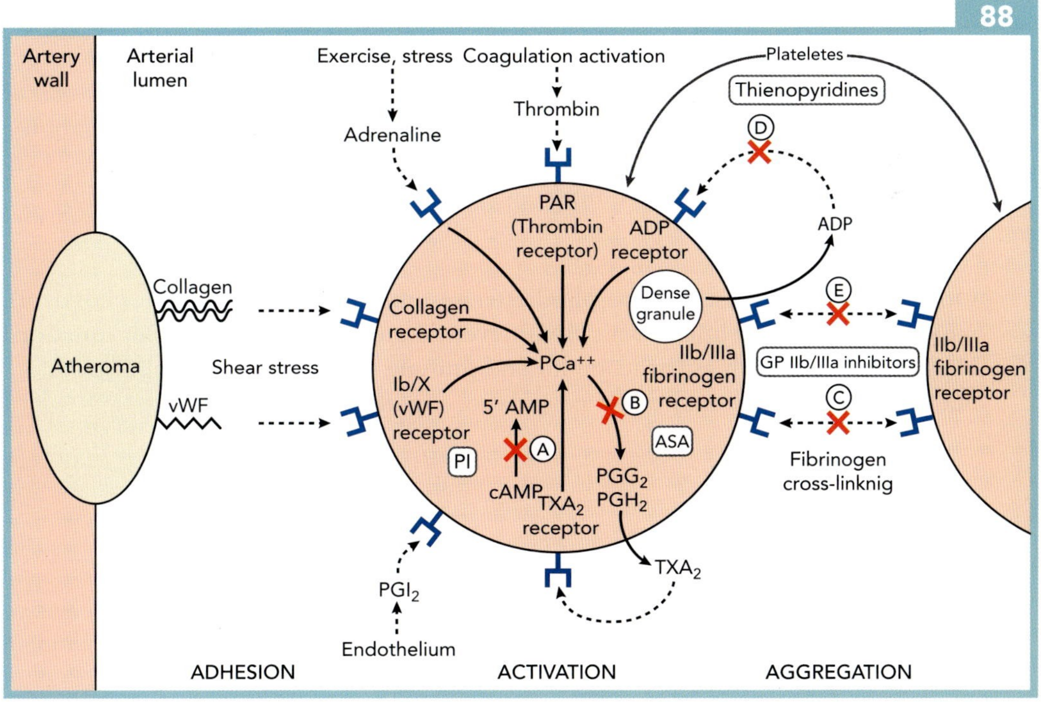

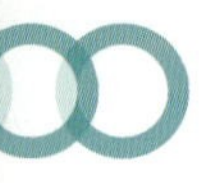

Answer 88

88 Platelets adhere to proteins on an exposed vessel endothelium (e.g. collagen and von Willebrand factor. Platelet agonists (shear forces, adrenaline, thrombin, ADP, thromboxane A_2) promote intraplatelet calcium, which enhances platelet activation.

- Drug A: aspirin. Irreversibly inhibits platelet and megakaryocyte prostaglandin H synthase (cyclo-oxygenase-1). Blocks formation of thromboxane A_2, a potent vasoconstrictor and platelet aggregant. Only acetylsalicylic acid has any significant effect on platelet function. Platelets are unable to regenerate cyclo-oxygenase so the antithrombotic effect remains for the lifespan of the platelet (8–10 days). After stopping aspirin, normal haemostasis is regained when 20% of platelets have normal cyclo-oxygenase activity.
- Drug B: prostacyclin. An alternative to IV heparin infusion. Augments intracellular cyclic AMP and reduces platelet aggregation.
- Drug C: dextrans. Complex sugars that prevent the adhesion of GP receptors to the vessel wall or other platelets. Cross-linking between platelets is inhibited and platelet aggregation prevented.
- Drug D: clopidogrel. A thienopyridine used for up to 12 months after non-ST elevation acute coronary syndromes or after coronary angioplasty/stenting. Main advantage is a decreased incidence of GI bleeding. Metabolised in the liver. Active compounds are formed that covalently bind and block ADP receptors on platelets, dramatically reducing platelet activation.
- Drug E: abciximab. Complicated myocardial events, such as non-ST elevation and acute coronary syndromes, can be treated in the short term with IIa/IIIb GP inhibitors (e.g. abciximab), which prevent fibrinogen cross-linking between platelets.

Other drugs of interest are phosphodiesterase inhibitors (dipyridamole, cilostazol), which elevate intracellular cyclic AMP levels, thereby inhibiting platelet function. Herbal remedies such as garlic, ginko and ginseng may also affect coagulation, but only extreme use may affect coagulation significantly.

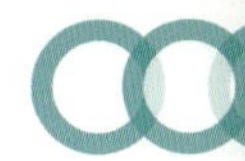

QUESTION 89

89 Consider the figures in the Table below statistically:

DATA TYPE		Measurement scale (nominal, ordinal, interval or ratio)? Parametric or non-parametric?
Female	Male	
Brunette	Blond	
Small	Large	
Cool	Feverish	
Short	Tall	
GCS = 10	GCS = 8	
5 ft	6 ft	
110 lb (50 kg)	220 lb (100 kg)	
37°C (98.6°F)	38°C (100.4°F)	
273° Kelvin	274° Kelvin	

i. Classify from this list each type of data in its appropriate measurement scale: (a) nominal or categorical; (b) ordinal or ranking; (c) interval; (d) ratio or absolute.

ii. Are the data parametric or non-parametric?

iii. Define each measurement scale listed above (a to d).

iv. Which of the four scales are parametric and which are non-parametric?

v. If parametric data are not normally distributed, is it acceptable to use a non-parametric test (e.g. Mann-Whitney U test)?

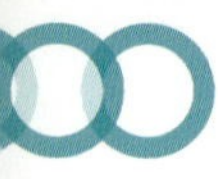

Answer 89

89i. The classification is shown below:

ii.

DATA TYPE		Measurement scale (nominal, ordinal, interval or ratio)? Parametric or non-parametric?
Female	Male	Nominal, non-parametric
Brunette	Blond	Nominal, non-parametric
Small	Large	Ordinal, non-parametric
Cool	Feverish	Ordinal, non-parametric
Short	Tall	Ordinal, non-parametric
GCS = 10	GCS = 8	Ordinal, non-parametric
5 ft	6 ft	Ratio, parametric
110 lb (50 kg)	220 lb (100 kg)	Ratio, parametric
37°C (98.6°F)	38°C (100.4°F)	Interval, parametric
273° Kelvin	274° Kelvin	Ratio, Parametric

iii. (a) Nominal or categorical scales are groups of data that do not bear any mathematical relationship to one another and are all 'equal' categories (e.g. one eye colour is not 'larger' or 'better' or ranked any differently from another eye colour).

(b) Ordinal or ranking scales (ranked from large to small, or small to large) are groups of data points that bear a mathematical relationship to one another (e.g. one subject is sicker, more traumatized, more dehydrated than another).

(c) Interval scales are measurements where the intervals (distances) between data points are fixed, linear and constant over the whole range of measurement. The size of the difference between 10 and 11 kg is the same as the difference between 100 and 101 kg.

(d) Absolute or ratio scales are data with an absolute zero point (e.g. lbs or kg weight). Temperature in degrees Kelvin has an absolute zero point, so it is an absolute scale. Temperatures in Celsius/Fahrenheit, have arbitrary zero points in each scale (0° Celsius is freezing, and 0° Fahrenheit is 32°F below freezing point). The term 'ratio scale' is also used because weight scales (ounces, kg) have true zero points. The ratio between any two points is independent of the unit of measurement (e.g. the ratio of 20 kg to 10 kg is 20/10 = 2). The ratio between the same mass in lbs is 44 lb/22 lb, also 2. The ratio of body temperature to room temperature in °C and °F are not the same. 37/20°C is 1.85 while in °F 98.4/60 is 1.64. Temperatures measured in °C and °F are interval not ratio scales.

iv. Categorical and ordinal scales are non-parametric.

v. Yes. 'Downgrading' data that requires fewer assumptions is acceptable but if data are downgraded, less information from the data set is used, so a statistical difference is more difficult to detect. Skewed data may be missed.

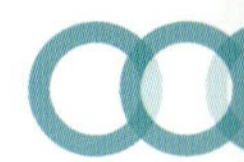

QUESTION 90

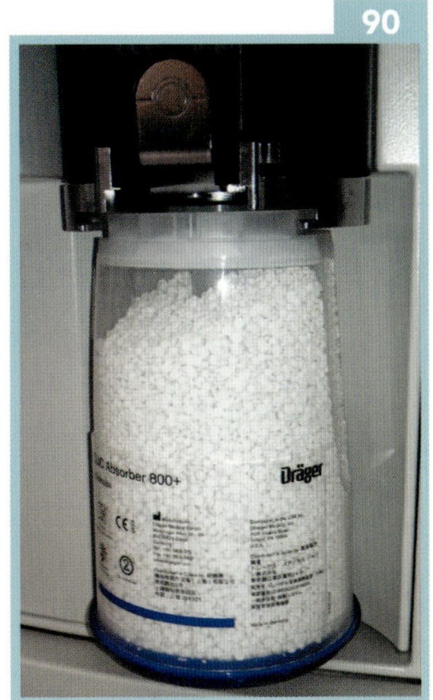

90

90i. What is the granular agent in the canister (**90**), and what does it do?

ii. Describe the chemical constituents of the agent and give the chemical equation for the reaction that takes place.

iii. What size are the granules?

iv. Describe the signs of exhaustion of this agent.

v. How can this agent produce carbon monoxide (CO)?

vi. Which volatile anaesthetic agents are chemically altered by interaction with this agent?

QUESTION 91

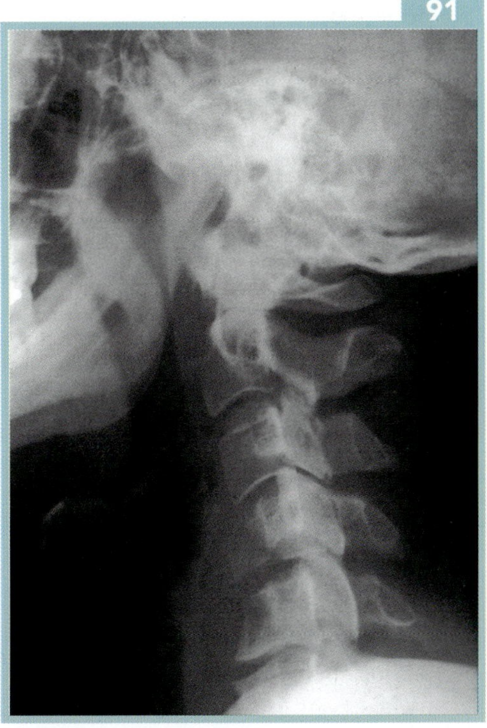
91

91i. Comment on this lateral cervical spine film (**91**).

ii. Is there a spinal injury shown and, if so, how do you recognise it?

iii. Why does an anaesthesiologist need to know this?

Answer 90

90i. Soda lime, used for CO_2 absorption in anaesthetic breathing systems.

ii. Soda lime contains calcium hydroxide (94%), sodium hydroxide (5%), potassium hydroxide (1%), silicates (for binding; <1%), dye indicators (see below) and 14–19% water. Exhaled gases enter the canister from the patient and CO_2 absorption takes place. Water and heat are produced and the warmed, humidified gas returns with fresh gas flow to the patient. The chemical reactions involved are:

$$CO_2 + 2NaOH \rightarrow Na_2CO_3 + H_2O + \text{heat}$$
$$Na_2CO_3 + Ca(OH)_2 \rightarrow 2NaOH + CaCO_3$$

iii. 4–8 mesh (i.e. granules will pass through a mesh of 4–8 strands per inch in each axis). Canisters are tightly packed to reduce channelling of gases through gaps in the granules.

iv. Exhaustion is indicated by dye colour change (from white to blue in the illustrated example and from pink to white in other products.

v. CO production can occur if desflurane, enflurane and/or isoflurane have prolonged contact with dry, warm soda lime. Excessive 'flushing' of the soda lime canister (e.g. overnight) has this effect.

vi. Soda lime decomposes trichloroethylene and chloroform to produce formic acid and phosgene, producing CO and leading to neurological damage. Sevoflurane is also decomposed to form Compound A (pentafluoroisopropenyl fluoromethyl ether [an olefin]), which is toxic in rats, causing renal, hepatic and cerebral damage. However, Compound A has not been found to harm humans.

Answer 91

91i. The examination is incomplete as it does not show the lower cervical spine, specifically the C7/T1 junction.

ii. There is a fracture diagonally across of the body of C4. This is highlighted by the loss of normal lordosis, replaced by a kyphosis, as C3 has moved forward on the fractured C4.

iii. When resuscitating trauma patients, immobilisation of the cervical spinal is mandatory until a cervical injury is radiologically excluded, especially when intubation is performed. This film shows signs (particularly the loss of lordosis) that an anaesthesiologist must recognise so that if intubation is required, the c-spine should be correctly immobilised by collar or manual in-line stabilisation to prevent spinal cord injury.

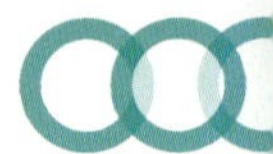

QUESTION 92

92 A femoral nerve catheter for infusion of regional anaesthesia is suggested for a patient with a mid-shaft fracture and surgical fixation of the right femur.

i. What structures, labelled A, B and C on **92a**, are used as landmarks to identify the approximate position of the femoral nerve?

ii. An ultrasound image of the groin, enabling accurate identification of the femoral nerve, is shown (**92b**). The position of the ultrasound probe is shown on the inset. What are the anatomical structures D, E and F?

iii. Why are these anatomical structures important, how would you identify them, and why should an anaesthesiologist know about them?

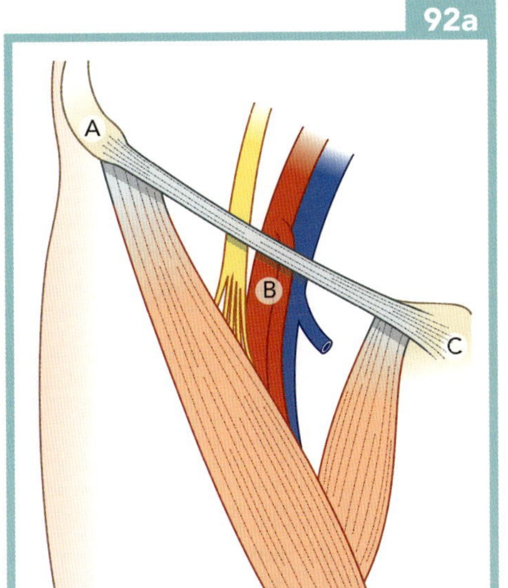

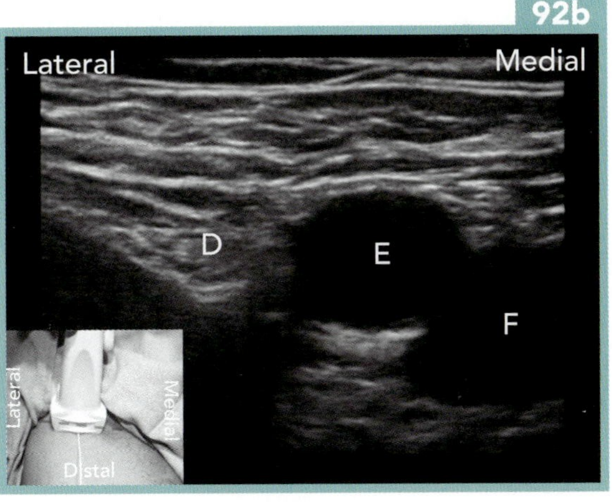

QUESTION 93

93i. Why is it important for anaesthesiologists to know about antiplatelet drugs?

ii. What are the recommended precautions needed to be taken when antiplatelet drugs are used around the time of surgery?

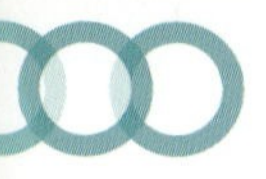

Answer 92

92i. The femoral nerve should be just lateral to the palpated pulse of the femoral artery (B) pulse and inferior to the inguinal ligament, which runs between the anterior superior iliac spine (A) and the pubic tubercle (C)

ii. D = femoral nerve; E = femoral artery; F = femoral vein. Ultrasound is performed to visualise the nerve and an insulated needle used to correctly place a catheter. Paraesthesia on insertion of the catheter may confirm correct positioning but is not always detected. Nerve stimulation with electrical current passed through the needle should be used to localise the nerve. The lower the current needed to get contraction of the quadriceps muscles (and in particular movement of the patellar tendon) the higher the success rate of the procedure.

iii. The femoral nerve enters the thigh, passing under the inguinal ligament, lateral to the femoral artery. Below the inguinal ligament it divides into anterior and posterior branches. The anterior (superficial) branch supplies sensation to the skin of the anterior and medial thigh and a posterior (deep) branch supplies the periosteum of the femur, the quadriceps muscles, the medial knee joint and the skin on the medial side of the calf and foot (via the saphenous nerve). The block should not be performed lower than the inguinal ligament as one of the branches may be missed. The anatomy of the femoral artery and vein should be known to enable cannulation for intra-arterial pressure monitoring or central venous access, respectively.

Answer 93

93i. Surgical risk of bleeding. Aspirin or other non-selective non-steroidals are supposedly not associated with increased risk of bleeding, but anecdotally they are often discontinued 1–2 days prior to surgery. Clopidogrel should be discontinued 7 days prior to surgery. Glycoprotein (GP) IIa/IIIb inhibitors should be discontinued 1–2 days prior to surgery. As GP inhibitors are used around the time of coronary events, the nature of the acute coronary syndrome will have a greater bearing on operative safety than the use of these drugs.

ii. Performance of regional anaesthetic techniques and specifically the avoidance of spinal haematoma. Due to the lack of sufficiently powered clinical trials, recommendations can only be made about the use of regional anaesthesia in anticoagulated patients. American practice is more conservative than European practice, as there appears to be an unexplained higher incidence of spinal haematomas in North America. With regard to the antiplatelet medications discussed above, the German and American societies of regional anaesthesia have concluded that spinal haematoma after antiplatelet drugs is very rare. The guidelines of the Association of Anaesthetists of GB and Ireland, which refer to the other international guidelines, are given in the Table (see Appendix, page 310).

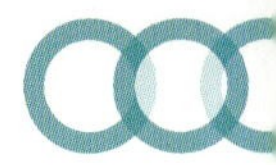

QUESTION 94

94 A non-smoking 56-year-old female with no respiratory history suffers sudden breathlessness 10 days after hysterectomy for uterine carcinoma. She is anxious, has a temperature of 37.6°C (99.7°F) and a respiratory rate of 32. She has no clinical signs and her O_2 saturations on air are 92%. Her pulse is 105 and BP 160/95.

i. What is the differential diagnosis?

ii. Determine the likelihood of this patient having a pulmonary embolus (by a scoring system)?

iii. What investigations are needed?

iv. What is **94**, and what does it show?

v. What treatment does this patient need?

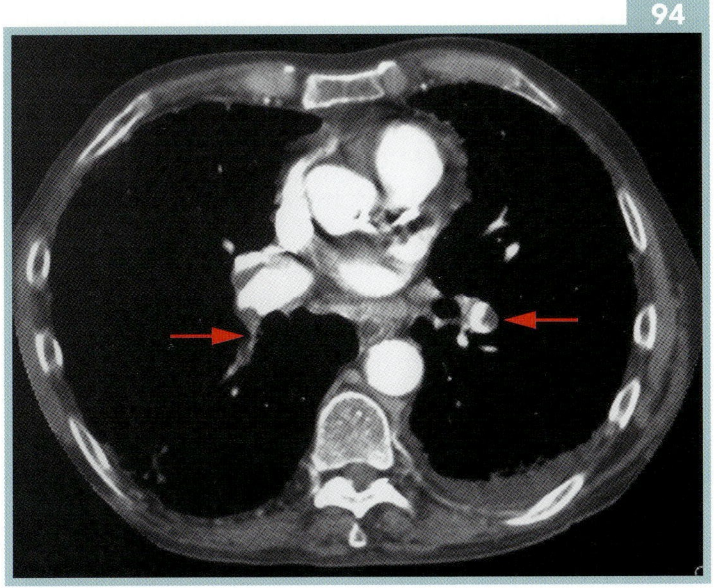

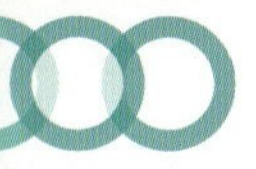

Answer 94

94i. Asthma, allergy, anaphylaxis, pneumothorax, pneumonia, pulmonary oedema, pulmonary malignancy/effusion, shock and pulmonary thromboembolus (PTE). The sudden onset suggests PTE, likely after abdominal or pelvic surgery. Prolonged immobility, old age, obesity, cancer and hypercoagulablity (e.g. antithrombin III deficiency, protein S or C deficiencies, thrombocytosis) are risk factors. Chest pain and haemoptysis are associated with PTE but often absent.

ii. The Wells score is used:
- Clinically suspected deep vein thrombosis (DVT) = 3 points;
- Alternative diagnosis is less likely than PTE = 3 points;
- Heart rate >100 = 1.5 points;
- Immobilisation (≥3 days) and/or surgery in previous 4 weeks = 1.5 points;
- Previous history of DVT or PTE = 1.5 points;
- Haemoptysis = 1 point;
- Malignancy (with treatment within 6 months) or palliative = 1 point.

A score of >4 makes PTE likely and a CTPA should be considered. A score of 4 or less makes PTE unlikely. Low D-dimers excludes PTE. High D-dimers are associated with many diagnoses and do not prove PTE.

iii. CXR, ECG, arterial blood gases, FBC (CBC), electrolytes, clotting and D-dimers. CTPA should be requested if the CXR is normal.

iv. The CTPA. Emboli are visible in the left and right pulmonary arteries (arrows). The white appearance is contrast in the pulmonary blood; the darker area is thrombus. Thrombus adherent to the vessel, as illustrated, is often not acute. A central round lesion in the vessel (Polo mint sign) is acute. There is a left pleural effusion posteriorly.

v. Further embolism/thrombus is inhibited by subcutaneous low molecular weight heparin (7,500–18,000 units, dependent on body weight). An alternative is 5,000–10,000 units heparin by IV bolus followed by a 1,000–2,000 units/hour infusion to maintain APTT between 1.5 and 2.5 times normal, but this risks haemorrhagic complications. Warfarin should commence but causes an initial hypercoagulable state and so must overlap heparin treatment. An INR of between 1 and 2 is acceptable and should be maintained for 3–6 months. Thrombolysis may help with haemodynamic instability or shock. Thrombolysis is monitored by thrombin time (2–4 times control). Cardiothoracic surgical intervention (pulmonary embolectomy) is of uncertain value. Vena cava filters may be inserted in patients who cannot receive anticoagulation or after pulmonary embolectomy.

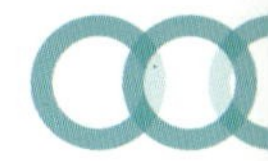

QUESTION 95

95 This device (**95a**) is an electronic version of a previously purely mechanical device that is essential for the safe running of an anaesthetic machine.

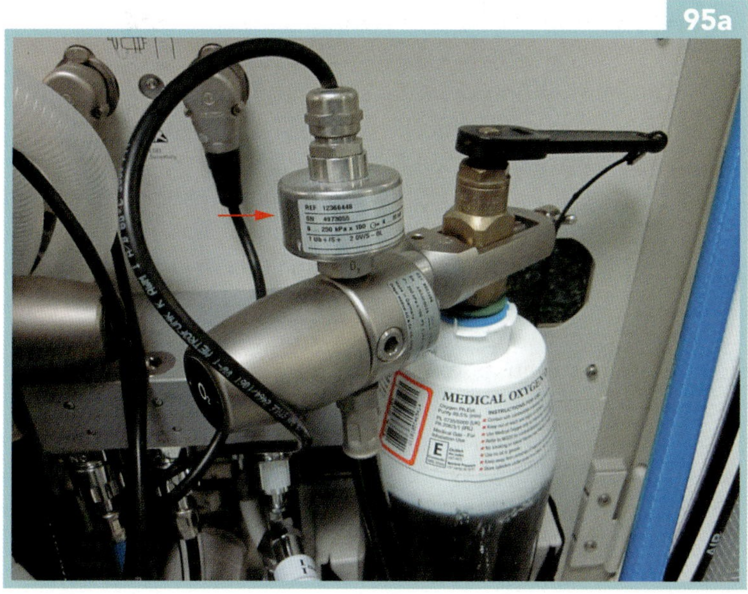

95a

i. What is this device?

ii. Draw a scheme of the interior of the mechanical version of the device, and explain how it works.

iii. Why are these devices used on the standard anaesthetic machine?

iv. Where are they located on a standard anaesthetic machine?

Answer 95

95i. An electronic pressure regulator or pressure reducing valve (PRV). In the past this device was purely mechanical and functioned utilising a diaphragm. Pressure is reduced from very high cylinder/pipeline pressure to a lower regulated constant value appropriate for the machine or equipment used.

ii. See **95b**. Continuous high pressure (labelled HP in) is exerted by the spring (S) on the diaphragm (D) attached to the valve (V). Gas flows out of the low-pressure chamber (light blue) (labelled LP out), reducing the pressure and allowing the diaphragm to displace the valve downwards to admit gas from the high-pressure chamber. As the low-pressure chamber pressure increases, the valve closes again as the diaphragm is pushed back. A screw (A) alters the force applied by the spring to the diaphragm so controlling the amount of gas entering the low-pressure chamber.

iii. Because the pressure within an oxygen cylinder is 137 atmospheres (bars), far too high to be safely administered to a patient. If unregulated, this pressure would certainly cause lung barotrauma. Excessive pressures also damage equipment. Flow control meters, valves and tubing are fine and accurate and could be damaged by pressure surges, leading to inaccurate gas flows delivered to patients. Pressure build-up could also occur, potentially causing the apparatus to fracture or explode. As a cylinder empties, a constant flow must be ensured and this is controlled by the regulator.

iv. Between the oxygen and other high-pressure gas tanks and between the back bar and the flowmeters.

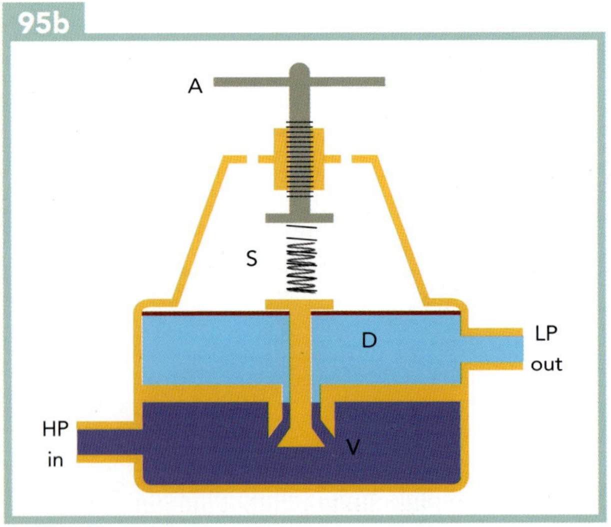

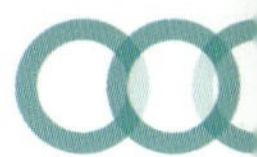

QUESTION 96

96 The soles of the feet of a man electrically burned via his perineum are shown (**96a**).

i. What does this tell you about this man's injury?

ii. His urine is very dark (**96b**). What should the anaesthesiologist do about this?

iii. Has this man been hit with direct current (DC) or alternating current (AC), and which of the two is more lethal?

iv. What factors influence electrical burns?

v. What are the commonest clinical features of electrical burns?

96a

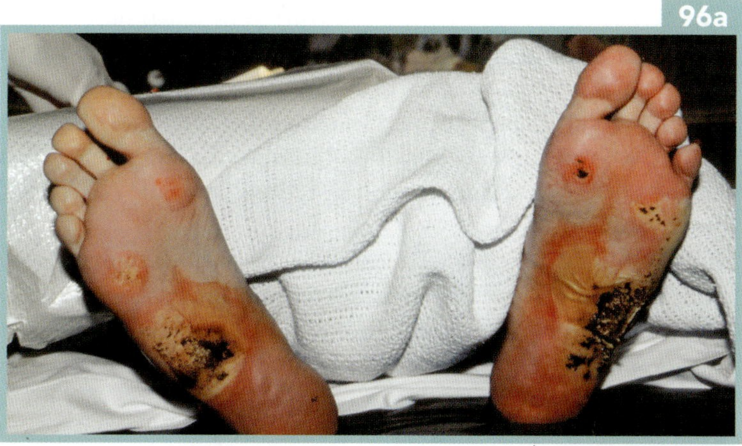

96b

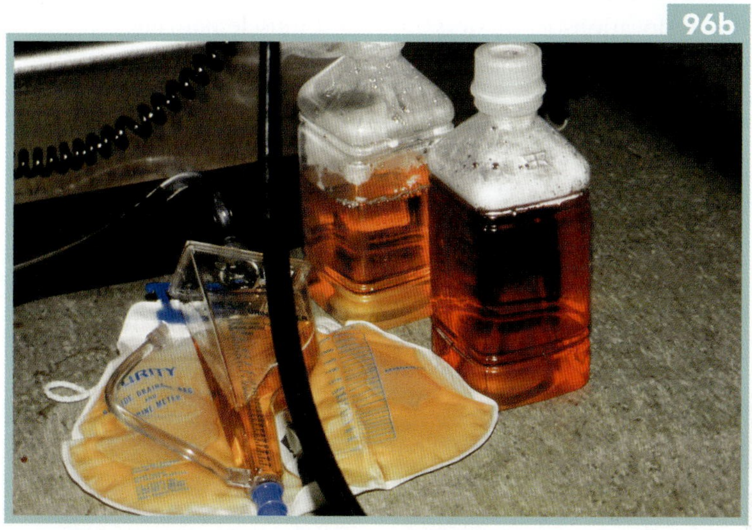

Answer 96

96i. The feet show characteristic exit burns from electrocution. Careful anaesthetic management of fluids, analgesia and nutrition (in ICU) is needed. Although current transited his perineal soft tissues (**96c**), his skin was largely spared. Extensive internal electrical burns may not show as external skin burns. Here, extensive subcutaneous damage, with muscle protruding from the incision, has occurred, requiring bilateral fasciotomies (**96d**) and debridement.

ii. This is myoglobinuria. High urine output with IV fluid loading and mannitol is required to promote diuresis. Renal failure and dialysis are likely with such extensive thermal trauma.

iii. Entry and exit burns do not occur with AC current, so this was DC injury. Domestic AC current is more dangerous than DC due to its 'tetanizing' effect (i.e. locking a victim's grasp to the current source and inducing ventricular fibrillation [VF]). The current did not arc through this man's chest, thus avoiding myocardial problems.

iv. Surface area of contact (increased area decreases the current density); duration of contact; pathway of the current (transthoracic is particularly dangerous); amperage (strength of the current); voltage; resistance; type of current (AC versus DC).

v.
- Arrhythmias. Immediate or late VF (up to 8 hours after injury).
- Myocardial damage and valve perforation. Transthoracic current passage can cause myocardial necrosis and valve and coronary artery damage.
- CNS damage. Seizures, unconsciousness, disorientation and hemiplegia can result. Later, headache, neuropathy, spinal cord transection, transverse myelitis, amyolytrophic lateral sclerosis and sympathetic dystrophies can occur.
- Musculoskeletal disorders. Sudden violent muscle contractions may result in fractures, dislocations (shoulders/hips) and muscle damage.
- Thermal burns. Usually skin is affected but here extensive coagulation necrosis of the leg muscles occurred, causing rhabdomyolysis and compartment syndrome.

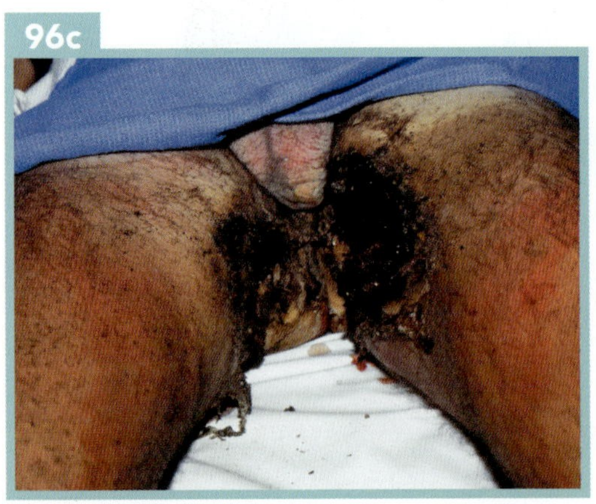
96c

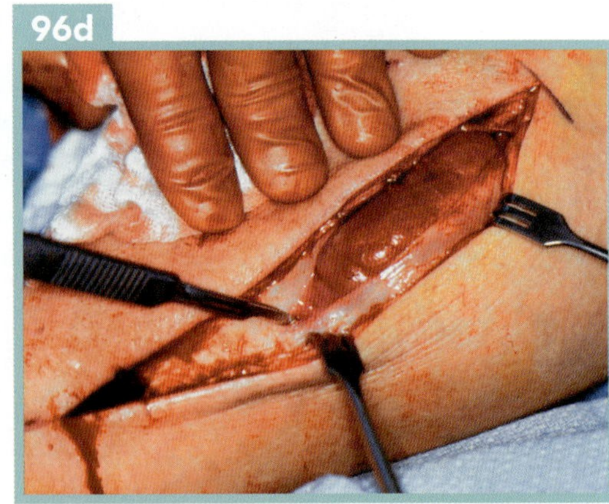
96d

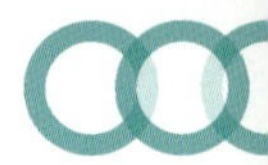

QUESTION 97

97 The relationship between intracranial pressure (ICP) and intracranial volume is shown (**97**). Consider this graph in the context of a slowly expanding intracranial lesion.

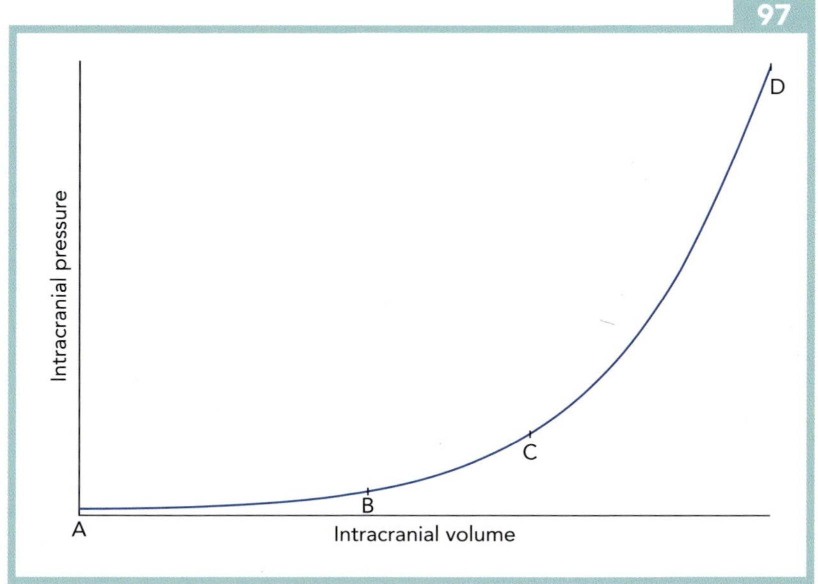

i. Explain what is occurring between points A and B and points C and D.

ii. What is normal ICP in an adult?

iii. What is cerebral perfusion pressure (CPP)?

iv. What influence does ICP have on CPP in a patient with a head injury?

v. What physiological parameters are important in control of CPP?

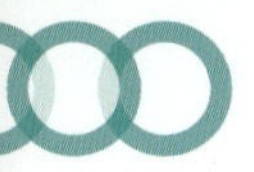

Answer 97

97i. This curve explains the importance of ICP on the injured brain or in the presence of an intracranial space-occupying lesion (e.g. haemorrhage, haematoma, tumour). Between points A and B, a negligible rise in ICP occurs despite increasing intracranial volume. Compensatory mechanisms, namely, displacement of intracranial CSF into the spinal sac, displacement of intracranial venous blood into the extracranial vascular space, reduction of CSF production and increasing CSF absorption all prevent an ICP increase. Between points C and D, a sudden rise in ICP occurs despite only a small increase in intracranial volume. All compensatory mechanisms have been exhausted at this point and ICP rapidly rises. At very high ICP, death from brainstem compression can result.

ii. Normal ICP in an adult is 7–15 mmHg in a supine position changing to a negative pressure of up to -10 mmHg in a standing position.

iii. CPP = mean arterial pressure (MAP) – ICP.

iv. Normally CPP is equivalent to MAP as ICP is low (–10 to +10 mmHg). With intracranial pathology, ICP may rise to 15–20 mmHg. Above 25 mmHg active measures should be taken to reduce ICP, as CPP will be reduced. CPP should not be allowed to fall below 70mmHg, as below this level secondary insults to the injured brain start to occur.

v. Hypoxia and hypercarbia must be prevented in brain injured patients as both increase cerebral blood flow and, therefore, volume. MAP should be maintained at a level of at least 90 mmHg (assuming that the ICP is <20 mmHg), as this will maintain the critical CPP of 70 mmHg.

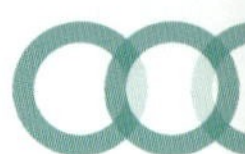

QUESTION 98

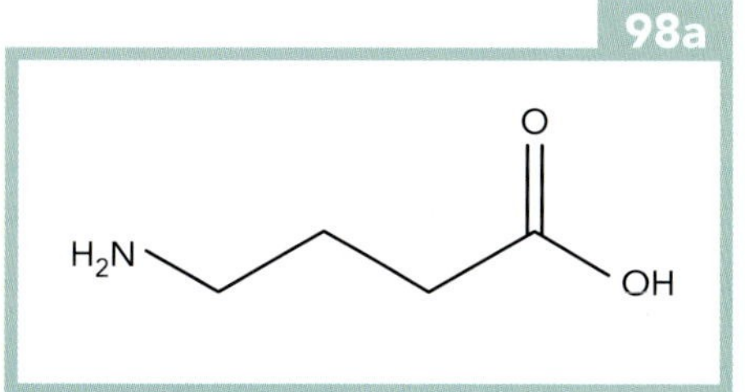

98i. What molecule is illustrated (**98a**)?

ii. How is this molecule produced?

iii. How does the molecule work on the human body?

iv. How is the molecule's receptor involved in promotion of GA?

QUESTION 99

99 With regard to the circle system shown (**99**):

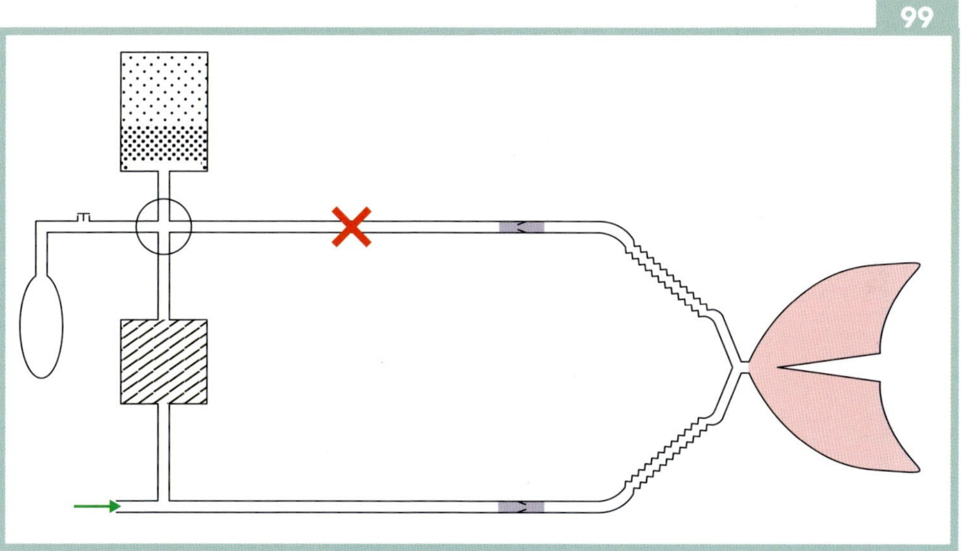

i. Why is the fresh gas flow (FGF) inlet situated on the side of the inspiratory limb? Why is it not placed at the position marked X?

ii. Why is the soda lime absorber situated after the connection that leads to the anaesthesia reservoir bag and the ventilator?

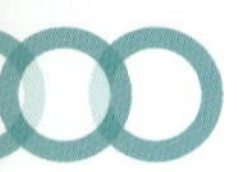

Answer 98

98i. Gamma-aminobutyric acid (GABA).

ii. GABA is synthesised from the anion salts of the amino acid glutamic acid by the action of glutamic acid dehydrogenase.

iii. $GABA_A$ receptors are pentameric subunits around a central pore and are linked to an intrinsic ion channel. They are the principle mediators of the fast inhibitory neurotransmitter in higher centres of the CNS, accounting for approximately 30% of all inhibitory synapses.

iv. These $GABA_A$ receptors have emerged as target for most anaesthetic agents (**98b**) and are sensitive to general anaesthetics, benzodiazepines and other neurodepressant drugs including ethanol. Many different proteins (including ion channels, enzymes, second messengers and transporters) integrate together as a result of $GABA_A$ receptor action. The end result is that these structures act as a 'gate' to ionic channels. $GABA_A$ activation causes inward movement of chloride ions, thus causing hyperpolarisation of the cell membrane, and augments inhibitory signals, thus promoting GA. $GABA_A$ receptors are particularly sensitive to modulation by the majority of anaesthetic agents (with the exception of ketamine and xenon).

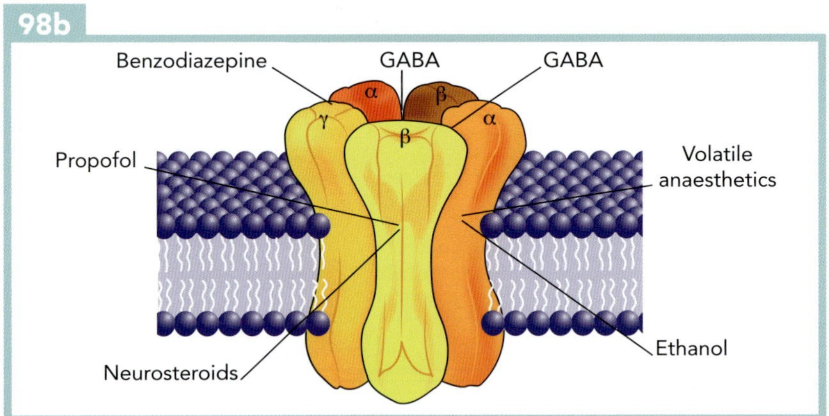

Answer 99

99i. The position of the FGF inlet (and the soda lime absorber) is dictated by reasons of economy. If the FGF inlet is placed prior to the take-off that leads to the scavenger, fresh gas may be exhausted (lost and wasted) to the scavenger before it reaches the patient.

ii. Similarly, it would be a waste of the soda lime if it is used to scrub exhaled gases, which will then be exhausted (lost and wasted) to the scavenger.

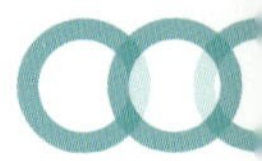

QUESTION 100

100i. What does CPET stand for when applied to testing patients prior to surgery?

ii. What threshold does it identify, what units are used to express this threshold, and how should this be interpreted?

iii. What are the contraindications for CPET?

iv. When should CPET be employed?

QUESTION 101

101i. What are the chemical compositions of the solutions shown (**101a, b**)?

ii. Why is the solution in **101a** preferable to that in **101b** for resuscitation of severe haemorrhagic shock?

iii. What other circumstances or techniques could lead to the same problem?

iv. Why does this happen?

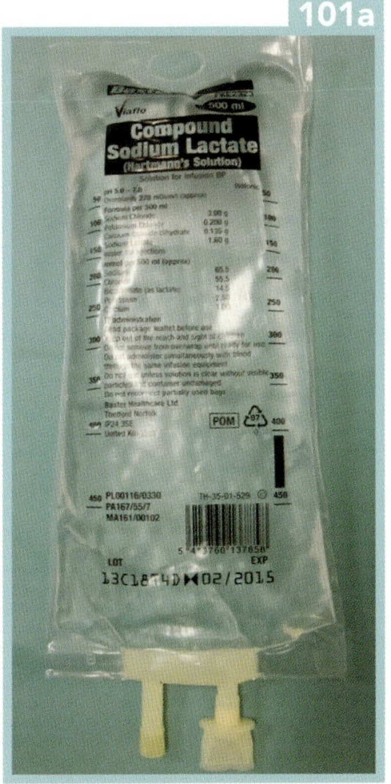

101a

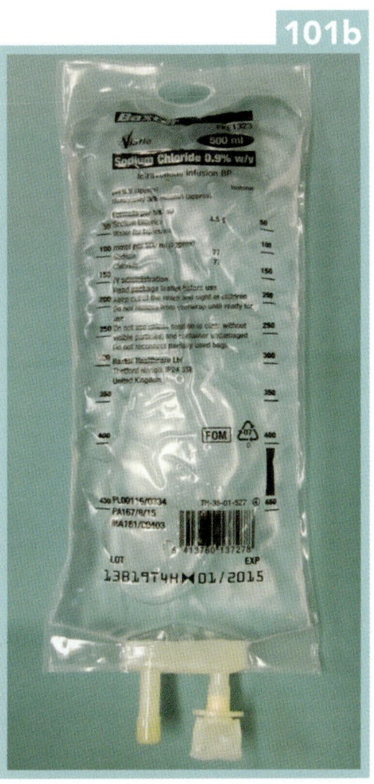

101b

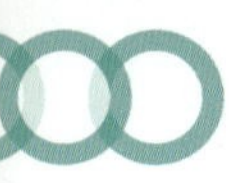

Answer 100

100i. Cardiopulmonary exercise testing (may also be abbreviated to CPX).

ii. CPET identifies patients at high risk of developing cardiorespiratory complications after surgery, primarily by identification of the anaerobic threshold (ml/kg/min). Major surgery increases postoperative oxygen demand, so evidence of impaired tissue perfusion when oxygen demands are increased suggests a poor outcome. The anaerobic threshold is the point at which lactate starts to be produced at a certain measured oxygen consumption. A value of <11 ml/kg/min (especially with associated ischaemic heart disease) confirms those patients at highest risk after surgery up to age 80. After 80 the data are unreliable.

iii. Contraindications are: acute myocardial infarct (within 7–10 days of transmural infarct or within 5 days if minor and uncomplicated); symptomatic uncontrolled arrhythmias causing haemodynamic compromise; left mainstem stenotic lesions in excess of 50%; malignant hypertension; pulmonary oedema; oxygen saturation <85% while breathing room air at rest; acute inflammatory conditions (pericarditis, myocarditis); unstable angina (patient should be pain free for 4 days before CPET); dissecting aneurysm; acute or recent pyrexial illness; thyrotoxicosis; syncope; thrombosis of lower extremities.

iv. CPET aids the surgical decision as to whether operative treatment is in the patient's best interests. If patients are found to be very high risk based on a CPET result, treatments other than surgery may be the best option.

Answer 101

101i. Hartmann's solution (**101a**) contains 131 mmol/l of sodium, 111 mmol/l of chloride ion, 29 mmol/l of lactate, 5 mmol/l of potassium ion and 4 mmol/l of calcium ion. (**Note:** All values in mmol/l are identical in mEq/l). Normal (0.9%) saline (**101b**) contains 154 mmol/l each of both sodium and chloride.

ii. Hartmann's solution is preferred because it is less likely to induce a state of hyperchloraemic metabolic acidosis.

iii. Whenever large volumes (usually over 6 litres over a 3–4 hour period) of resuscitation fluids are given, hyperchloraemic metabolic acidosis can occur. This can easily happen, for example, during cases that require large amounts of fluid use, such as acute normovolaemic haemodilution, diabetic ketoacidosis resuscitation, cardiopulmonary bypass, septic shock, burns and hepatic failure/transplantation.

iv. The conventional explanation is that a simple dilution of extracellular bicarbonate (HCO_3^-) by large volumes of non-HCO_3^--containing fluid occurs. Stewarts strong ion theory is also quoted as an explanation (see case **217**).

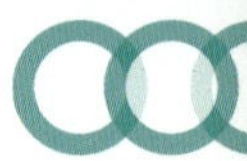

QUESTION 102

102i. What theory of anaesthesia does this graph illustrate (**102**)?

ii. What is the explanation for the theory?

iii. Why is this not universally true, and what other theory has replaced it?

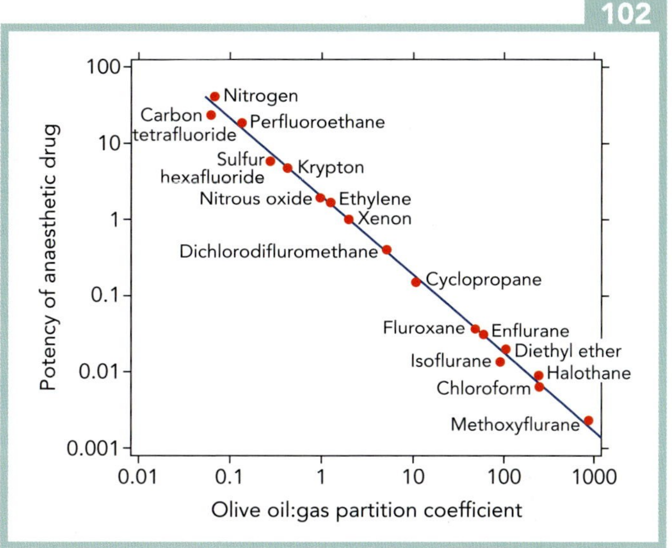

QUESTION 103

103i. What is the main abnormality depicted in this ECG (**103**)?

ii. What treatment is required if this rhythm occurs during GA for a laparotomy?

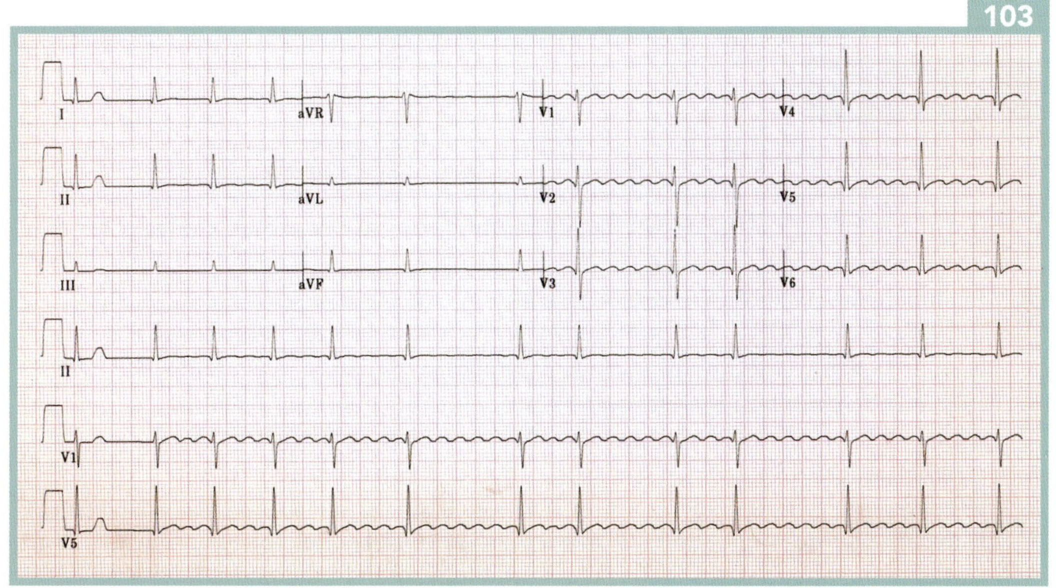

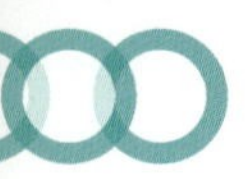

Answer 102

102i. The Meyer-Overton (MO) theory, which describes the correlation between lipid solubility of inhaled anaesthetics and minimal alveolar concentration.

ii. The MO theory suggests:

- That anaesthesia occurs when a sufficient number of inhalational anaesthetic molecules dissolve in the lipid cell membrane, causing normal functioning of neuronal membranes to be disrupted, leading to loss of consciousness.
- The number of molecules dissolved in the lipid cell membrane causes anaesthesia, not the type of inhalational agent.
- Why combinations of different inhaled anaesthetics may have additive effects at the level of the cell membrane.

iii. The MO theory was the first significant step towards identifying the way anaesthetic agents work, but does not hold true in all circumstances. Some halogenated alkanes (predicted to be potent anaesthetics based on their lipid solubility) fail to anaesthetise. *In vitro*, general anaesthetics alter the structure of lipid membranes with a simple temperature rise of 1°C. This obviously does not induce anaesthesia. Anaesthetic agents can be overcome by a protein, luciferase, suggesting strongly that general anaesthetics work by interaction with membrane proteins. The protein theory of action postulates that general anaesthetics involve certain soluble proteins in central nervous tissue. Enantiomers of some anaesthetic agents (mirror images of isomers of the same compound) have profoundly different clinical effects despite having identical physicochemical properties (e.g. the R isomer of etomidate is 10 times more potent than the S form). This suggests that the primary source of anaesthetic action is not the lipid bilayer in cells but a stereoselective binding site within proteins.

Answer 103

103i. Atrial flutter with a variable ventricular response at an average of 74 bpm. Note that the flutter waves in this ECG are hardly visible in the peripheral leads.

ii. Exclude hypoxia and hypercarbia, as with any anaesthetic emergency. Ask the surgeon to desist from any peritoneal traction or other vagal stimulus that may have precipitated the rhythm change. If the arrhythmia has never happened before, rubbing the neck beside the carotid body rub can sometimes terminate it, but this manoeuvre can dislodge plaque from the carotid artery in elderly or vasculopathic patients and cause a stroke. Caution is advised. Electrical cardioversion is usually effective, otherwise IV adenosine or beta blockade may terminate the arrhythmia. If the rhythm does not revert to sinus, there is a risk of clot formation in the atria and embolic phenomena. Referral to cardiology after awakening is advisable as electrophysiological studies and ablation of an ectopic focus may be required.

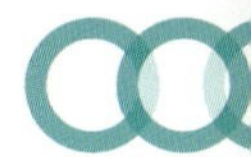

QUESTION 104

104i. What is the oxygen cascade, and what equation summarises it?

ii. A graph illustrating this cascade from dry air to tissues via the airway and blood stream is shown (**104**). Why does the anaesthesiologist need to know this, and how can anaesthesia influence the cascade?

iii. What effect does humidifying the inspired air have on the oxygen content?

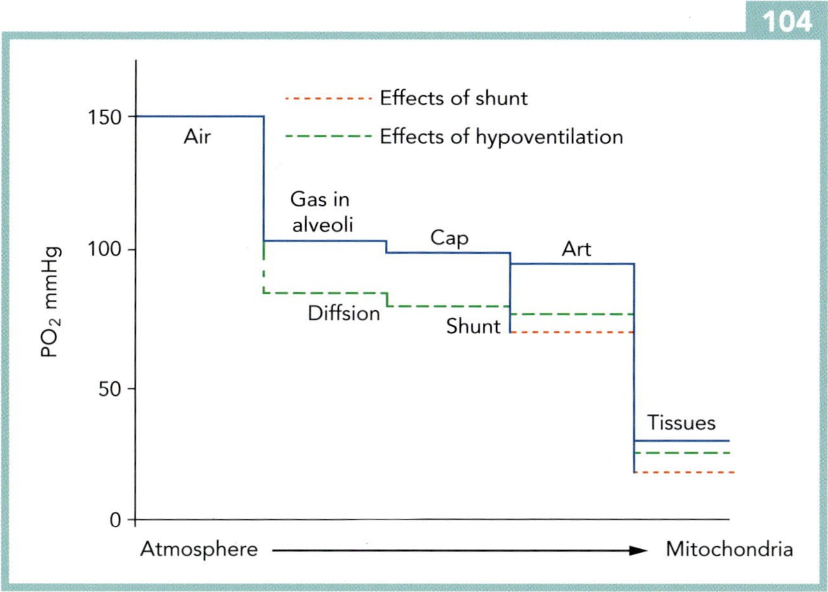

Answer 104

104i. It is the oxygen tension gradient from the atmosphere to cells. It comprises alternating stages of mass transport (pulmonary ventilation and blood flow) and diffusion (within the alveoli, across the alveolar capillary membrane and between the capillary and the site of utilisation, the mitochondrion). The cascade is described by the alveolar gas equation:

$$P_AO_2 = FIO_2 - (P_aO_2 - P_aCO_2)/R$$

P_AO_2 = partial pressure of alveolar oxygen; FIO_2 = fraction of inspired oxygen; P_aO_2 = partial pressure of oxygen dissolved in arterial blood; R = respiratory quotient (ratio of the volume of CO_2 produced to the volume of oxygen consumed per unit of time).

ii. Alveolar PO_2 is lower than inspired PO_2 due to CO_2 production displacing alveolar oxygen and oxygen absorption into the blood, so the anaesthesiologist should supply supplemental oxygen to the unconscious patient (typically 30% or above). Alveolar ventilation greatly affects the inspired/alveolar PO_2 difference and must be maintained with adequate ventilation. Increased oxygen consumption with low alveolar ventilation leads to catastrophic falls in P_AO_2 (e.g. postoperative shivering with poor respiratory effort). In healthy conscious subjects the A-a gradient (alveolar gas to arterial blood) is only a few kilopascals (or mmHg). A significant A-a gradient may result when ventilation and perfusion are not well matched (shunt), which can occur under anaesthesia or in the ICU. From arterial blood to cells, the oxygen cascade varies between organs and also within differing parts of an organ. There is a progressive fall in oxygen tension depending on the relationship of oxygen consumption to blood flow. Blood flow must be facilitated under anaesthesia by good blood volume and cardiac output.

iii. Water vapour contributes 6 kPa (47 mmHg at 37°C) of partial pressure to inspired air, so inspired gas always has a lower PO_2 than atmospheric gas. At atmospheric pressure of 100 kPa (760 mmHg), oxygen contributes 21% or 21 kPa (160 mmHg), reduced to 19.7 kPa (150 mmHg) by saturation with water vapour.

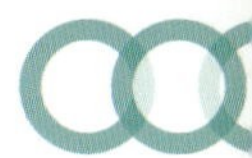

QUESTION 105

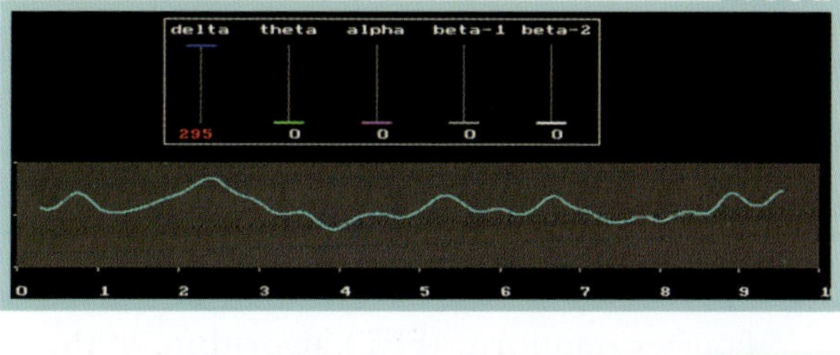

105a

105i. List the frequency ranges in Hz for each of the following EEG waves: delta, theta, alpha and beta.

ii. The typical frequency range for the spontaneous depolarisation of the frontalis muscle is above 30 Hz. With regard to the simulator generated signals in **105a** (delta waves), **105b** (theta waves) and **105c** (alpha waves), which of these waves will experience the most interference from the spontaneous EMG signals from the frontalis muscle?

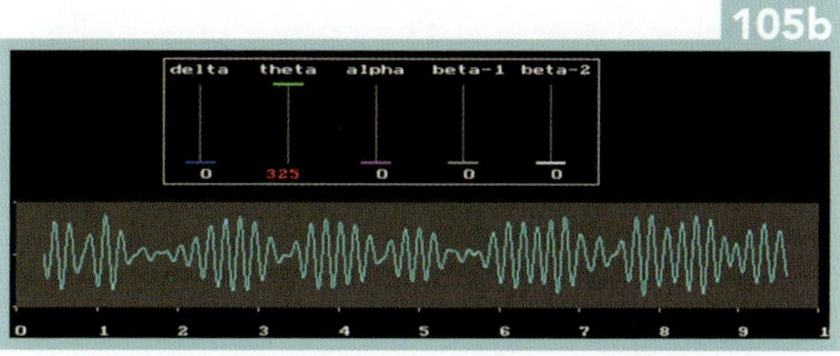

105b

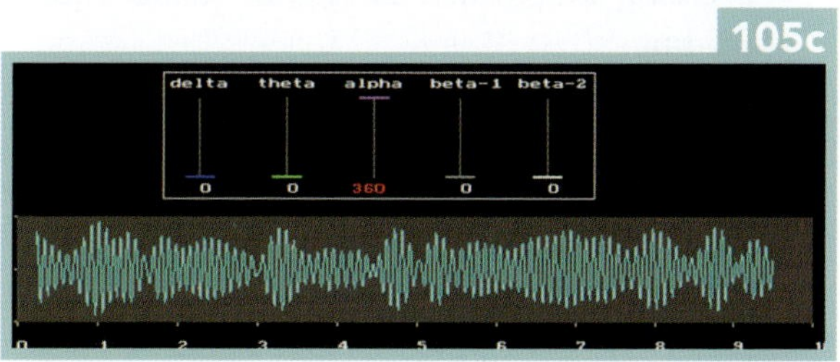

105c

iii. Which are the dominant wave forms creating the shape of the EEG signal in **105d**? What mathematical technique is demonstrated in **105d**?

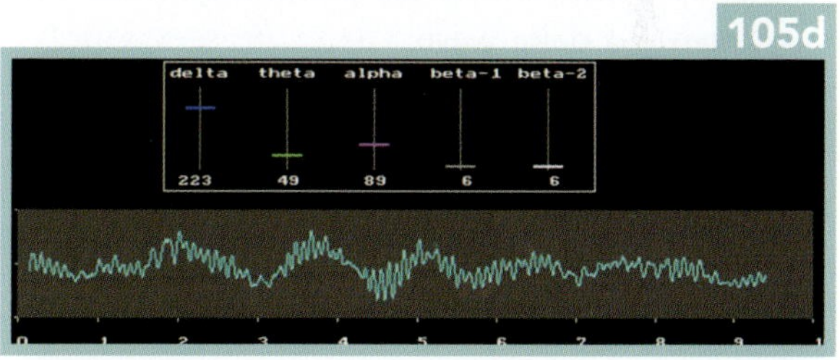

105d

iv. How does the BIS (bispectral) monitor indicate to the user that there is interference from (1) the EMG from the frontalis muscle, (2) electrical interference such as the diathermy ('Bovie')?

v. What are the typical voltages of the EEG and ECG signals? Explain why the EEG is so much more prone to electrical interference.

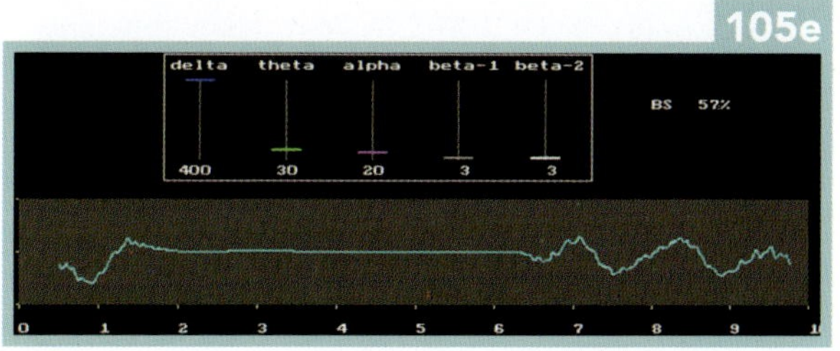

105e

vi. What EEG phenomenon (related to a deeper level of anaesthesia) is demonstrated in **105e**? What is the predominant EEG wave form seen in **105e**?

Answer 105

105i. Delta = 0.1–4 Hz; theta = 4–8 Hz; alpha = 8–13 Hz; beta = 14–30 Hz.

ii. The spontaneous high frequency EMG depolarisations will interfere with the highest frequency components of the EEG (i.e. the beta waves).

iii. **105d** demonstrates a simulation of the mathematical combination, using a fast Fourier transform (FFT) algorithm, of the fundamental wave form as well as the higher harmonics. The relative power of each of the harmonics is indicated in the sliding scales above the EEG wave form.

iv. The BIS monitor indicates interference from the high frequency components by indicating the EMG strength on a sliding scale. A high EMG value indicates an unreliable (typically false high) BIS reading due to high power in the high frequency components. The BIS monitor indicates general electrical interference by a sliding scale called the signal quality index (SQI.) A high SQI indicates a reliable reading.

v. The typical voltage for the EEG signal is in the microvolt range. The typical voltage for the ECG signal is in the millivolt range. The small stray currents in the environment (such as the operating room) have a much greater influence on the smaller EEG signal.

vi. **105e** demonstrates the phenomenon of 'burst suppression'. The predominant wave form is a delta wave.

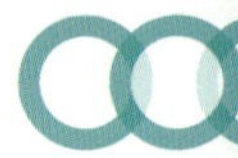

QUESTION 106

106i. Draw a schematic diagram of the brachial plexus.

ii. On your diagram show how the roots, trunk, divisions, cord and branches lie in relation to the bony landmarks of the neck and shoulder.

QUESTION 107

107 With regard to this ECG (**107**):

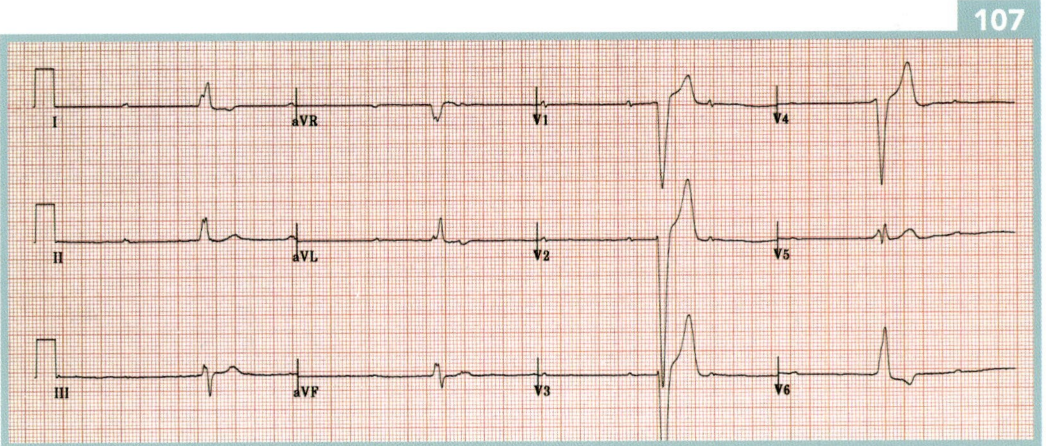

i. What is the rate of the P waves, and how constant is this rate?

ii. What is the rate of the QRS complexes, and how constant is this rate?

iii. Is there a fixed relationship (time interval) between the P waves and the QRS complexes?

iv. What is the diagnosis?

Answer 106

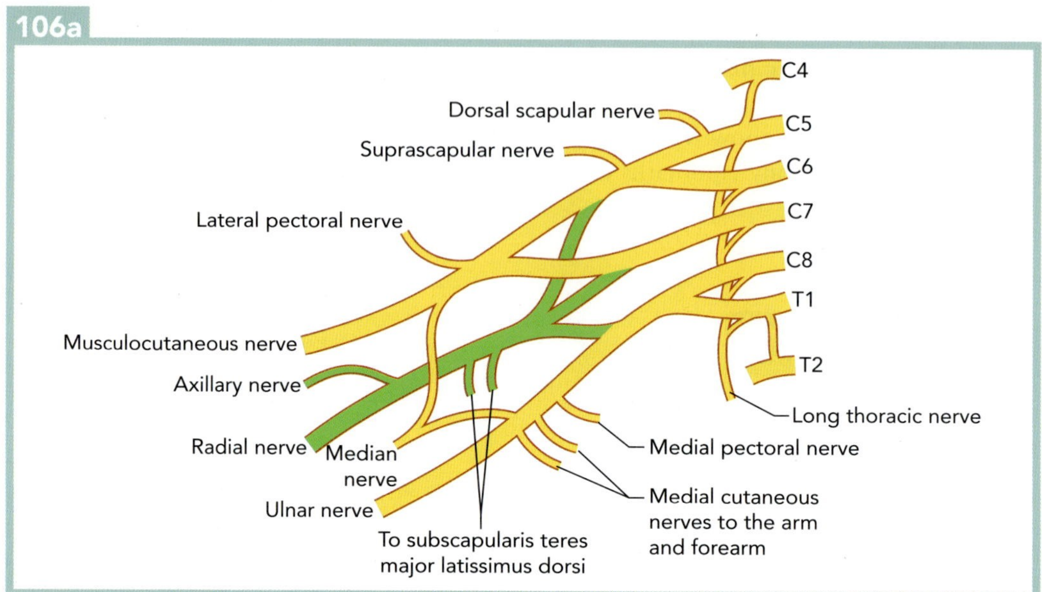

106i. Shown in **106a**.
ii. Shown in **106b**.

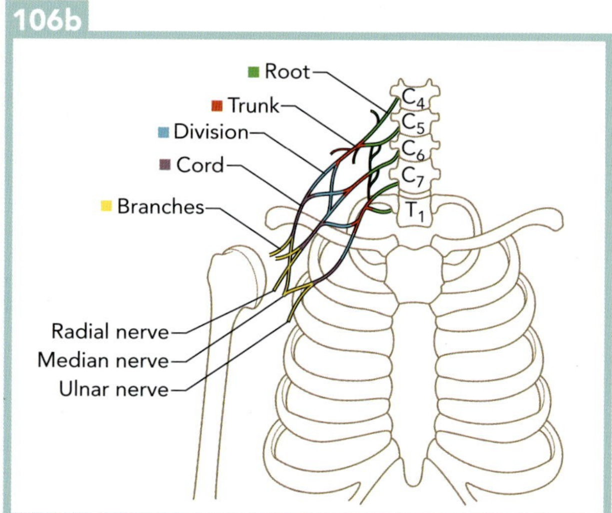

Answer 107

107i. Approximately 75 bpm. (Divide 300 by the number of large blocks to calculate the frequency of the event.) The rate is fixed and relatively constant.

ii. Approximately 25 bpm. This rate is also relatively constant.

iii. No.

iv. Third-degree (complete) heart block.

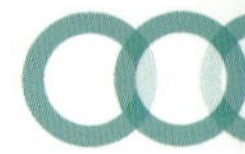

QUESTION 108

108 A trauma patient requires urgent surgery for a ruptured spleen. No history is available. The patient's CXR is shown (**108a**) and a prior median sternotomy is noted as well as placement of a 'pacemaker'.

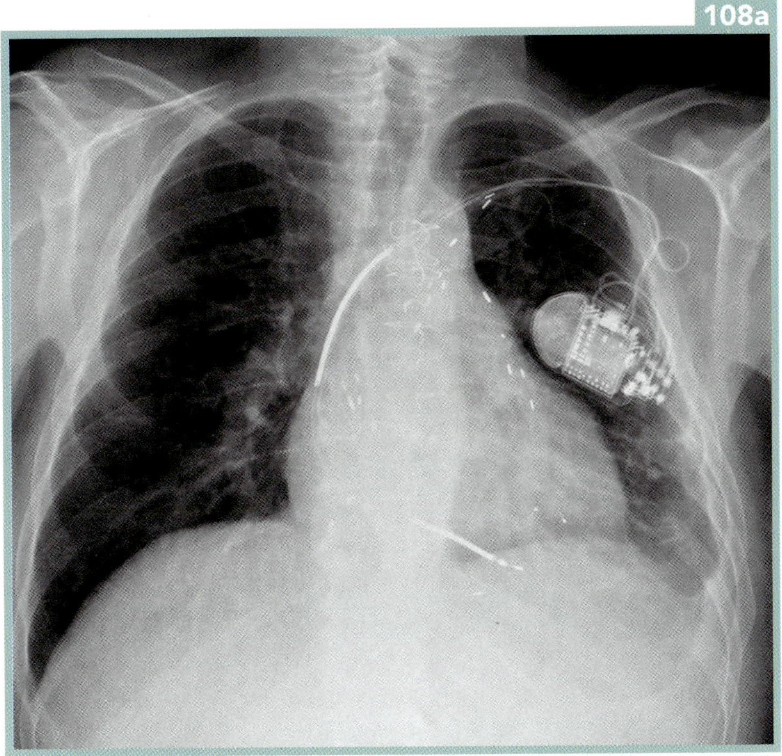
108a

i. How many cardiac leads from the pacemaker are visible on the CXR?

ii. Why are some leads thicker?

iii. What is the most likely type of pacemaker, given the number and sizes of the pacemaker leads? What are the advantages of this type of pacemaker?

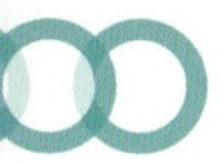

Answer 108

108i. Three (see **108b**).

ii. The leads used for cardiac defibrillation are typically thicker (red arrows in **108b**) than the leads used only for pacing (yellow arrow).

iii. Given the thicker leads, the device has the capability for defibrillation (automated internal cardioverter defibrillator [ACID]). Given the 3rd lead, which is typically placed in the coronary sinus, the device is most likely used for cardiac resynchronisation therapy (CRT). The advantages of a CRT pacemaker are that the left ventricle can be paced at a point when the right ventricle is still ejecting, thereby maintaining the septum as a more rigid structure, preventing shift of the cardiac septum and improving left ventricular output.

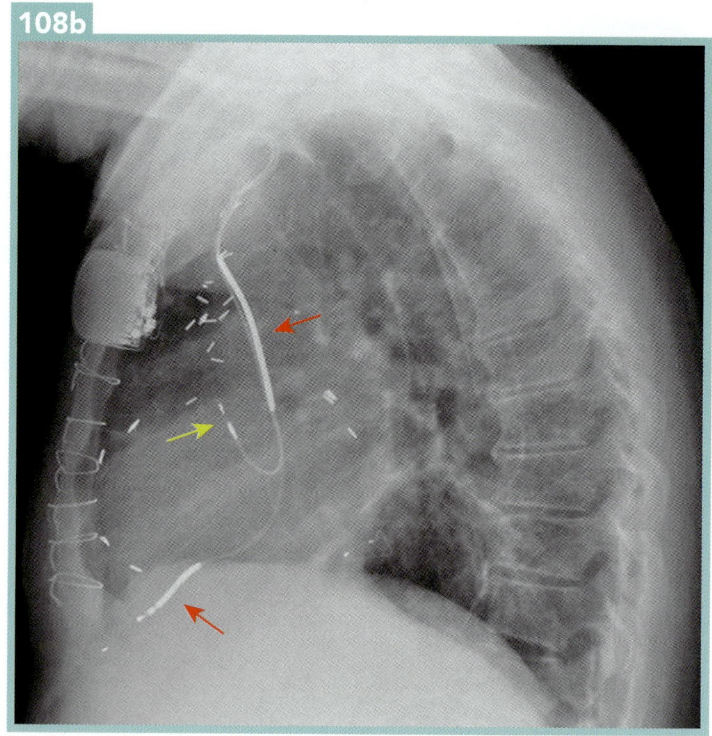

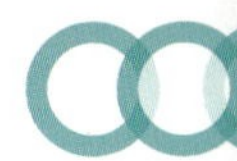

QUESTION 109

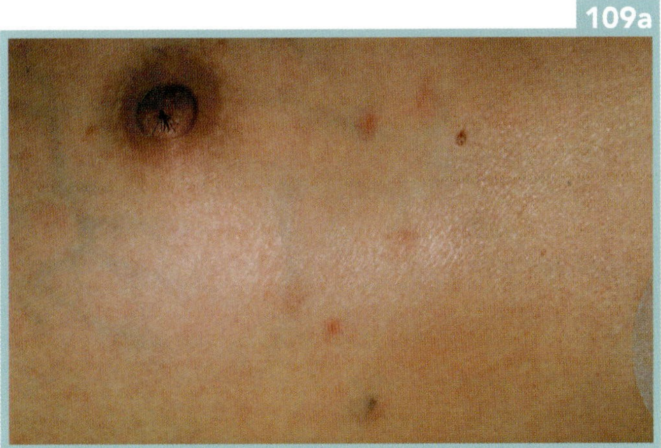

109 The chest of a previously fit and well 18-year-old woman with a 24-hour history of a flu-like illness and increasing pain in her joints is shown (**109a**). She is conscious but confused. She has a pulse rate of 130 beats per minute, a temperature of 39.5°C (103°F), a respiratory rate of 30 and a BP of 75/40.

i. What might be the diagnosis?

ii. Is it serious?

iii. What is important to know about this condition?

iv. What immediate treatment is required?

QUESTION 110

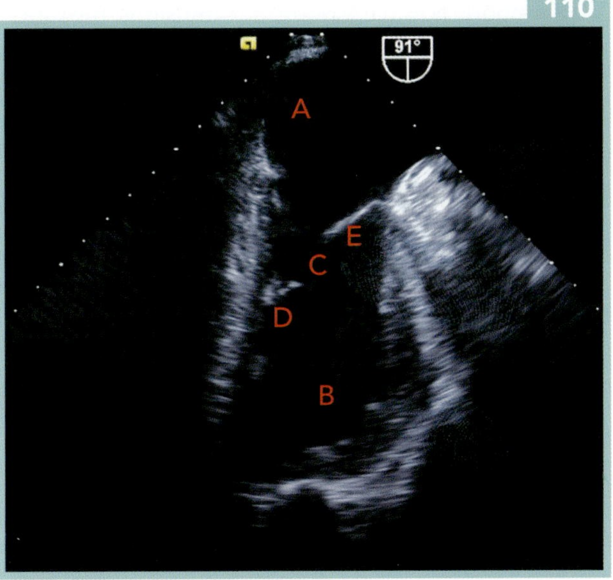

110 A TOE image is shown (**110**).

i. What is this view called?

ii. Which chambers are indicated by A and B?

iii. What opening is indicated by C?

iv. What structures are indicated by D and E?

Answer 109

109i. This patient has the characteristic rash of meningococcal septicaemia and is infected with *Neiserria meningitides*. An acute vasculitis could look similar but would not usually be accompanied by such a high fever.

ii. Meningococcaemia kills very rapidly and thus anaesthesiologists should be aware of this condition. This case is particularly serious because of the associated organ failure (confusion, high respiratory rate, tachycardia and hypotension).

iii. Transmission is via respiratory secretions, the human upper respiratory tract being the only known reservoir. Cutaneous manifestations can be the most dramatic aspect of the disease. The rash is non-blanching when a glass is applied to it. The limbs are often affected first but trunk involvement is also common. Lesions may develop a gunmetal grey appearance as well as classical red petechiae. The woman's leg 6 days after presentation is shown (**109b**). She survived but spent 3 weeks in critical care, 5 weeks in hospital, needed multiple skin grafts and lost some of her toes. The contacts of meningococcal patients need to be screened and treated with antibiotics. Vaccination against some strains of the disease is also possible. Meningitis must be notified to public health authorities.

109b

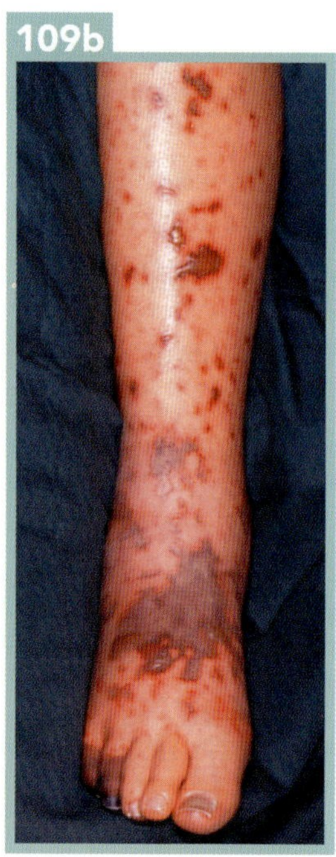

iv. IV third-generation cephalosporins should be used immediately a diagnosis is suspected (i.e. systemic illness and rash). Management of systemic illness and hypotension must also be rapidly done with supplemental O_2, IV fluid support, possible vasopressor infusions, measurement of lactate and urine output (catheter) and urgent referral to critical care. Blood cultures should be performed after initial antibiotic treatment.

Answer 110

110i. A mid-oesophageal two-chamber view.

ii. A is the left atrium, B is the left ventricle.

iii. C indicates the mitral valve.

iv. D is the posterior (PML) and E is the anterior (AML) leaflet of the mitral valve (MV).

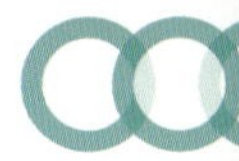

QUESTION 111

111 The CXR of a 73-year-old man 2 days after an emergency laparotomy is shown (**111**). A right hemicolectomy with end-to-end anastomosis was performed for a perforated colonic adenocarcinoma. His respiratory rate is 35 and O_2 saturations are 88% on oxygen via a trauma mask. He denies chest pain and has no cardiac history. He has a normal ECG. His troponin level is 0.09 ng/l.

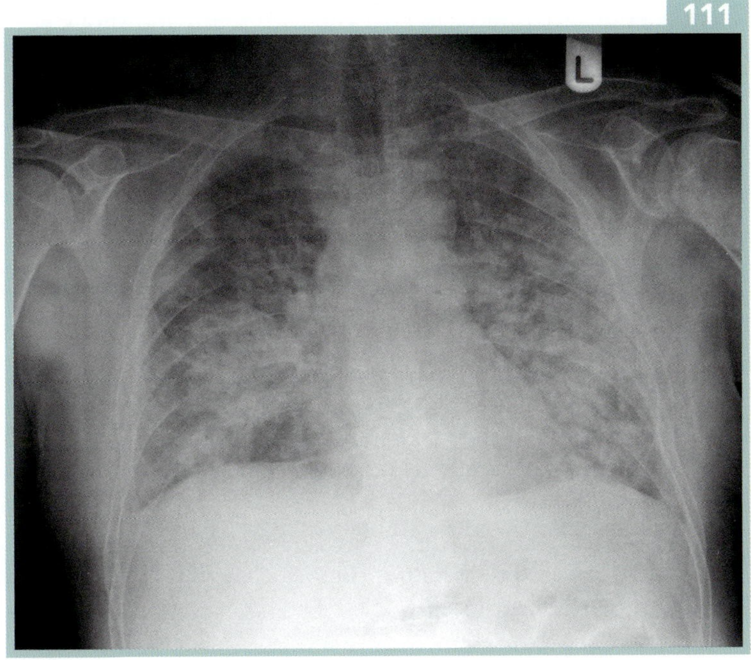

i. What does the CXR show?

ii. What could have caused this chest pathology?

iii. What further investigations are necessary?

iv. Define your CXR diagnosis accurately with an internationally recognised definition.

v. How should this man's condition be treated?

Answer 111

111i. Non-cardiogenic pulmonary oedema.

ii. Two diagnoses are possible: acute respiratory distress syndrome (ARDS) or acute pulmonary oedema due to cardiac decompensation. The patient has had no chest pain or arrhythmias and has a normal ECG, so a cardiac event is unlikely. The troponin also indicates no cardiac damage as <0.5 ng/l is normally considered normal. (**Note:** High troponins can co-exist with sepsis and shock.)

iii. This man's colonic perforation led to intra-abdominal spillage of faeces. Even though the operation was technically competent, intra-abdominal sepsis can still develop. Anastomotic breakdown of the end-to-end anastomosis may have occurred, leading to further peritoneal soiling. CT is necessary to look for any indications for further surgery.

iv. ARDS is defined as:

- Bilateral diffuse infiltrates on CXR.
- Intractable hypoxia with a PaO_2 /FIO_2 ratio of less than 200 mmHg (26.3 kPa) (i.e. even on 100% oxygen PaO_2 remains below 200 mmHg).
- A pulmonary artery (PA) occlusion pressure less than 18 mmHg (where a PA catheter is in place). As PA catheters are now rarely used, another non-invasive measure of cardiac filling (e.g. echocardiography), to show a lack of heart failure, is required.
- ARDS must also have a precipitating cause such as sepsis, major trauma, fat embolus, burns or pancreatitis.

v. ARDS is challenging to treat and may last 6 weeks or more. Intra-alveolar oedema collects due to the effects of cytokines released during the inflammatory process, in this case intra-abdominal sepsis. This oedema is obligatory as it occurs because of a proteinaceous leak across the alveolar membrane causing an osmotic pressure gradient into the alveolus. It is not removed by diuretics and excessive diuresis will cause renal failure. The treatment is supportive ICU management including low volume/low pressure ventilation (or possibly ECMO) until the ARDS resolves.

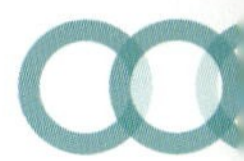

QUESTION 112

112i. In the graph shown **(112)**, which lung volumes are represented by each of the letters A, B, C, and D, and what is the approximate size of each of the lung volumes?

ii. When going from two-lung ventilation (10 ml/kg for a 70 kg patient) to one-lung ventilation (e.g. with a double lumen endotracheal tube), the total tidal volume of 700 ml is delivered to one lung. Based on your understanding of the lung volumes, is this a safe practice?

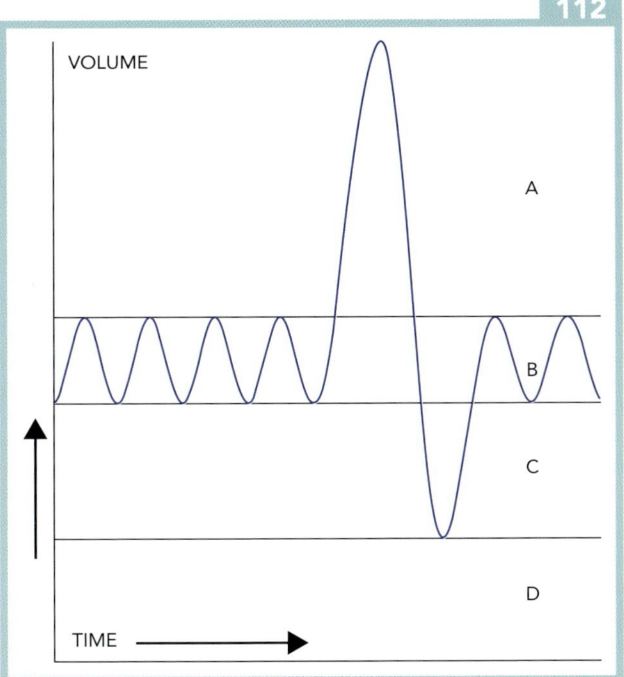

QUESTION 113

113 This patient (**113**) presents for repair of a supraumbilical hernia. List 11 points that you would inspect in this patient during the airway examination: teeth and jaw (4 points); inside the mouth and pharynx (2 points); mandibular space (2 points); and focus on the neck (3 points).

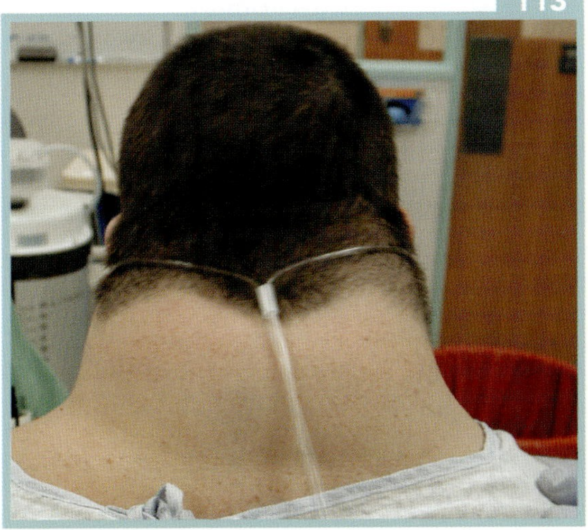

Answer 112

112i. For practical purposes, consider the lung volumes as multiples of 1,200 ml. The varied published ranges are given in parentheses:
A = residual volume (RV) = 1,200 ml.
B = expiratory reserve volume (ERV) = 1,200 ml (1,000–1,500 ml).
C = tidal volume (VT) = 500 ml.
D = inspiratory reserve volume (IVR) = 2,400 ml (3,000–3,300 ml).

ii. The answer to this question lies in an understanding of the relationship between the typical VT (used for two lungs) and the inspiratory capacity of a single lung. It is acceptable in the average patient as the VT (700 ml for two lungs) is less than the available volume (inspiratory capacity) of the single lung for which it is destined: half of 500 ml (VT) plus half of 1,200 ml IRV = 850 ml available to contain the 700 ml VT.

Answer 113

113
- Teeth and jaw. (1) Length of the upper incisors. (2) Prominent and/or overriding incisors ('buck teeth'); missing upper incisors (laryngoscope drops into this slot, with no space (to manoeuvre) to introduce the ET tube). (3) Whether prognathia is possible (i.e. can lower teeth be moved anterior to the upper teeth). (4) Mouth opening (normal is around 5–6 cm [2–2.4 in]).
- Inside the mouth and pharynx. (5) Size of the tongue in relation to the size of the pharynx (Mallampati classification). (6) Height and width of the arch of the palate (lateral volume, side-to-side, of the oropharynx, 'small mouth').
- Mandibular space. (7) Position of the larynx, described by the thyromental distance: length of the mandibular space (normal 6 cm [2.4 in] or 3 fingerbreadths). (8) Compliance of the mandibular space; might be non-compliant, non-distensible, stiff, especially after radiation for neck cancer; the larynx might be fixed, hard and indurated, causing difficulty in 'flipping up' and/or 'lifting up' the epiglottis during intubation.
- The neck. (9) Length of the neck. (10) Thickness of the neck. (11) Range of motion of the neck (cervical range of motion); evaluate the ability to assume the sniffing position; is 15° neck flexion on the chest possible? Is there 85–90°extension of the neck at the atlanto-occipital joint?

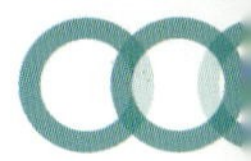

QUESTION 114

114 After 1 month of therapy in randomly selected patients, all of whom have starting pain scores of 9 to 10 (on a 10 point pain scale), the data in the Table below are calculated.

	Average daily pain score (scale 0–10)	
	Average	± Standard deviation
Medication A	6	±2.11
Medication B	3	±2.12

i. A researcher makes this statement: 'The pain score is exactly halved, therefore the pain intensity is also exactly halved'. Is the researcher's statement correct?

ii. The Student's t-test applied to the above data shows a statistically significant difference with a p-value of less than 0.05. The researcher suggests that the Student's t-test is appropriate, because we are working with numbers (and numbers are automatically parametric data because 6 is exactly twice as large as 3). Are pain scores parametric data?

iii. List four other examples of numbers used in clinical practice that are not parametric data.

QUESTION 115

115 Consider a patient undergoing 'free flap' reconstructive surgery following resection of a floor of mouth tumour.

i. Describe the important issues relating to the anaesthetic management of free flap surgery.

ii. How do the blood vessels in the flap differ from those in other tissues, and how could this impact on blood flow?

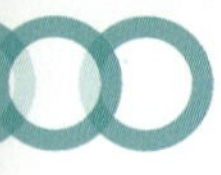

Answer 114

114i. No. It is neither accurate nor correct.

ii. Student's t-test is only appropriate for parametric data. Pain scores are not parametric data. They are non-parametric and are specifically measured on an ordinal or ranking scale.

iii. Include: APGAR score, GCS, recovery scores in recovery room such as Aldrete score, sedation scores in the ICU and trauma severity scores (e.g. APACHE, ISS).

Answer 115

115i. Although microvascular plastic surgery is widely used to transfer free vascularised tissue, hypoperfusion and subsequent necrosis of tissue remain important problems. Success or failure of a 'free flap' depends mainly on surgical skill, but anaesthetic management is also important.

Although seen in young trauma victims, free flap excision of malignancy in older patients is commoner. Ischaemic heart disease, peripheral vascular disease and COPD due to smoking may affect this latter group and anaesthetic technique must consider these factors. A long operating time is usual and GA is required. Positioning is critical and all pressure areas must be padded. IV lines and catheters must be readily accessible and the ET tube should be carefully secured. Haemodynamics and regional blood flow should be optimised in conjunction with advanced haemodynamic monitoring (a-line, CVP and Doppler/cardiac output/TOE). If the patient is warm, has a good blood volume, adequate arterial pressure and cardiac output is maintained (if necessary with inodilators such as dobutamine), blood flow to the transferred tissue should be optimal. Vasoconstriction should be avoided by preventing hypocapnia and providing good analgesia. Hypervolaemic haemodilution is practised but requires careful monitoring. Haematocrit, checked periodically throughout surgery, should be approximately 35%, as this increases cardiac output and improves microcirculatory flow. Induced hypotension, used to minimise blood loss, is not recommended as blood flow may not be adequate to the flap.

ii. 'Free flap' blood vessels are denervated so have no sympathetic tone with maximal vasodilation. Systemic pharmacological vasodilatation (used to reduce systemic vascular resistance) may preferentially affect normal innervated tissues and thus cause a 'steal phenomenon', resulting in enhanced flow to normal tissue and hypoperfusion of the flap.

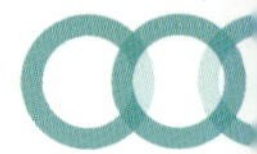

QUESTION 116

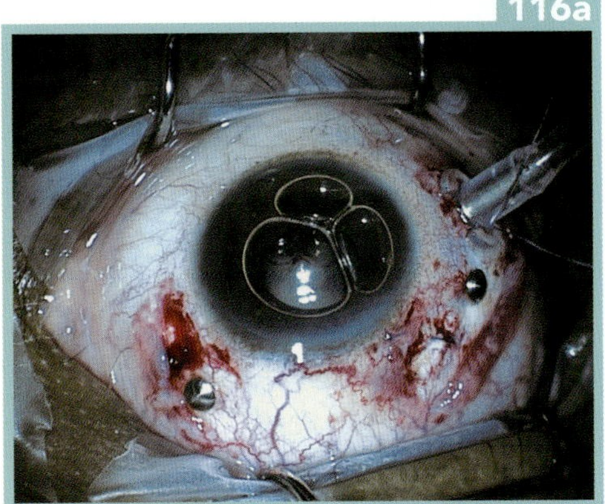

116a

116 This eye operation is about to start. Puncture wounds are sealed by metal studs on the exterior of the eye shown (**116a**). These will be used for a light source and microsurgical instruments to be inserted into the eye. The interior of the eye (**116b**) clearly shows the cutting instrument and the light source as viewed through a microscope by the ophthalmic surgeon. The pathological scarring can be seen as a white veil across the bottom of the screen.

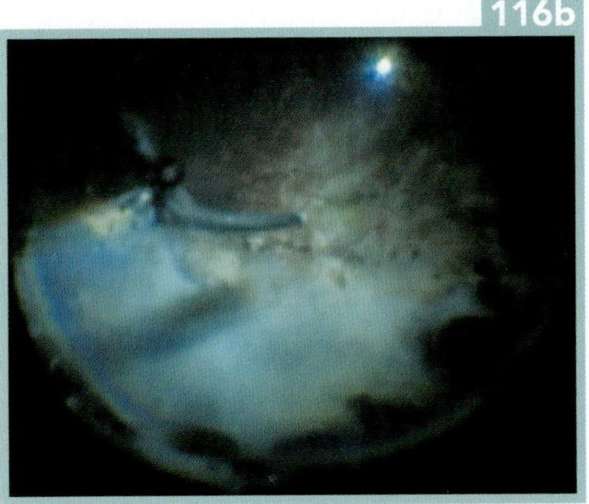

116b

i. What is this operation, and why is it performed?

ii. What problems must the anaesthesiologist anticipate with this kind of surgery when done under LA with or without sedation?

iii. Why can GA be preferable? Describe a suitable technique.

QUESTION 117

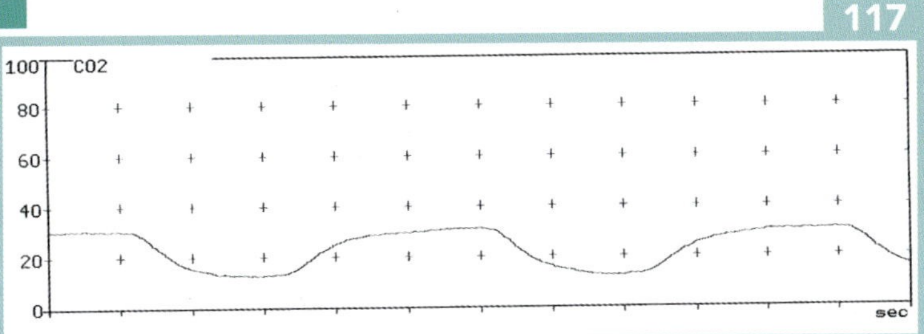

117

117 This capnography strip (**117**) indicates an increased inspired CO_2 concentration while using a circle breathing system.

i. Given a slow, spontaneous respiratory rate with an adult patient, give three reasons for such an occurrence.

ii. Would a low fresh gas flow (e.g. 300 ml per minute) be a cause for an increased inspired CO_2 concentration in a normally functioning anaesthetic machine and normal circle system?

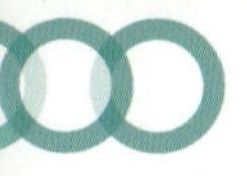

Answer 116

116i. Vitrectomy (VR) with laser surgery. The sclera is punctured and microsurgical instruments and a fibreoptic light source are inserted. A fluid infusion maintains the eye's shape during surgery and instruments and/or laser remove the pathological vitreous. Heavy oil can also be introduced into the eye to weigh down a detached retina and encourage reattachment. The back of the eye can contain pathological blood, debris or scar tissue, causing blurred vision by obscuring light as it passes to the retina. VR can also alleviate pathological retinal traction exerted by vitreous humour causing retinal distortion. Common reasons for vitrectomy include: diabetic retinopathy; macular hole; retinal detachment; preretinal membrane fibrosis; intraocular/vitreous haemorrhage; injury or infection; effects of previous eye surgery. Laser surgery stops bleeding from tiny retinal vessels and a small gas bubble may be placed intraocularily to help seal a macular hole.

ii. VR may be performed under LA but the patient must remain still. Due to the variable response with sedation, LA with sedation (e.g. midazolam, target-controlled IV propofol) can cause problems such as airway obstruction, movement of the head should the patient fall asleep or disinhibition/sudden awakening causing excessive movement or desterilisation of the operating field.

iii. GA is needed for patients with claustrophobia, tremor, intractable cough or those unable to lie still. Intubation and paralysis prevents movement. Mean arterial pressure should be maintained above 65 mmHg in a well hydrated patient to avoid any compromise to retinal blood flow.

Answer 117

117i. Exhausted soda lime; malfunctioning one-way valves; incomplete flushing of dead space, for instance with a laryngeal mask airway.

ii. A low fresh gas flow does not lead to an increased inspired CO_2 concentration given a fully functional anaesthetic machine.

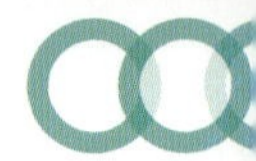

QUESTION 118

118i. What settings on the anaesthetic machine can be adjusted to help differentiate the causes of a slow, spontaneous respiratory rate in an adult (see the capnography trace in case **117**)?

ii. Given a rapid respiratory rate in a small child breathing spontaneously through a laryngeal mask airway (LMA), what would be a common explanation for the increased inspired CO_2?

QUESTION 119

119 Cerebral blood flow (CBF) on the y axis against mean arterial pressure (MAP) on the x axis (mmHg values are in brackets) is shown (**119**) Two other curves are shown.

i. What does curve A represent?

ii. What does curve B represent?

iii. What concept does the flat portion between 8 and 18 kPa represent?

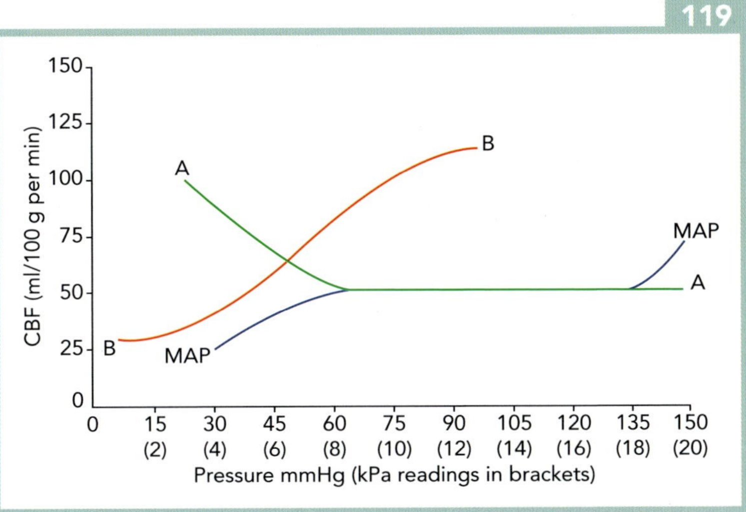

iv. Explain the concepts illustrated by the graph. How is the graph modified by the effects of underlying hypertension and age?

v. Why is an understanding of this graph essential for the practice of anaesthesia? Are there any other organs within the body that have similar autoregulatory mechanisms, and if so what are they?

Answer 118

118i. Increase the fresh gas flow (10 litres/min) so that all the exhaled gas goes to the scavenger: in the case of exhausted soda lime, the inspired CO_2 concentration will approximate zero. With malfunctioning one-way valves, the inspired CO_2 concentration will not go to zero, nor will it in the case of a small tidal volume.

Increase the tidal volume by hand: in the case of too small a tidal volume this will assist in flushing the dead space; the inspired CO_2 will greatly decrease.

ii. The most common reasons include the capnograph not being able to follow the rapid respiratory rate (the flush-out rate or time constant of the CO_2 analysis cell is too long) or the tidal volume of the child being too small to fully flush out the dead space, especially with an LMA.

Answer 119

119i. Curve A shows the relationship between arterial O_2 tension and CBF. O_2 only influences CBF if pO_2 is <8 kPa. Avoiding hypoxia prevents secondary brain insult after head trauma but has little effect on CBF at normal O_2 levels. Excess (100%) O_2 can reduce CBF by up to 10%.

ii. Curve B shows the linear relationship between CBF and arterial CO_2 between values of 3 and 10 kPa. This is important when intracranial space-occupying lesions (SOLs) (e.g. head injury, cerebral oedema, other brain pathology) cause limited intracerebral compliance. A low normal $PaCO_2$ (between 4.0 and 4.6 kPa [30 and 35 mmHg]) temporarily reduces CBF, preventing brain swelling and increased ICP. Prolonged mild hyperventilation, however, alters cerebrospinal bicarbonate and CBF increases again 6–12 hours after any change of pCO_2.

iii. It shows cerebral autoregulation. CBF, at 45–60 ml/100g brain tissue/min, is maintained at a constant level between MAPs of 60 and 30 mmHg. (CBF grey matter approx. 80 ml/100g/min; CBF white matter approx. 20 ml/100g/min). Outside this range, flow varies passively with pressure. Without autoregulation, brain perfusion is susceptible to sudden fluctuations in arterial BP caused by changes in posture and/or environmental stresses.

iv. Hypertension and increasing age cause a long-term change in the relationship between BP and CBF, shifting the curve to the right.

v. Cerebral and renal autoregulation are comparable but renal blood flow (RBF) is regulated more by the microcirculation (i.e. glomerular afferent and efferent arterioles). RBF and CBF, when compared across physiological BPs, are very similar.

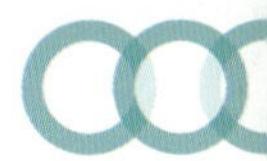

QUESTION 120

120i. What clinical sign is shown in **120a** and **120b**?

ii. How is this thought to come about?

iii. List the causes.

iv. Schamroth's sign may be helpful in confirming this diagnosis. What is Schamroth's sign?

v. Why does this matter to the anaesthesiologist?

120a

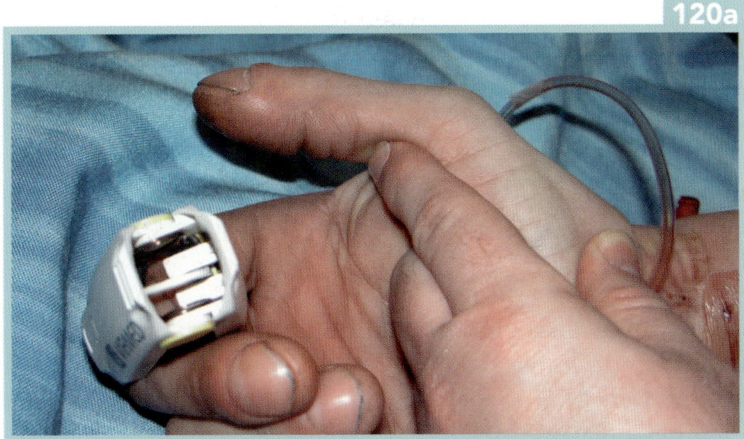

120b

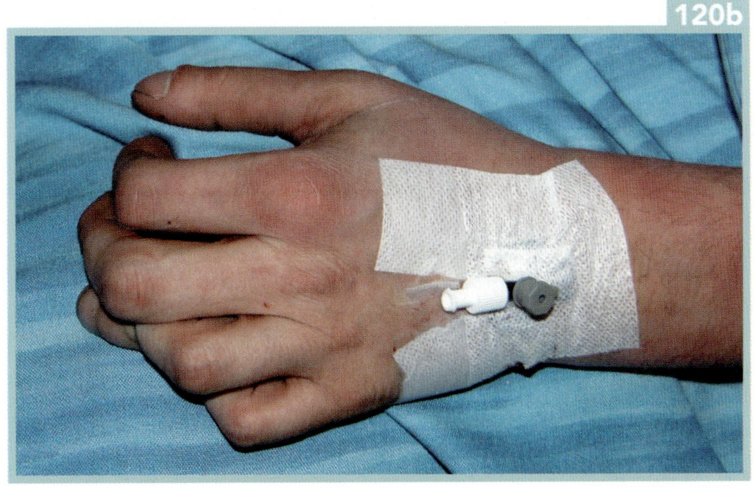

Answer 120

120i. Digital clubbing, an enlargement of the distal segments of the fingers (which can also affect toes).

ii. Clubbing is usually pathological and associated with pulmonary and cardiovascular diseases. The pathogenesis is thought to be dilatation of peripheral vessels causing megakaryocytes or platelet clumps to stimulate connective tissue overgrowth in the digital stratum. This is promoted by platelet-derived growth factor and/or hepatocyte growth factors associated with some types of malignancy. Hypoxaemia is associated with clubbing in respiratory disease. Clubbing does not occur in COPD or asthma and if present in these patients, underlying malignancy should be excluded.

iii. Pulmonary: bronchiectasis; chronic interstitial lung disease; chronic lung infection; cystic fibrosis; lung abscess; lung cancer. Cardiovascular: cyanotic congenital heart disease; infective endocarditis. Other: cirrhosis of the liver; thyrotoxicosis; inflammatory bowel disease; congenital.

iv. Schamroth's sign is elicited by placing the dorsal surfaces of the terminal phalanges on opposite fingers together. The normal diamond-shaped aperture is absent, as illustrated in **120c**.

v. Many serious pathological processes cause clubbing, any of which could have serious consequences for anaesthesia. In this 27-year-old patient's case his clubbed hands and toes were present as a child and he had had no health problems or pathological heart defects.

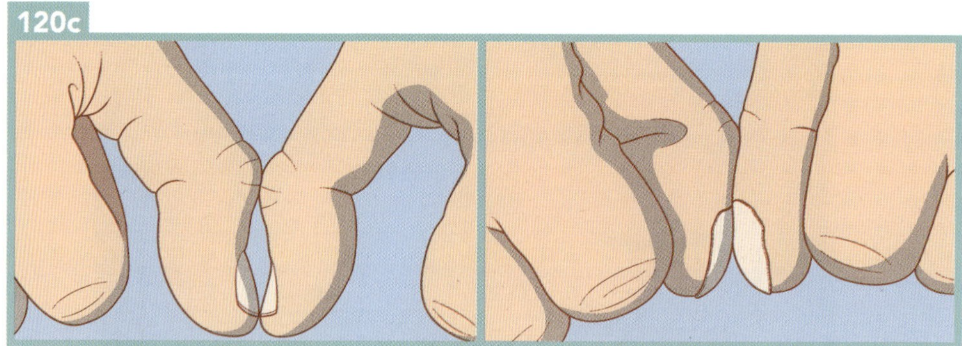
120c

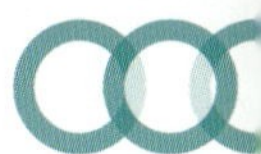

QUESTION 121

121i. What are the indicators of left ventricular hypertrophy (LVH)?

ii. Are they present in this ECG (**121**) of a 68-year-old man?

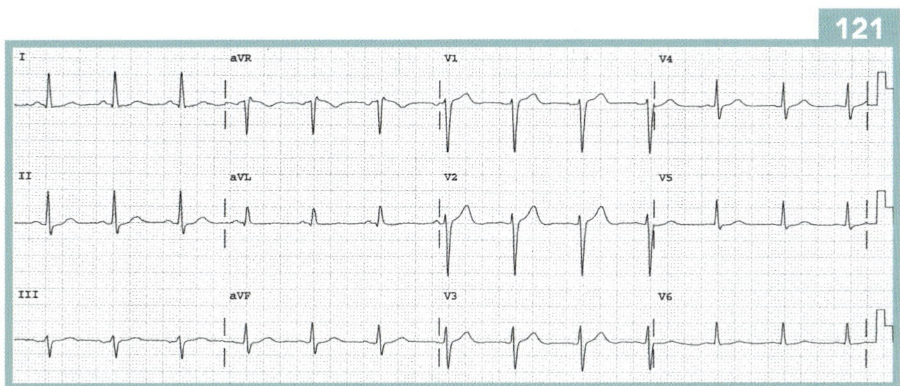

QUESTION 122

122 The physicochemical properties of some volatile and gaseous anaesthetic agents are shown in the Table below. BP = boiling point.

i. Fill in the gaps in the Table.

	MW (Dalton)	BP (°C)	SVP @ 20°C (kPa)	MAC (%)	Blood:gas solubility	Oil:gas solubility	% Metabolised
Sevoflurane	200	58.5	22.7				
Desflurane	168		89				
Halothane	197	50.2	32		2.4	224	
Enflurane	184	56.5	23		1.8	98	2
Isoflurane	184						
N_2O	44		5,200	105	0.47	1.4	

ii. Why is the MAC of N_2O above 100%? How is it possible to calculate and/or determine a MAC value above 100%?

iii. Complete the following sentences related to potency and onset of action:

The higher the oil:gas solubility the .... potent the agent.

The higher the blood:gas solubility the .... the onset of action of the agent.

Answer 121

121i. The ECG voltage criteria (Cornell) for LVH are an S wave in V_3 and an R wave in aVL >28 mm (men) or an S in V_3 and an R wave in aVL >20 mm (women). The ECG shows left ventricular strain, as indicated by the flattened T-wave in V6.

ii. Note the calibration of the ECG at the right-hand side. The stepped calibration indicates that the voltage on the ECG has been halved (each calibration step indicates 1 milli-Volt (mV). The normal calibration is 1 mV per 1 cm (10 mm). In this case, 1 mV is represented by 0.5 cm (5 mm or 5 little blocks - vertically), so the ECG is calibrated to enable the ECG to fit onto the paper and is truly showing LVH.

Answer 122

122i. See Table below.

	MW (Dalton)	BP (°C)	SVP @ 20°C (kPa)	MAC (%)	Blood:gas solubility	Oil:gas solubility	% Metabolised
Sevoflurane	200	58.5	22.7	2.0	0.7	80	3.5
Desflurane	168	23.5	89	6.6	0.45	29	0.02
Halothane	197	50.2	32	0.75	2.4	224	20
Enflurane	184	56.5	23	1.7	1.8	98	2
Isoflurane	184	48.5	33	1.2	1.4	98	0.2
N_2O	44	–88	5,200	105	0.47	1.4	<0.01

ii. N_2O has an MAC of >100% (>760 mmHg) because it is too weak to anaesthetise a patient at <100%. It is obviously not possible to administer 100% N_2O, as this is a hypoxic concentration. The theoretical MAC of N_2O is 105%.

This value can be obtained by extrapolating the non-hypoxic concentrations of the gas to above 100%, to reveal the theoretical MAC of 105% (+/- 800 mmHg). Alternatively, the MAC can be determined in a hyperbaric chamber. For instance, at 2 ATA (1,520 mmHg) a mixture of 25% oxygen (355 mmHg) and 75% N_2O (1,115 mmHg) could be used to determine the MAC of N_2O.

iii. The higher the oil:gas solubility the *more* potent the agent.

The higher the blood:gas solubility the *faster* the onset of action of the agent.

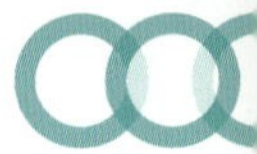

QUESTION 123

123i. What is illustrated (**123**)?

ii. What lung volume is represented by the red arrow?

iii. What lung volume is represented by the black arrow?

iv. Why is adding A to B an important anaesthetic concept?

v. Explain this concept in terms of how anaesthesia and patient factors influence it.

123

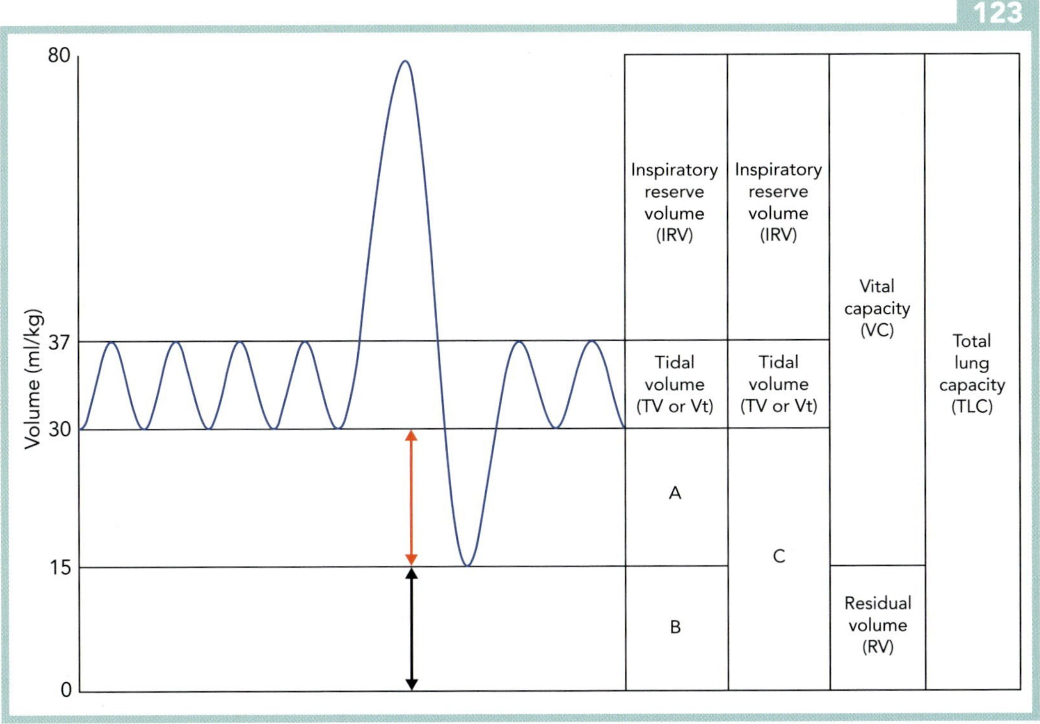

Answer 123

123i. A spirometry trace. Quiet breathing with normal tidal volumes (TV) changes when a maximal inspiration is taken, then maximal exhalation and returning to normal breathing. The maximal inspiratory/expiratory manoeuvre allows calculation of the various different lung volumes (absolute values) and capacities (the product of two or more volumes).

ii. The expiratory reserve volume (A).

iii. The residual volume (B).

iv. The sum of A and B is the functional residual capacity (FRC) (C), the volume of air left in the lung at the end of a normal tidal exhalation. The FRC is the resting lung volume at the end of exhalation. It contains the volume of the lung that provides gas exchange, irrespective of the tidal volume. Changes in the FRC can be diagnostic for specific lung diseases. If distal airways 'close off' (e.g. atalectasis/consolidation), this can reduce FRC, reducing lung efficiency to make hypoxia more likely. Due to the pressure of abdominal contents on the diaphragm, FRC is greatest when a patient is erect, less when supine and least in a head-down position. Amelioration of this reduction in FRC by anaesthesia is difficult. PEEP prevents some atalectasis. Prone positioning increases FRC.

Anaesthesia and opiates will also reduce FRC, which is one of the reasons why supplemental oxygen under anaesthesia is recommended. Elderly patients also have a relatively reduced FRC due to an increase in their closing volume. The closing volume is that value of lung volume at which some airway closure occurs. This is known to increase in elderly patients, and when it encroaches significantly on FRC the efficiency of gas exchange is dramatically reduced. This is especially likely in patients who have long-standing COPD or other respiratory disease.

v. Understanding FRC is one of the basic principles of respiratory physiology vital to the understanding of anaesthesia.

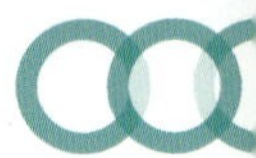

QUESTION 124

124i. Fill in the gaps in this Table.

	MW (Dalton)	Density (kg/m³)	Viscosity (mPas)	BP (°C)	Critical temperature (°C)	Critical pressure (kPa)
O_2		1.43				
N_2O						7,250
CO_2		1.98	0.014		31	7,400
Helium	4	0.18	0.018	–269	–268	200

BP = boiling point

ii. What does the term critical temperature mean?

iii. Why is this important to understand?

iv. What does the term critical pressure mean?

v. What are the full cylinder pressures, at room temperature, of the following: O_2, N_2O, CO_2, air, Entonox, Heliox.

QUESTION 125

125i. What is a transducer?

ii. What is the technology in the device shown (**125**), which is used to convert the pressure waveform in an arterial line into an electrical reading that can be seen on a monitor?

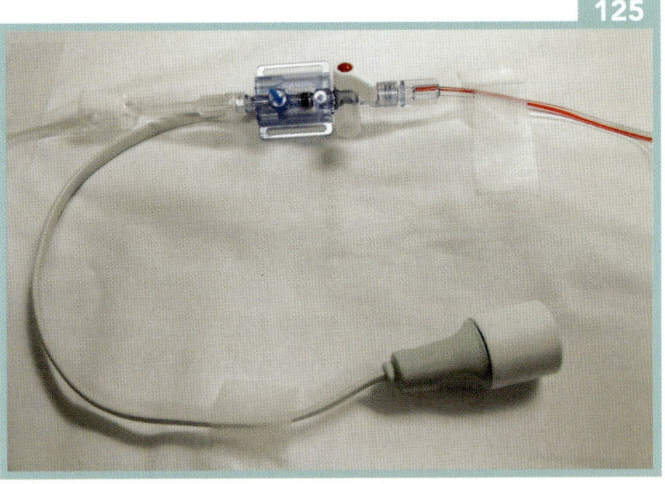
125

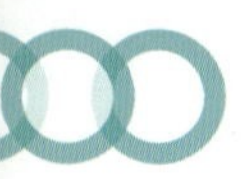

Answer 124

124i. See Table below.

	MW (Dalton)	Density (kg/m³)	Viscosity (mPas)	BP (°C)	Critical temperature (°C)	Critical pressure (kPa) (psi)
O_2	32	1.43	0.0196	–183	–118	5,100 (740)
N_2O	44	1.98	0.014	–89	36.4	7,250 (1,052)
CO_2	44	1.98	0.014	78.5	31	7,400 (1,073)
Helium	4	0.18	0.018	–269	–268	200 (29)

ii. It is the temperature at which a gas cannot be liquefied by pressure alone.

iii. A substance above its critical temperature will always be a gas irrespective of the ambient pressure. Oxygen is a gas above -118°C and thus not liquid in cylinders used for anaesthesia (at room temperature.) N_2O, however, is a vapour at room temperature as, when pressurised, some of it will liquify. This is important when N_2O is combined with oxygen to give Entonox, as N_2O may liquefy at the bottom of an Entonox cylinder when ambient temperature is $<$36.4°C. If Entonox is used under these circumstances, oxygen can be released from the cylinder first, followed by the vapour from the liquid N_2O at the bottom of the cylinder, leading to a hypoxic mixture of pure N_2O. Entonox cylinders must be regularly inverted in cool environments and stored at room temperature or above.

iv. Critical pressure is the pressure exerted by a volume of gas at its critical temperature. This is also its saturated vapour pressure (at that temperature) (i.e. equilibrium between gaseous and liquid forms).

v. O_2 = 13,700 kPa (1,900 psi): N_2O = 4,400 kPa (638 psi): CO_2 = 5,000 kPa (725 (psi): air = 13,700 kPa (1,900 psi); Entonox = 13,700 kPa (1,900 psi); Heliox = 13,700 kPa (1,900 psi).

Answer 125

125i. A device that converts one form of energy into another.

ii. A strain gauge, which is created as part of a Wheatstone bridge electrical circuit. These originally consisted of wire strain gauges, but now a silicon crystal diaphragm replaces the wire. The principle of operation is the same (see also case **126**).

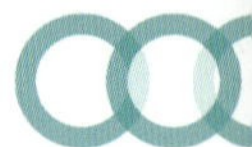

QUESTION 126

126i. With regard to the device illustrated in case **125**, describe the system schematically and explain how it functions with the equation that describes the electrical resistances in the circuit.

ii. Why is it necessary for the device to be temperature compensated, and how is it made resistant to temperature changes?

QUESTION 127

127 With regard to the circle system shown (**127**):

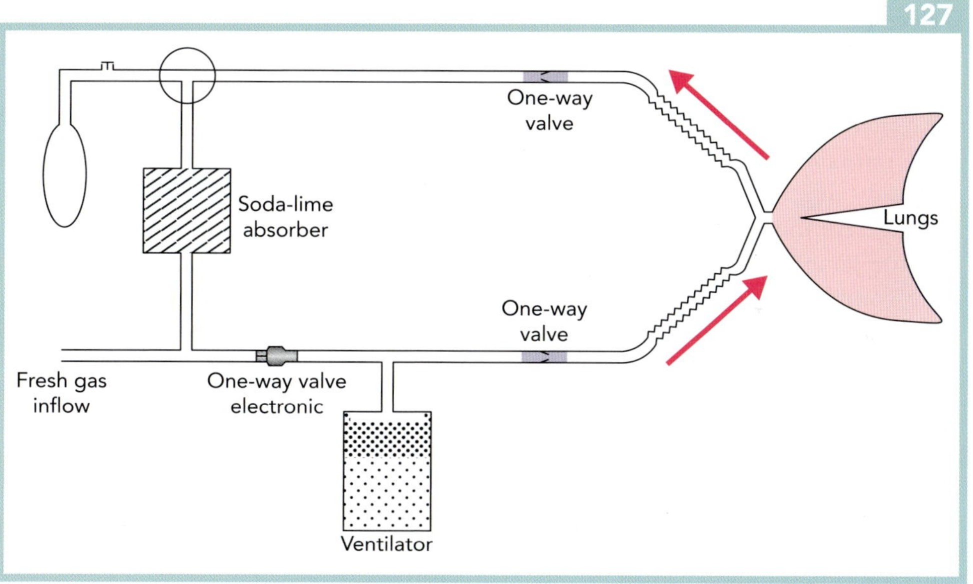

i. Why is the anaesthesia reservoir bag on the side of the inspiratory limb? (Compare with a classical anaesthesia system where the reservoir bag is on the side of the expiratory limb – see case **196**).

ii. What do we mean when we say that an anaesthetic machine has 'fresh gas flow compensation'?

iii. List two methods in anaesthetic machine design used to provide 'fresh gas flow compensation'.

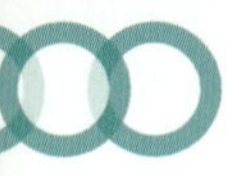

Answer 126

126i. When the silicon crystal diaphragm is stretched, its electrical resistance increases as a function of the atomic structure of the crystal. This can be utilised as part of an electrical circuit (a Wheatstone bridge as shown in **126**). The central device marked G is a galvanometer. The current passing through the galvanometer should be zero if the resistances are equal due to the equation below:

$$R2/R1 = R3/Rv$$

When the diaphragm distorts because of the arterial pressure waveform, the resistance in the crystal changes (variable resistance, Rv) and a current passes through the galvanometer and registers an electrical signal. This is processed and displayed on a monitor as the electrical waveform. This is how the energy of the pressure waveform is converted into electrical energy that can be displayed on the monitor.

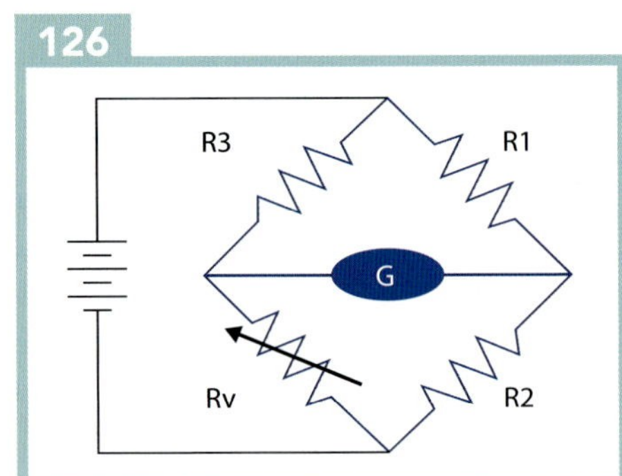

ii. An increase in temperature increases the resistance in a metal conductor. This would cause calibration errors in the bridge. All the tiny resistors are exposed to the same temperature changes, which are compensated by stretching two of the resistors and compressing the other two.

Answer 127

127i. It is on the side of the inspiratory limb so that it can store the fresh gas flow during the inspiratory phase of the ventilator.

ii. Fresh gas flow compensation means that changes in the fresh gas flow (or duration of inspiration) will not affect the tidal volume. The anaesthetic machine compensates for variations in fresh gas flow during inspiration as well as for variations in the duration of inspiration at a constant fresh gas flow.

iii. (1) A reservoir is added to the inspiratory side of the anaesthetic breathing system. A separate (hidden) reservoir may be used or the anaesthesia reservoir bag may be used (this explains why the reservoir bag moves on some anaesthetic machines during controlled ventilation). Extra valves are needed to isolate the reservoir bag from the ventilator during the inspiratory phase (see device labelled 'One-way valve – electronic' in **127**). (2) The amount of driving gas delivered to a 'bag-in-a-bottle' may be varied to compensate for the amount of fresh gas flowing during inspiration.

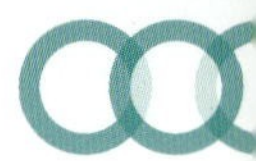

QUESTION 128

128i. How would gas flow be described in the simplest terms?

ii. Name three different types of flow that can occur in anaesthetic breathing systems?

iii. Write the equation that describes the easiest type of flow to quantify mathematically.

iv. What is Reynolds number, and what is its significance?

v. Why are these concepts of interest when considering patients breathing through anaesthetic breathing systems or tracheostomy tubes?

QUESTION 129

129 Identify these four anaesthetic agents based on their structures as shown (**129**).

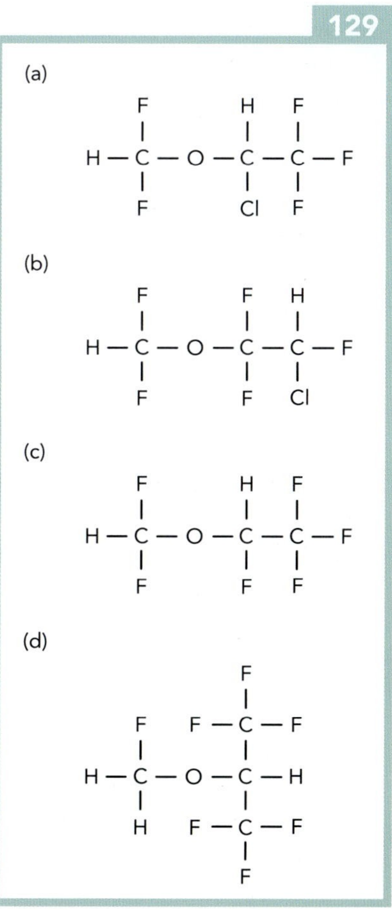

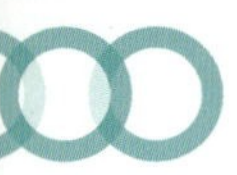

Answer 128

128i. Flow is the volume of a mass of gas passing a point in unit time as per the equation:

$$\dot{Q} = \frac{\Delta P}{R}$$

$\dot{Q}$ = flow; ΔP = pressure change across the point of flow; R = resistance.

ii. Laminar, turbulent and transitional.

iii. The easiest to describe mathematically is laminar flow, which can be described by the Hagen-Poiseuille equation:

$$\dot{Q} = \frac{\Delta P \times \pi \times r^4}{8 \times \eta \times 1}$$

$\dot{Q}$ = flow; ΔP = the pressure difference across the anaesthetic circuit; η = viscosity of the gas in the circuit; l is the length and r is the radius of the circuit.

iv. Flow changes from laminar to turbulent, via transitional flow, if certain parameters are exceeded. Transitional flow does not follow the mathematical predictions for either laminar or turbulent flow, but Reynolds number describes when flow becomes turbulent. If Reynolds number exceeds 2,000 turbulence, it is described thus:

$$Re = \frac{\upsilon \times \eta \times r}{L}$$

ν = velocity of the gas; η = viscosity; r = radius of the tube; L is gas density.

v. When attempting to deliver gases at high velocity, turbulent flow is more likely and, if this happens, paradoxically a lower gas velocity results. This is because more energy is required to deliver turbulent gas than laminar gas. In anaesthetic systems, a patient's work of spontaneous breathing depends heavily on flow being turbulent or laminar. This is important when weaning from ventilation or tracheostomy tubes. Tracheostomy tubes, despite their short length, can be more difficult to breathe through than similarly sized ET tubes because the tracheostomy tube shape leads to turbulence. A size 8 ET tube of 23 cm length has approximately the same resistance to breathing as a standard size 8 tracheostomy tube.

Answer 129

129 (a) = isoflurane; (b) = desflurane; (c) = sevoflurane; (d) = halothane.

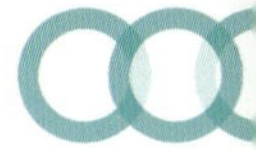

QUESTION 130

130i. What is the purpose of the mask shown (**130**)?

ii. How does it work, and why must it be used with a leak in the circuit?

iii. Define sleep apnoea,and describe the pathophysiology of the syndrome.

iv. What makes it worse?

v. Describe what preoperative investigations should be done and how they should be interpreted.

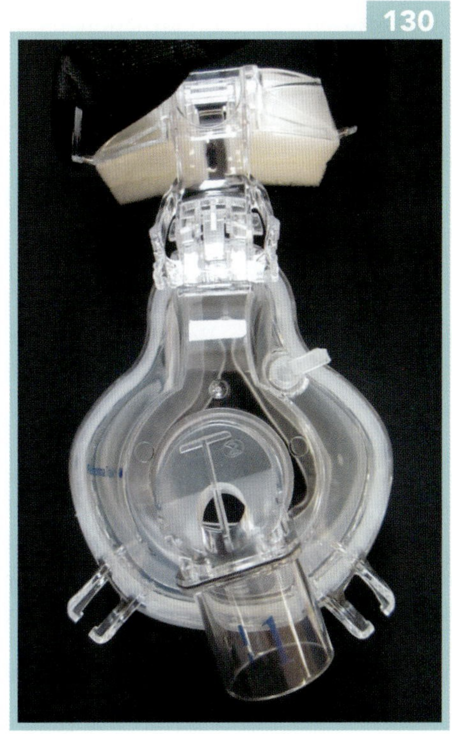

130

Answer 130

130i. To provide nasal continuous positive airway pressure (nCPAP) to treat sleep apnoea.

ii. Positive pressure is applied to the nose, splinting open the upper airway to prevent pharyngeal collapse during sleep. The sleep apnoea patient then sleeps continuously and avoids the problem of intermittent wakening ('sleep fragmentation') associated with airway obstruction. A minimum mask fixed leak prevents CO_2 retention, although often a small leak around the mask seal/patient's mouth occurs anyway.

iii. Sleep apnoea is recurrent nocturnal apnoea and hypoxaemia during sleep causing undue daytime hypersomnolence. It affects adults (4% reported in middle age) or children (3% aged 2–5). In adults, obesity and snoring are common presentations. Snoring arises from palatal/nasopharyngeal obstruction, retroglossal/hypopharyngeal obstruction or failure of the upper airway dilator muscles to stabilise the airway during sleep. The pathophysiological consequences of the condition can result in pulmonary and systemic hypertension, right and left heart failure, polycythaemia and, sometimes, respiratory failure. Children may suffer from sleep apnoea due to hypertrophy of tonsils/adenoids or congenital abnormalities (Down's, Pierre Robin syndrome). Surgical correction of the cause of obstruction is effective in selected cases.

iv. Obesity, ageing, tissue oedema (caused by the vibration of snoring), nasopharyngeal carcinoma or mandibular abnormalities. Benzodiazepine, alcohol or other drug dependence, brainstem infarcts, polio or respiratory muscle disorders such as myasthenia, myotonia or diaphragmatic paralysis also make sleep apnoea worse.

v. A sleep apnoea laboratory measures a combination of apnoeic episodes during sleep per hour (known as the apnoea hypopnoea index, AHI) and/or the lowest O_2 saturations during an apnoeic event. These factors (AHI >10, saturations <80%) are significant risk factors predictive for development of perioperative airway complications (e.g. difficult/failed intubation and post-extubation upper airway obstruction).

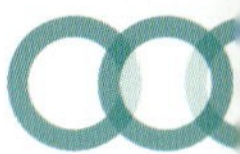

QUESTION 131

131 The middle section (labelled Lung volumes) of **131** shows the four static lung volumes (indicated as A, B, C and D), which do not overlap. The right-hand section (labelled Lung capacities) shows the four static lung capacities (indicated as E, F, G and H) where each lung capacity consists of two or more lung volumes.

i. What are the four lung volumes marked A, B, C, and D in the middle graphic of **131**?

ii. What four lung capacities are indicated by E, F, G and H in **131**?

iii. Which three lung volumes are measured with a flow–volume loop?

iv. Which of the four static lung capacities are measured by the flow–volume loop?

v. Which of the four lung capacities include the residual volume?

vi. Are any of the lung capacities that include residual volume measured by a flow–volume loop?

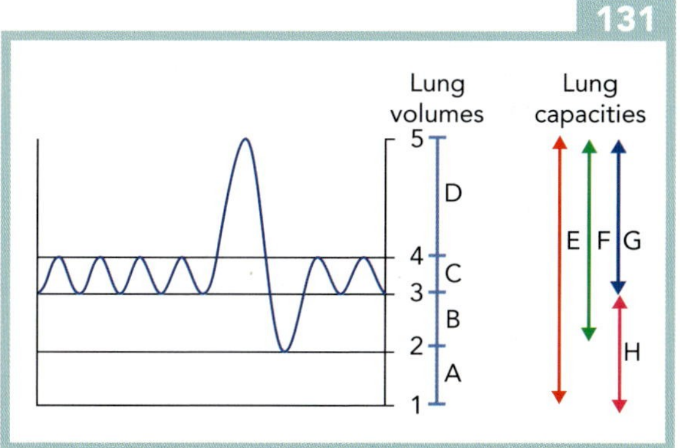

QUESTION 132

132 A spirometry trace is shown (**132a**).

i. With regard to the y-axis (ordinate) above the zero point, which point indicates the higher flow values: ⋆ or %?

ii. With regard to the y-axis (ordinate) below the zero point, which point indicates the higher flow values: # or &?

iii. With regard to the x-axis (abscissa), in which direction are the higher values: left side or right side: @ or $?

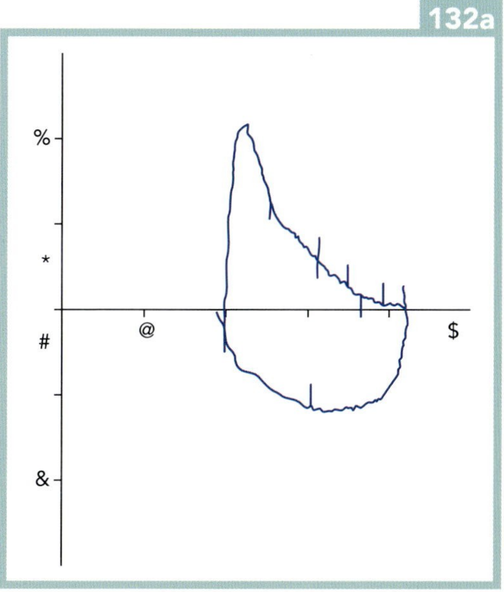

Answer 131

131i. A = residual volume; B = expiratory reserve volume; C = tidal volume; D = inspiratory reserve volume.

ii. E = total lung capacity; F = vital capacity; G = inspiratory capacity; H = functional residual capacity.

iii. Inspiratory reserve volume, tidal volume and expiratory reserve volume.

iv. The vital capacity and the inspiratory capacity can be measured with a flow–volume loop.

v. The total lung capacity and the functional residual capacity include the residual volume and therefore cannot be measured with a flow-volume loop.

vi. No.

Answer 132

132i. The expiratory values on the y-axis increase (blue arrow on **132b**) in the vertical upwards direction (i.e. % represents a higher flow rate than *).

ii. The values of inspiratory flows increase (red arrow) from the zero value in a downwards direction (i.e. & has a higher flow rate [value] than #). This is not a 'negative' flow, but just represents the inspiratory flow, which is in the opposite direction than exhalation.

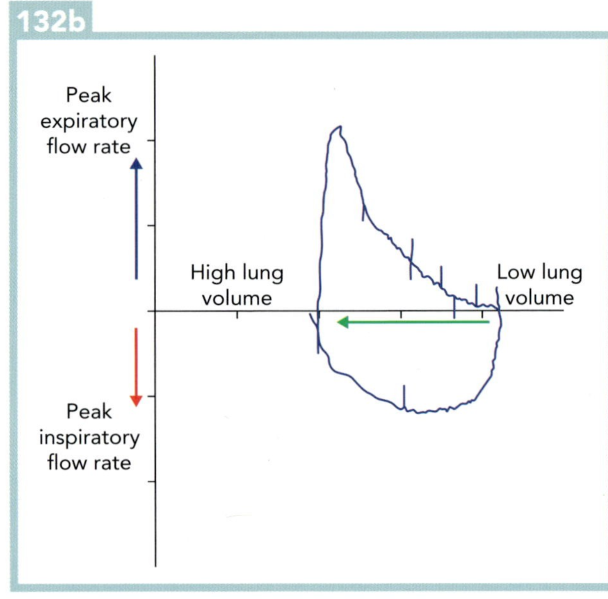

iii. The values on the x-axis represent an empty lung on the right-hand side ($ = lower lung volumes), with the values on the left-hand side representing increasing (larger) lung volumes (green arrow) and a 'full' lung (@ = higher lung volumes).

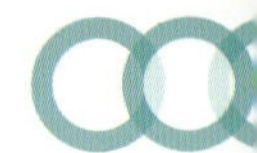

QUESTION 133

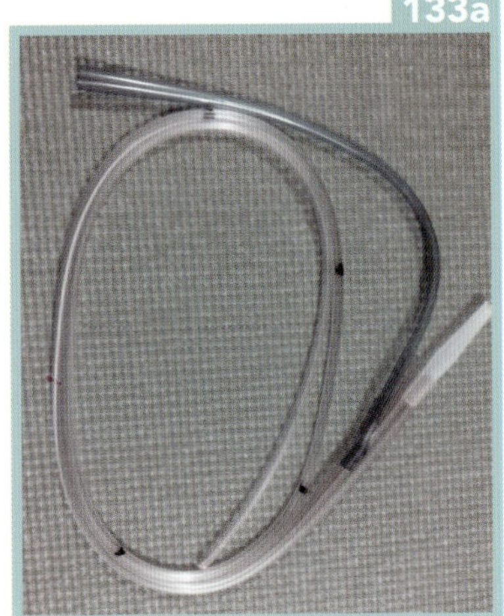
133a

133 Some nasogastric (NG) tubes have four black lines on them. A 'Ryles' tube, designed for short-term drainage of the stomach of air or gastric contents, is shown (**133a**). It is not a feeding tube because its large size may result in pressure necrosis of the nares (external opening of the nose).

i. What distances are indicated by these four lines?

ii. From which end of the tube are these distances measured?

iii. Which line should be at the nares when used as an NG tube?

iv. Some NG tubes have centimetre (cm) markings on them (**133b**). What depth marking should be at the nares when this metric tube is used?

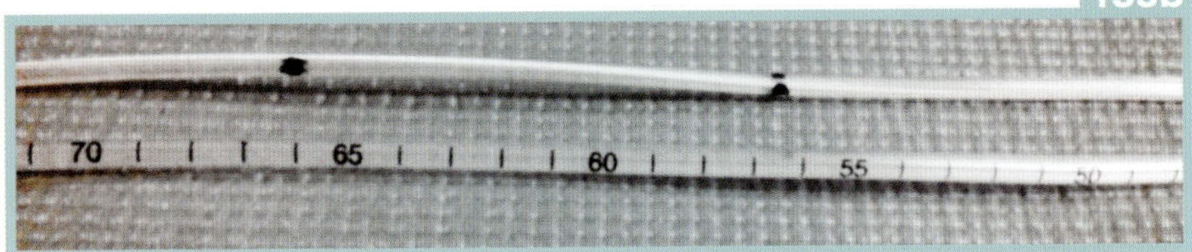

133b

QUESTION 134

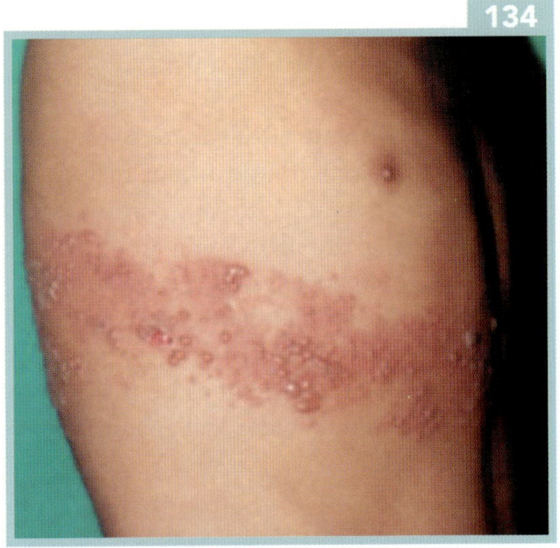
134

134 A patient presents with this rash (**134**). Three months later he is seen at the chronic pain clinic with allodynia affecting the same area.

i. What is this rash?

ii. What is allodynia?

iii. Explain what has happened at three months.

iv. Discuss techniques that can reduce the severity of the chronic condition.

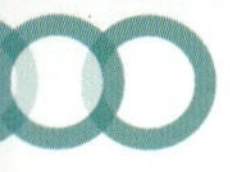

Answer 133

133i. In the US the four black lines are placed at 18, 22, 26 and 30 inches from the tip (stomach end) of the NG tube. In Europe, markings are usually placed on the NG tube at 5 cm intervals between 40 and 70 cm.

ii. The distances are measured from the end of the tube that is placed in the stomach.

iii. Typically it is stated: 'Two-and-a-half lines should be in, and two-and-a-half lines should be out'. This means that the tube would be at 24 inches or 65 cm.

iv. The typical distance for the NG tube in cm is 60–65 cm.

Answer 134

134i. *Varicella zoster* (shingles) infection.

ii. A sensation that differs from the one expected (e.g. pain from light touch).

iii. Post-herpetic neuralgia has developed. Viral infiltration of the dorsal root ganglion of the sensory nerves has occurred, with destruction of the cell bodies and deafferentation of the dorsal horn or trigeminal nucleus. This is also associated with ingrowth into the dorsal horn or nucleus of sympathetic nerve fibres that synapse with the deafferentated dorsal horn cells. The result is an area of skin with abnormal sensation (e.g. numbness, loss of fine sensation, allodynia, altered sensation to hot and cold or persisting crawling or itchy sensations). The pain is exacerbated by cold and eased by warmth.

iv. Early treatment of the acute phase with analgesics and antiviral agents is important. Early oral antiviral treatment may prevent or shorten the duration of post-herpetic neuralgia. If pain continues 2 weeks after the onset of the rash, targeted neuronal, particularly sympathetic blockade (for facial pain stellate ganglion block) dramatically reduces the intensity and duration of continuing neuralgia. Interventional sympathectomy and local anaesthetic techniques are much less effective if initiated later (e.g. after 3 months). The burning or dysaesthetic itch sensations can sometimes be treated with local application of capsaicin, a substance 'p' depletor, or with local anaesthetic creams.

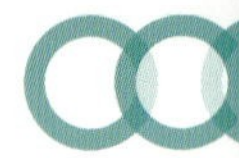

QUESTION 135

135 Describe how the condition in case **134** is treated pharmacologically when it has developed.

QUESTION 136

136 This is a TOE image (**136**).

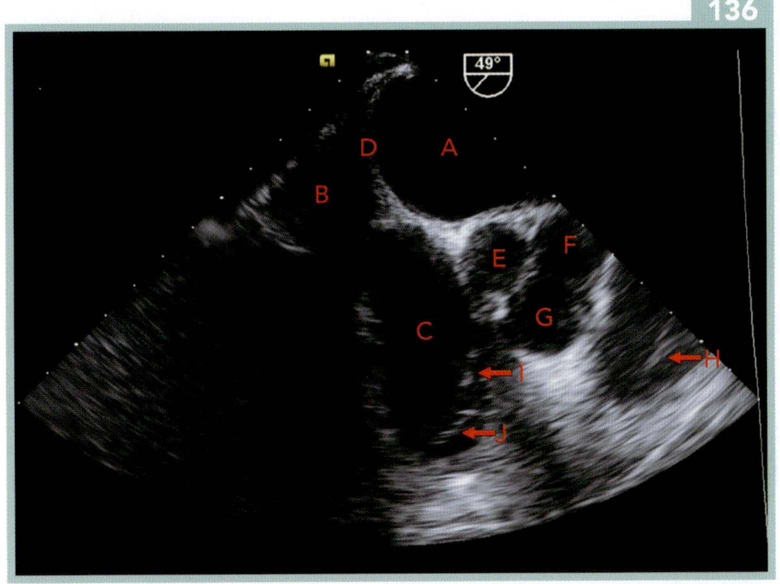

i. What is this view called?

ii. Which chamber is indicated by A?

iii. Which chambers are indicated by B and C?

iv. What structure is indicated by D?

v. What structures are indicated by E, F and G?

vi. What structure is indicated by H?

vii. What structures are indicated by I and J?

Answer 135

135 See the algorithm (**135**).

135

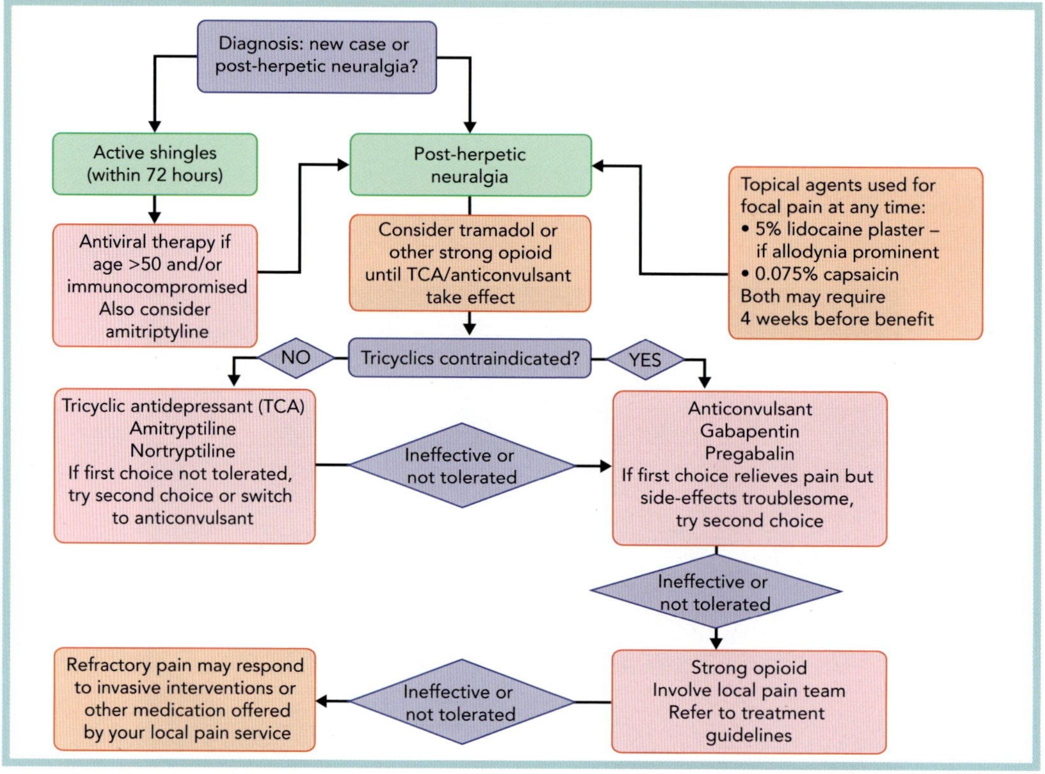

Diagnosis: new case or post-herpetic neuralgia?

Active shingles (within 72 hours)

Antiviral therapy if age >50 and/or immunocompromised
Also consider amitriptyline

Post-herpetic neuralgia

Consider tramadol or other strong opioid until TCA/anticonvulsant take effect

Topical agents used for focal pain at any time:
- 5% lidocaine plaster – if allodynia prominent
- 0.075% capsaicin

Both may require 4 weeks before benefit

Tricyclics contraindicated?

NO

YES

Tricyclic antidepressant (TCA)
Amitryptiline
Nortryptiline
If first choice not tolerated, try second choice or switch to anticonvulsant

Ineffective or not tolerated

Anticonvulsant
Gabapentin
Pregabalin
If first choice relieves pain but side-effects troublesome, try second choice

Ineffective or not tolerated

Strong opioid
Involve local pain team
Refer to treatment guidelines

Ineffective or not tolerated

Refractory pain may respond to invasive interventions or other medication offered by your local pain service

Answer 136

136i. The mid-oesophageal, aortic valve, short-axis (SAX) view.

ii. A is the left atrium.

iii. B and C are both parts of the right atrium.

iv. D indicates the septum.

v. E is the non-coronary cusp, F the left coronary cusp and G the right coronary cusp.

vi. H indicates the pulmonary valve.

vii. I and J indicate the leaflets of the tricuspid valve.

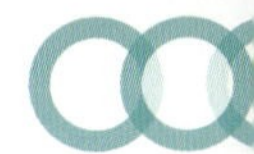

QUESTION 137

137i. What is the correct name of the device shown (**137a**)?

ii. How does this device work?

iii. List its safety features.

iv. What does 'TEC' stand for, and how is this achieved?

137a

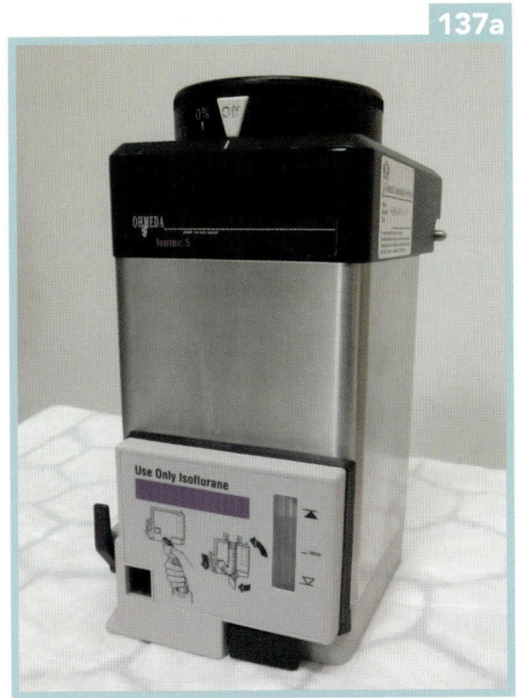

Answer 137

137i. A plenum vaporiser (TEC Mk1-6). Plenum vaporisers deliver accurate concentrations of anaesthetic vapour. Because of their high internal resistance they must be operated using a constant positive pressure and also be correctly mounted on the anaesthetic machine.

ii. It accurately splits gas into two streams (**137b**). Stream 1 flows through a bypass channel; stream 2 (a smaller amount) is diverted into the vaporising chamber. The proportion of gas in each stream is called the splitting ratio. The gas streamed to the vaporising chamber is fully saturated with volatile anaesthetic and then mixes with gas from the bypass channel. Gas then leaves the vaporiser at the desired anaesthetic vapour concentration.

iii. (1) Specific labelling and colour coding for each agent. (2) A clear indictor to show the filling level of the agent. (3) An anti-spill mechanism within the vaporiser. (4) The Selectatec system (this back bar mounting requires a locking lever to be engaged to allow the vaporiser dial to move) allows only one vaporiser to be used at a time. (5) The anaesthetic concentration dial cannot be turned without pressing a button at its back. (6) An 'MAC scale' is attached to the dial or side of the vaporiser.

These features prevent operator dependent errors (e.g. allowing the vaporiser to run dry, tip over or deliver insufficient anaesthesia). Additionally, a plenum vaporiser is unidirectional so cannot be connected in reverse (if this happened, much larger volumes of gas would enter the vaporising chamber and deliver excessive vapour concentrations). Filling with the wrong agent is difficult as agent-specific filling ports are built into their design. Accidental mixing of volatile agents is also prevented.

iv. TEmperature Compensated and is achieved by:

- A heavy (5 kg) metal jacket (or sometimes a mass of metal with a high density, high specific heat capacity and a high thermal conductivity [e.g. copper] is built into the base of the vaporiser) equilibrates with room temperature, providing a source of heat.
- Admission of gas into the vaporising chamber is controlled by a valve with a bimetallic strip. As the chamber cools, more gas is admitted to compensate for the loss of evaporation at the cooler temperature.

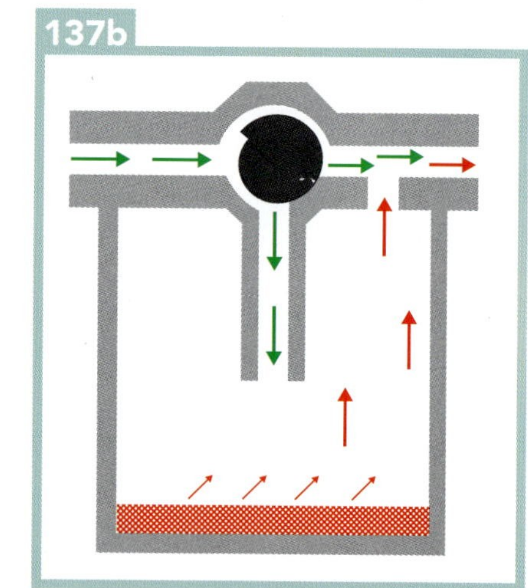

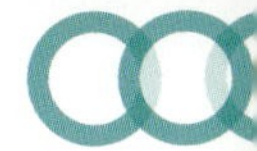

QUESTION 138

138 This patient (**138**) suffered a minor fracture in her right wrist 3 months prior to presentation to the chronic pain clinic with severe pain in her hand.

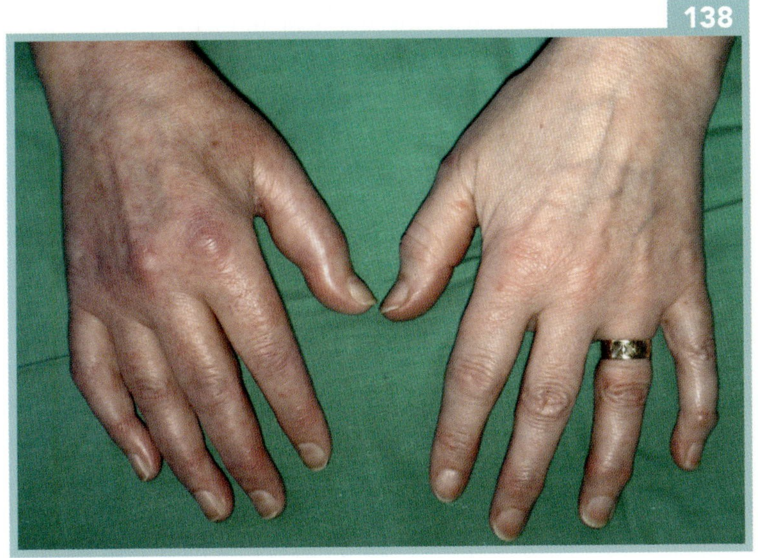

i. What is this syndrome?

ii. Describe the characteristic signs and symptoms.

iii. What are the pathological reasons for this condition?

iv. How is it treated?

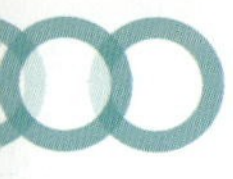

Answer 138

138i. Complex regional pain syndrome (CRPS) type II affecting the right hand (aka reflex sympathetic dystrophy or Sudek's atrophy).

ii. Blotchy discolouration, swelling, dystrophic nail and hair changes and disuse muscle atrophy. Severe incapacitating pain aggravated by cold (known as cold allodynia) results.

iii. Injury to a peripheral nerve is the cause. If the site of injury can be identified, the syndrome is known as CRPS I. Pathophysiological changes include expression of noradrenaline receptors on the injured nerve and/or growth of sympathetic fibres into the affected area, with increased sympathetic input into the dorsal horn of the spinal cord. Exaggerated sensitivity of vascular modulation results, leading to swelling, colour and temperature changes.

iv. Single agent pharmacological treatment is insufficient and multidisciplinary 'biopsychosocial' pain management is needed. Physiotherapy and occupational therapy treat CRPS (but it may be intolerably painful). A Bier's block, using guanethidine, blocks local sympathetic ganglia and outlasts the duration of the local anaesthetic, alleviating sympathetically-mediated pain and vascular symptoms, and may help physiotherapy to start. Quantifying the components of pain by the effect of IV drug challenges can be used. A high dose of a chosen medication is given IV to establish whether a therapeutic effect is possible using the same drug orally without intolerable side-effects. Specific receptors (or components of cellular function) are targeted using the medications listed:

- Noradrenaline receptors, (phentolamine).
- Sodium channels (lidocaine).
- μ receptors (fentanyl).
- NMDA glutamate receptors (ketamine).
- The calcium channel modulator gabapentin is not available as an IV dose, but has such a well-tolerated side-effect profile that an oral trial is easily conducted.
- Tricyclic antidepressants act on the descending inhibitory pathways of the spinal cord but have limited effect.

Psychosocial stress factors should be addressed with appropriate cognitive behavioural therapy.

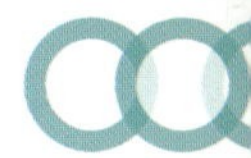

QUESTION 139

139i. What condition is this patient (**139a, b**) most likely to have?

ii. Describe the condition in detail.

iii. When anaesthetising a patient with this condition, what history and examination findings might be expected?

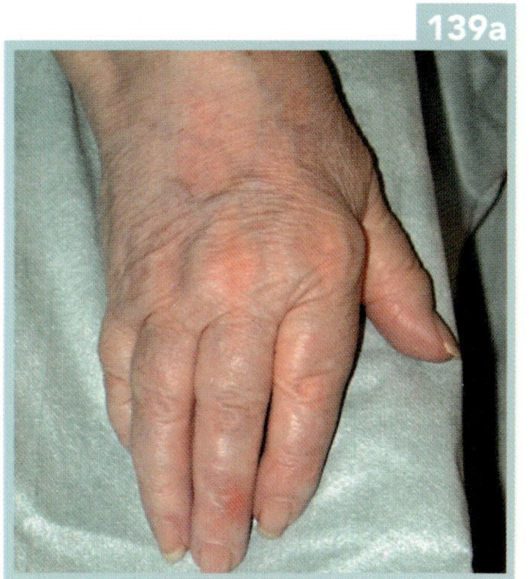
139a

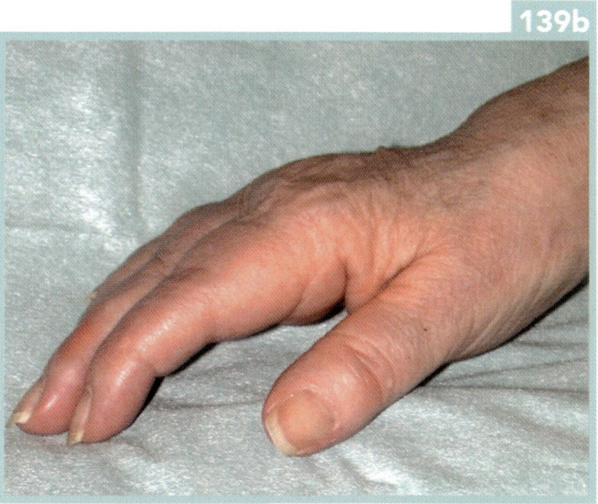
139b

QUESTION 140

140 A pressure time curve from a standard volume controlled ventilator breath is shown (**140**).

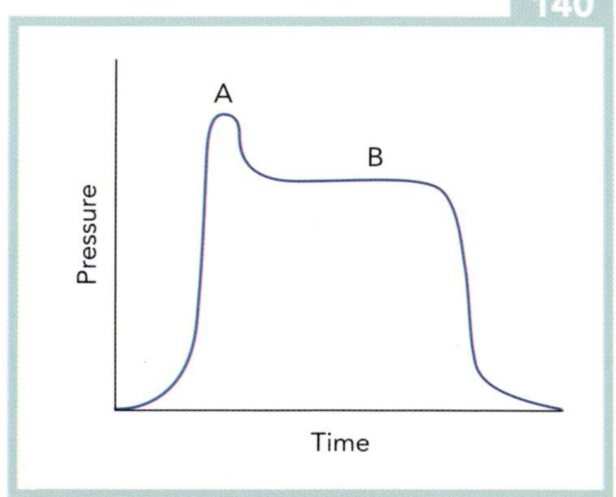

140

i. What pressures are represented by points A and B?

ii. What is the cause of pressure A.

iii. What is the cause of pressure B.

iv. Why does pressure decrease from point A to point B?

v. What is the clinical value to the clinician of knowing pressure A, pressure B, and their difference?

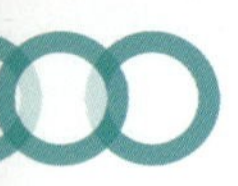

Answer 139

139i. Rheumatoid arthritis.

ii. This chronic inflammatory disease of unknown aetiology is characterised by remissions and exacerbations, most often starts between the ages of 25 and 55 and is three times commoner in females. Patients suffer from polyarthritides affecting one or more of the following: temporomandibular joint (TMJ), cricoarytenoid joint, costochondral junctions, cervical spine, shoulders, elbows, hips, knees, feet and hands. The disease can also involve heart, lungs, eyes, skin, blood vessels (vasculitis) and kidneys.

iii. Cardiorespiratory compromise is common. Exercise tolerance, sometimes difficult to assess because of inflamed joints, is important. If exercise is not possible, a 'dobutamine stress test' helps determine any cardiovascular limits. Side-effects from antirheumatic drugs should be sought. Aspirin, non-steroidals, corticosteroids, gold salts and penicillamine may cause anaemia, pancytopenia, platelet dysfunction and hepatic dysfunction. Chronic anaemia is common. Careful airway evaluation is important. Patients with throat fullness, tightness or foreign body sensations, hoarseness, stridor, dysphagia or pain radiating to the ears are likely to have TMJ and/or cricoarytenoid joint involvement. Neck range of movement is also important and symptoms or vertebrobasilar insufficiency or neurological deficits on neck flexion or extension influences head positioning. Preventing potential neurovascular or skeletal damage occurring because of faulty positioning under anaesthesia is essential.

Answer 140

140i. Point A is the peak inspiratory pressure; point B is the plateau pressure or inspiratory pause pressure.

ii. The peak inspiratory pressure gives a measure of two phenomena: airway resistance and the total lung compliance plus chest wall compliance ('recoil').

iii. The plateau pressure is a measure of only the total lung compliance.

iv. The pressure decreases from the peak inspiratory pressure to the plateau pressure because inspiratory flow has stopped at point A, and there is no further flow resistance generating pressure. Only the static lung compliance (static recoil) is creating the pressure.

v. The peak inspiratory pressure is an indication of two forces (airway resistance as well as compliance), while the plateau pressure is an indication of only the compliance (recoil). The difference between the peak and plateau pressures is an indication of airway resistance. All three values are therefore needed to obtain a 'pure' measure of airway resistance.

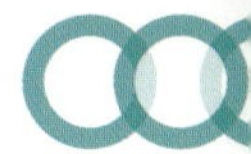

QUESTION 141

141i. What does this CT scan show (**141**)?

ii. What surgical intervention is needed?

iii. What goals should be aimed for, and how should they be achieved when anaesthetising the patient with this CT?

141

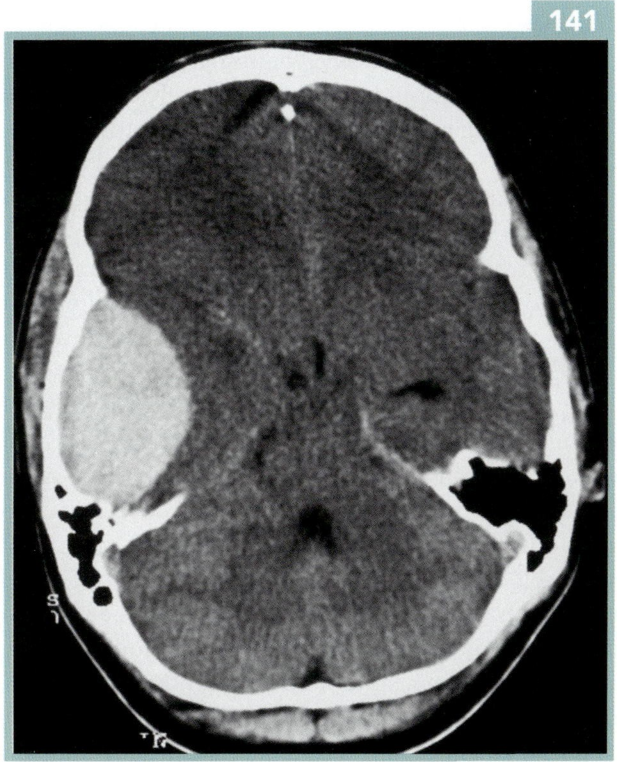

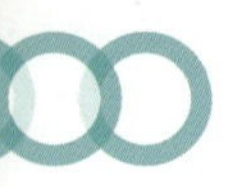

Answer 141

141i. Raised intracranial pressure (ICP) with midline shift as a result of an extradural haematoma (EDH).

ii. Immediate evacuation of this lesion with surgical control of middle meningeal artery bleed is required, particularly if signs of raised ICP are present (e.g. a unilateral fixed dilated pupil proceeding to bilateral pupillary dilation). The prognosis for EDH is excellent (>99% full recovery) if operated on within 1 hour.

iii.
- Maintain a safe airway, optimise oxygenation, maintain normocapnia. Anaesthesia with tracheal intubation should occur immediately if GCS is $\leq$8 or has deteriorated by more than 2 points from baseline. Monitoring should include ECG, SaO_2, FiO_2, $ETCO_2$, temperature and peripheral nerve stimulation. Non-invasive blood pressure should be performed at 2–3 minute intervals. Invasive arterial pressure monitoring is preferable, but setting it up must not delay surgery. Avoid dextrose IV solutions, which worsen brain swelling.
- Avoid hyper/hypotension as exacerbation of brain swelling or decreased cerebral perfusion occur, respectively. Remifentanil/alfentanil infusion or fentanyl boluses are used intraoperatively for analgesia. Remifentanil use requires additional analgesia to be given 15 minutes prior to termination of the infusion. Anaesthetic drugs that compromise cerebral perfusion pressure (CPP) should be avoided. Propofol can cause hypotension (reducing CPP) and should be carefully titrated. Adequate fluid loading is essential and vasopressors used if required.
- Avoid increasing ICP. Mild hyperventilation (to a PCO_2 of no greater than 4 kPa or 30 mmHg) will temporarily control intracranial hypertension as will an appropriate IV bolus of mannitol. Fifteen degrees head-up tilt ensures cerebral venous drainage without compromising cerebral blood flow. Flexion/rotation of the neck and tying the tracheal tube in too tightly may obstruct cerebral venous drainage and increase ICP.
- Use agents such as propofol and remifentanil infusions that allow a rapid postoperative recovery.

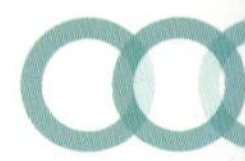

QUESTION 142

142 Describe a system for blood gas interpretation.

QUESTION 143

143 Two days previously this patient fell 10 metres (33 feet) onto concrete. The area behind her right ear is shown (**143**).

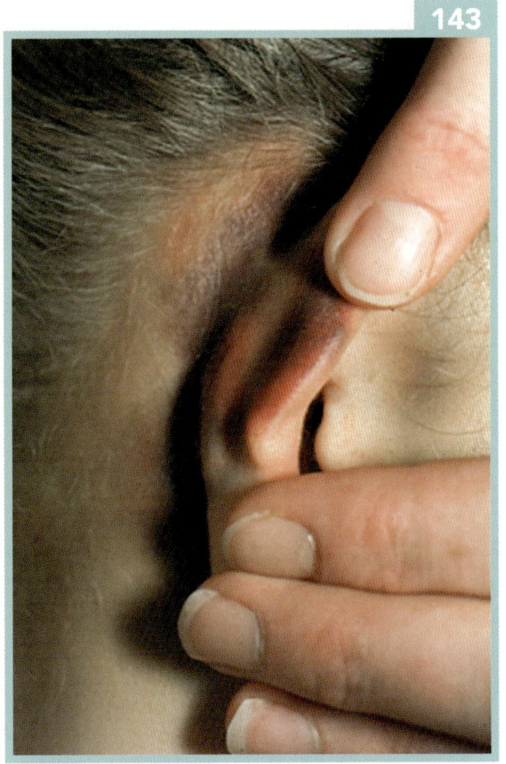
143

i. What is this sign called?

ii. What is its clinical significance?

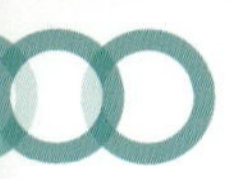

Answer 142

142 Blood gases should be read systematically, as suggested below, to be correctly interpreted and avoid omissions.

- Technical factors. FIO_2 and history from patient to allow interpretation.
- Hypoxia or not? Normal partial pressure of arterial oxygen (PaO_2) = 10–13 kPa (76–100 mmHg).
- Acidotic or alkalotic? Normal pH is 7.4 ± 0.05 (H^+ is 45–55 nmol/l).
- Respiratory or metabolic acidosis or alkalosis? Normal bicarbonate level (HCO_3^-) is 22–28 mmol/l (varies between laboratories), base excess 0 ± 5 mmol/l. Look first at the arterial partial pressure of carbon dioxide ($PaCO_2$) to determine the respiratory component to the acidosis/alkalosis. If CO_2 is above the normal range (4.6–6 kPa [35–45 mmHg]), the acidosis is due to CO_2 retention. If CO_2 low, there is respiratory alkalosis (or possible respiratory compensation for a metabolic acidosis). If the HCO_3^- is high, a metabolic alkalosis is present, also manifested by an excess of base or positive base balance. If HCO_3^- is low, a metabolic acidosis is likely. Either pathological blood acids (e.g. lactic acid) 'tie up' bicarbonate or, occasionally, HCO_3^- production is too low (having the same effect of producing acidosis). A low HCO_3^- to compensate for alkalosis is unusual unless acetazolamide has been used (e.g. for mountain sickness).
- Anion gap. Serum electrolytes allow calculation of the anion gap (A^-), which is the difference between the total concentration of measured cations (sodium and potassium) and that of measured anions (chloride and HCO_3^-). This is normally about 15–20 mmol/l.

$$[Na^+] + [K^+] = [HCO_3^-] + [C1^-] + [A^-]$$

- Where anion gap exceeds these levels, this can explain the cause of the acidosis. Possible causes are too little HCO_3^- (e.g. renal failure) or too much ketone or lactate in keto- and lactic acidosis, respectively. Ingestion of poisons such as methanol or ethylene glycol can also cause an abnormal anion gap.
- A summary and diagnosis completes the interpretation.

Answer 143

143i. 'Battle's sign'; mastoid bruising due to fracture of the skull base. This sign is concealed by the ear and/or long hair and must be specifically sought. It usually appears 1 or 2 days post trauma and cannot be expected to be seen immediately.

ii. Base of skull fractures can be difficult to diagnose, even with thin section CT, and Battle's sign may be the only indication of this injury. Passing nasogastric or nasotracheal tubes should be avoided in any cases of suspected base of skull fracture for fear of either tube entering the intracranial vault.

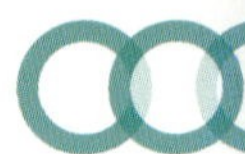

QUESTION 144

144 This patient (**144**) has severe recurrent trigeminal neuralgia.

i. What technique is being carried out?

ii. Why does it work?

iii. Describe the anatomy of where the needle tip needs to lie and how this is safely achieved.

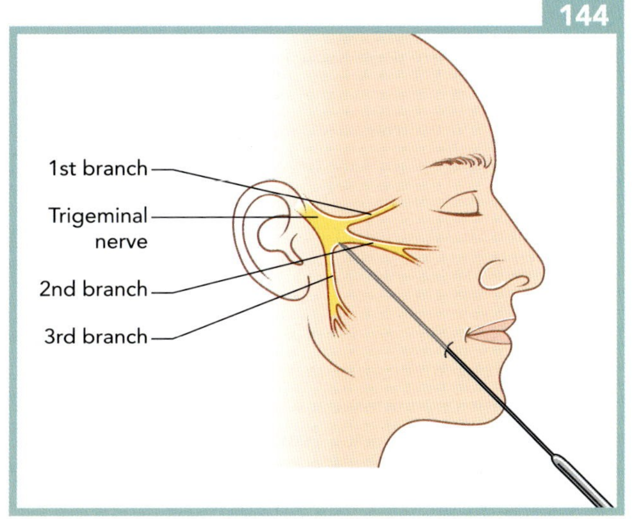

QUESTION 145

145i. What congenital abnormality is shown by this ECG (**145**) in a healthy 58-year-old patient?

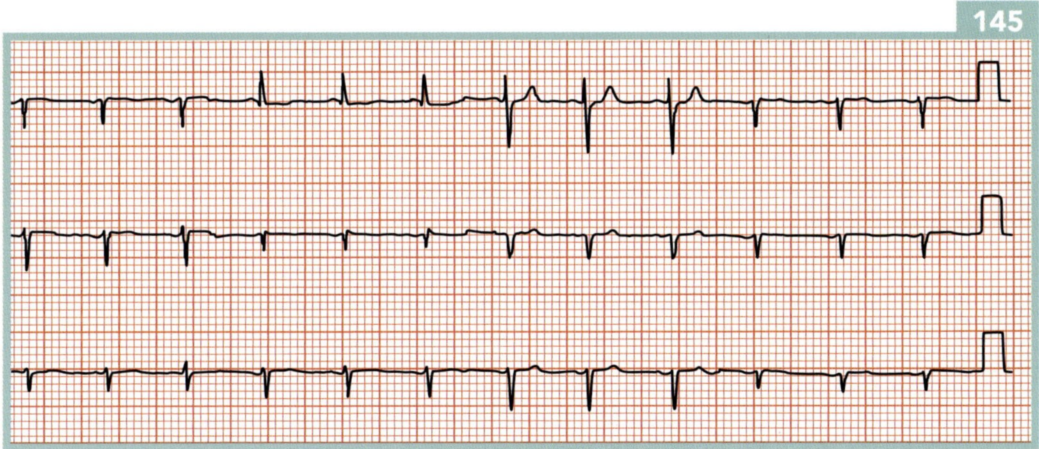

ii. Are the ECG leads correctly placed?

iii. What ECG features are typical of this condition?

iv. How can one tell that this has not come about by erroneous placement of the leads?

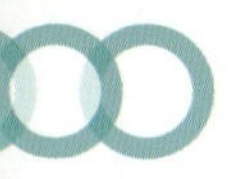

Answer 144

144i. The trigeminal nerve is being blocked, also known as blocking the Gasserian ganglion.

ii. It effectively anaesthetises the whole of the trigeminal nerve and all its roots. This is a treatment of last resort for severe trigeminal neuralgia. The technique can be carried out with a local anaesthetic to evaluate its effectiveness and this can be sufficient to ameliorate the neuralgia. If the block is successful, a permanent block with phenol can be performed, but this is irreversible.

iii. The Gasserian gangloin is formed from two roots starting along the ventral surface of the brainstem at the mid-pontine level. The roots pass forward and laterally within the posterior cranial fossa across the superior border of the petrous temporal bone. They enter a recess called Meckel's cave, which is formed by an invagination of the dura mater of the posterior cranial fossa. In this recess lies the ganglion of the trigeminal nerve and from its anterior border the three divisions of the nerve (ophthalmic, maxillary, mandibular) arise.

The block must be carried out utilising X-ray control and with the head slightly extended. The midpoint zygomatic arch is marked. Approximately 1 inch (2.5 cm) lateral to and slightly above the corner of the mouth on the involved side, a wheal of local anaesthetic is raised. A 4 inch (10 cm) 22 gauge needle with stylet in place is inserted so that it will pass through the substance of the cheek, travelling just medial to the ramus of the mandible in a cephalad and medial direction towards the pupil of the eye. The needle tip should then encounter the base of the skull at a point somewhat anterior to the foramen ovale; radiological verification is necessary. The needle is then redirected posteriorly until the foramen is entered. If the patient experiences paraesthesia of the mandibular nerve, the needle should be reinserted without paraesthesia. One to 3 ml of local anaesthetic is injected slowly until the desired clinical effect is reached.

Answer 145

145i. The ECG is indicative of situs inversus – the patient has dextrocardia.

ii. Yes, the leads are correctly placed.

iii. The typical features of dextrocardia are: right axis deviation; positive QRS complexes (with upright P and T waves) in aVR; lead I: inversion of all complexes (this can be known as 'global negativity' [i.e. inverted P wave with a negative QRS and an inverted T wave]); R-wave progression is not seen in any chest leads and there are dominant S waves throughout.

iv. Reversal of the left and right arm electrodes produces a similar picture in the limb leads, but the precordial leads will have a normal appearance.

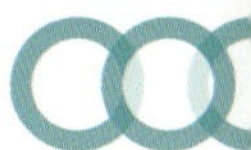

QUESTION 146

146 A TOE image is shown (**146**).

i. What is this view called?

ii. Which chamber is indicated by A?

iii. What structure is indicated by B?

iv. What structure is indicated by C?

v. What structures are indicated by D, E and F?

vi. What structure is indicated by G?

vii. What structure is indicated by H?

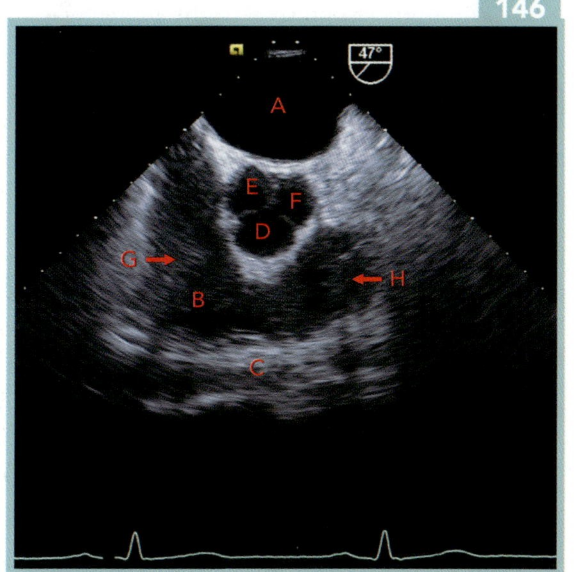

QUESTION 147

147 This is a graphic representation of the alveolar gas equation showing alveolar minute ventilation on the x-axis and PO_2 on the y-axis (**147**). The effects of increasing the alveolar minute ventilation on the PO_2 are also demonstrated. A convenient way to interpret the graphic is to identify the normal FIO_2 line (21%) where it crosses the normal minute ventilation, and then move along the x-axis (on this line), increasing and decreasing the minute ventilation.

i. Using the graphic, explain why hypoventilation on room air causes hypoxia.

ii. Explain why hypoventilation on an increased FIO_2 does not lead to hypoxia (until the hypoventilation is quite marked).

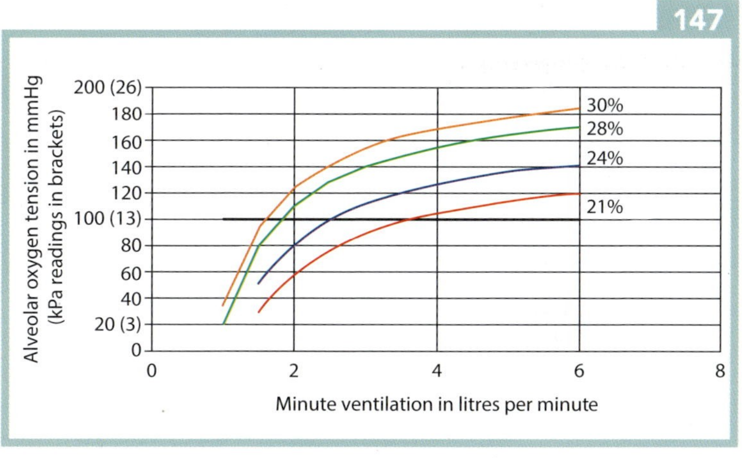

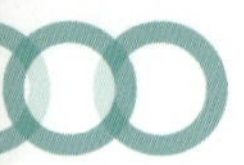

Answer 146

146i. The mid-oesophageal, right ventricular, inflow-outflow view.

ii. A is the left atrium.

iii. B indicates the right ventricle.

iv. C indicates the free wall of the right ventricle.

v. D, E and F are the cusps of the aortic valve: D is the right coronary cusp, E is the non-coronary cusp and F is the left coronary cusp.

vi. G indicates the position (shadow) of the tricuspid valve.

vii. H indicates the position of the pulmonary valve.

Answer 147

147i. When breathing room air (PO_2 = 21.2 kPa/159 mmHg), three factors decrease the alveolar partial pressure of oxygen while the minute ventilation replenishes oxygen in the functional residual capacity: (1) the water vapour dilutes the oxygen; (2) the CO_2 also dilutes the oxygen; (3) the blood removes oxygen from the inspired gas. The result is an oxygen partial pressure of 105 mmHg in the alveoli while breathing room air. With hypoventilation on room air, replenishment of alveolar oxygen is not sufficient to replace removal of oxygen from the alveolar space by uptake into the circulation, and the PO_2 decreases, leading to hypoxia.

ii. When breathing an increased FIO_2, even after removal of oxygen from the alveolar space, there is sufficient oxygen remaining to maintain normoxia.

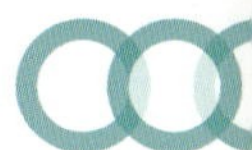

QUESTION 148

148 Three tracings of relevance are shown (**148**): impedance pneumogram ('impedance') signal indicating chest movement; pneumotachogram ('airflow') indicating flow through the nose and/or mouth; and saturation (SpO_2).

i. What type of apnoea is indicated by this tracing (i.e. does this patient show central or obstructive apnea)? Explain your answer.

ii. How can these principles be applied to clinical practice such as 'conscious sedation' and/or 'monitored anaesthesia care'?

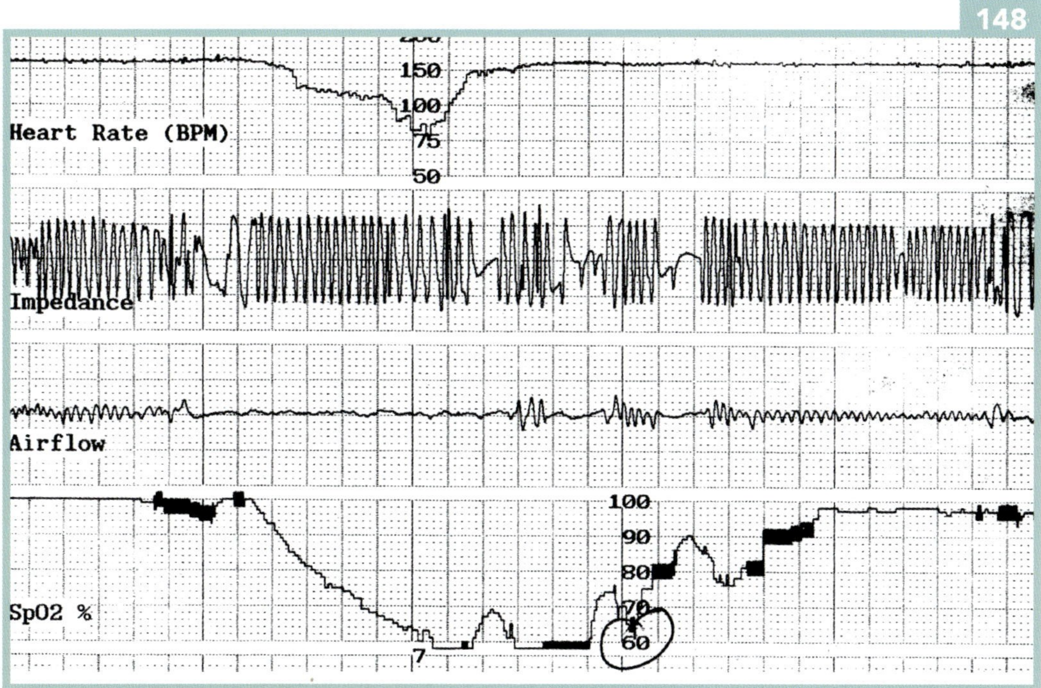

QUESTION 149

149 Describe the key ways in which the fetal circulation differs from the adult circulation.

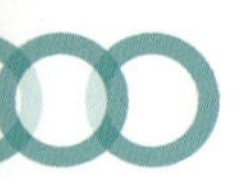

Answer 148

148i. The existence of chest movement (evidenced by the excursions of the signal of the 'impedance pneumogram') in the tracing indicates that the apnoea is obstructive (lack of excursions in the 'airflow' signal) and therefore probably not of central origin.

ii. By monitoring the 'impedance pneumogram' (chest movement) plus the nasal CO_2, it is possible to determine: (a) obstructive apnoea (loss of CO_2 signal, with continued chest movement), in which case the airway must be opened; in contrast to (b) central apnoea (loss of both the CO_2 signal as well as loss of the chest movement signal ('impedance pneumogram' becoming 'flat'). In this case ventilation should be temporarily supported and anaesthetic depth and/or narcotic concentration decreased.

Answer 149

149i. The placenta, the site of fetal gas exchange, receives deoxygenated blood via the umbilical arteries and returns oxygen-rich (saturations 80–90%) blood to the fetal systemic arterial circulation via the umbilical vein. Fifty to 60% of oxygenated placental blood flows through the ductus venosus, bypassing the hepatic circulation to enter the inferior vena cava (IVC). At the junction of the IVC and the right atrium is the Eustachian valve, which directs this blood across the foramen ovale into the left atrium, left ventricle and ascending aorta. The myocardium and brain therefore receive the most highly oxygenated blood. Desaturated blood (saturations 25–40%) returning from the superior vena cava and coronary sinus is directed across the tricuspid valve and into the pulmonary artery, which has a very high resistance. This high resistance means that only about 12% of the desaturated blood goes to the lung and 88% crosses the ductus arteriosus to the descending aorta and the lower extremities. These circulatory adaptations are known as intracardiac and extracardiac shunts and fetal circulation is referred to as 'shunt-dependent'. These shunts mean that the stroke volume of each ventricle differs, with 65% of venous return entering the right ventricle. Fetal cardiac output is a combined ventricular output (CVO) and 45% goes to the placenta. CVO is high in order to maintain tissue oxygen delivery despite low oxygen partial pressures.

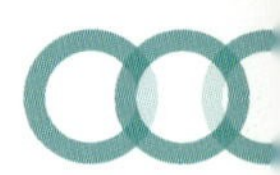

QUESTION 150

150i. Draw an illustration of fetal circulation to illustrate the points described in case **149**.

ii. How does this change at birth?

QUESTION 151

151 This flow–volume loop (**151**) is from a 40-year-old female presenting with dyspnoea with even mild exercise.

i. What is the normal range for the peak expiratory flow rate (PEFR)?

ii. What is the PEFR in this figure?

iii. What is the peak inspiratory flow rate (PIFR) in this figure?

iv. What type of pathology causes both the expiratory and the inspiratory flow rates to be greatly decreased?

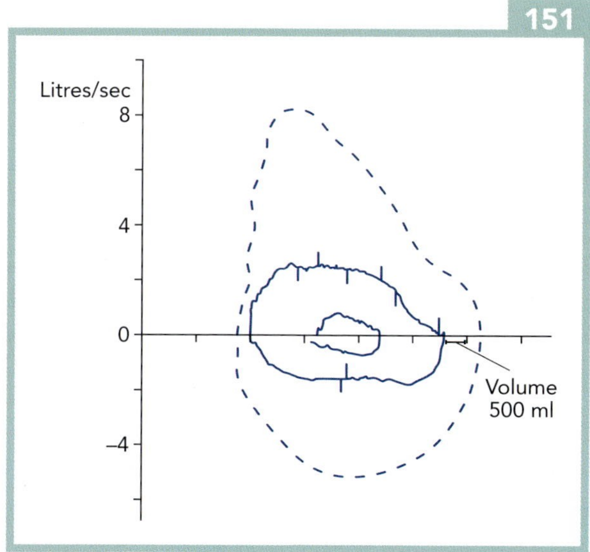

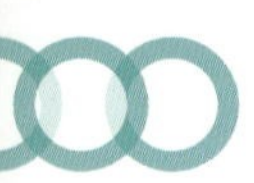

Answer 150

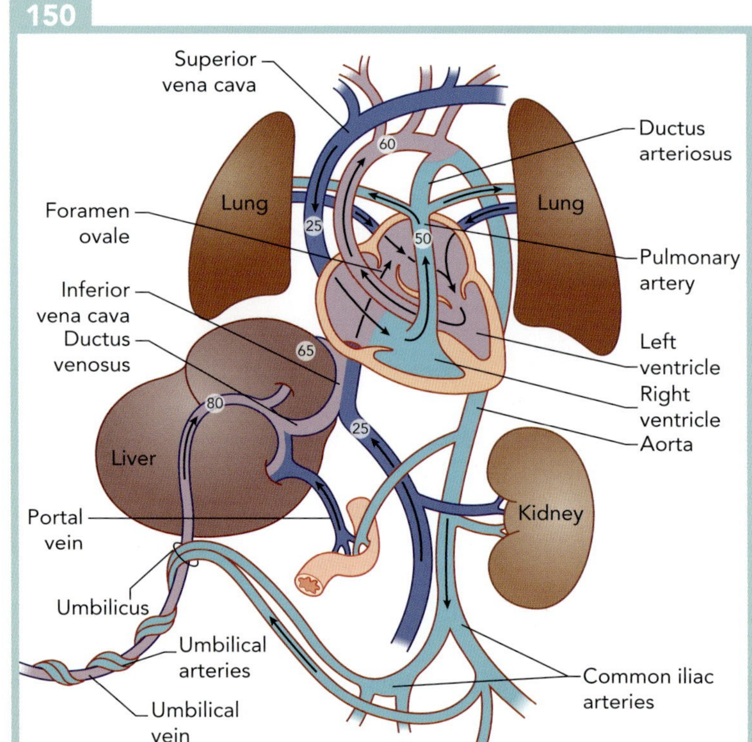

150i. See **150**.

ii. Catecholamines, hormones and locally released vasoactive substances influence the fetal circulation at differing gestational ages. Fetal to neonatal transition involves acute changes in pulmonary and systemic vascular resistance. Fetal lungs are collapsed and the ductus arteriosis (DA) remains open until, at birth, higher blood oxygen and sudden reduction of prostaglandins promote closure. After DA closure, pulmonary circulatory resistance falls, the left and right ventricles receive equal venous return and the adult circulatory anatomy prevails.

Answer 151

151i. The normal range for PEFR is around 200–300 litres per minute.

ii. The y-axis is marked in litres per second. The PEFR in this case is less than 2 litres per second or less than 120 litres per minute. The x-axis is marked in litres – the hash marks are at 1 litre intervals.

iii. The PIFR for this patient is also markedly decreased at less than 2 liters per second or 120 litres per minute.

iv. Simultaneously decreased PEFR and PIFR are typically caused by a 'fixed airway obstruction' such as a large thyroid or tracheal stenosis.

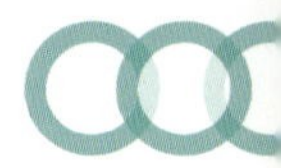

QUESTION 152

152 This Table represents the solubilities of the commonly used inhalational anaesthetic agents.

Agent	Blood:gas	Brain:blood	Fat:blood
N_2O	0.47	1.1	2.3
Desflurane	0.45	1.3	27
Sevoflurane	0.65	1.7	47
Isoflurane	1.4	1.6	45
Halothane	2.5	1.9	51

i. How does this information help predict the onset and recovery time of these agents? What would you expect the speed of onset and recovery of these agents to be?

ii. Does the duration of the anaesthetic exposure affect the relative speed of recovery?

iii. How does the solubility of an agent affect its titratability at low fresh gas flow rates?

QUESTION 153

153 A TOE image is shown (**153**).

i. What is this view called?

ii. Which chambers are indicated by A and B?

iii. What structure is indicated by C?

iv. What structure is indicated by D?

v. What structure is indicated by E?

vi. What structure is indicated by F?

vii. What structure is indicated by G?

viii. What structure is indicated by H?

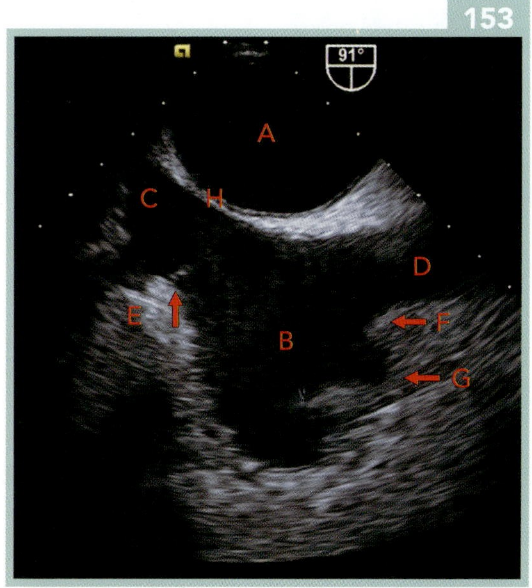

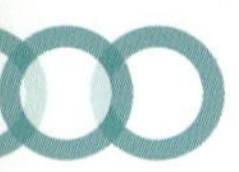

Answer 152

152i. Agents that are less blood:gas soluble quickly create a therapeutic partial pressure in the alveolus, blood and brain because they do not dissolve well. Lung/brain equilibration is therefore faster than with more soluble agents. Therefore, N_2O, desflurane and sevoflurane reach therapeutic levels at the effect site sooner than isoflurane. Although isoflurane has a slightly lower brain:blood solubility than sevoflurane, it reaches brain therapeutic levels more slowly. Its higher blood:gas solubility delays the rise in blood partial pressure, slowing onset. N_2O has the fastest onset time because of its very low solubility in both blood and brain.

ii. Despite a similar onset time to desflurane, sevoflurane has a fat:blood solubility similar to isoflurane. Over time, sevoflurane is stored in body fat, which serves as a reservoir to release the drug as anaesthesia is discontinued, thus prolonging awakening time. This is directly related to the duration and dose of anaesthetic and sevoflurane recovery is noticeably slower after 2 MAC-hours. All potent soluble inhalational agents have longer recovery times than N_2O at all time points.

iii. Lower solubility provides a faster equilibration between the concentration set on the vaporiser and the alveolar concentration at all flow rates. Relatively insoluble agents show a therapeutic effect sooner at low flow rates than more soluble agents. Therefore, N_2O, desflurane and sevoflurane respond to changes in stimulus faster at low flow rates that conserve heat, humidity and drugs. At flow rates of 2 l/min or less, isoflurane and halothane vaporisers must be set to 2–3 times the MAC value ('overpressure'), otherwise equilibration might be too slow to cope with a required change in anaesthetic depth.

Answer 153

153i. The mid-oesophageal, bicaval view.

ii. A is the left atrium, B is the right atrium.

iii. C indicates the inferior vena cava.

iv. D indicates the superior vena cava.

v. E indicates the Eustachian valve, which is of pre-natal importance.

vi. F indicates the crista terminalis of the right atrium.

vii. G indicates the position of the right atrial appendage.

viii. H indicates the atrial septum.

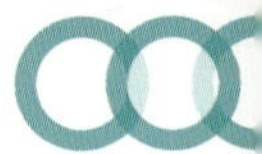

QUESTION 154

154 A patient presents for intracranial (posterior fossa) surgery in the sitting position. A decision is made to place a central venous catheter in the middle of the right atrium to enable removal (suctioning) of any entrained air. Two sequential ECG strips are shown (**154a, b**), recorded during positioning of the central line using a 'long-arm CVP' catheter from the ante-cubital fossa in the arm. **154a** shows the ECG with the tip of the catheter at the level of the clavicle. **154b** was recorded with the tip of the catheter presumed to be in the right atrium, (with large, biphasic P waves the same size as the QRS complex), and then being withdrawn to confirm the correct positioning by analysing the changes in the ECG pattern. A wire inside the CVP catheter is connected to ECG lead II.

i. Where (which part of the right atrium) is the tip of the CVP catheter at the start of ECG strip **154b**?

ii. Give an explanation for the size of the p-wave decreasing, and the shape changing, as indicated in ECG strip **154b**.

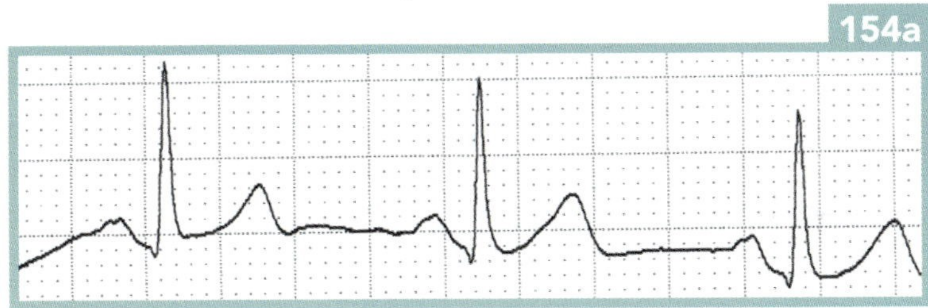

154a

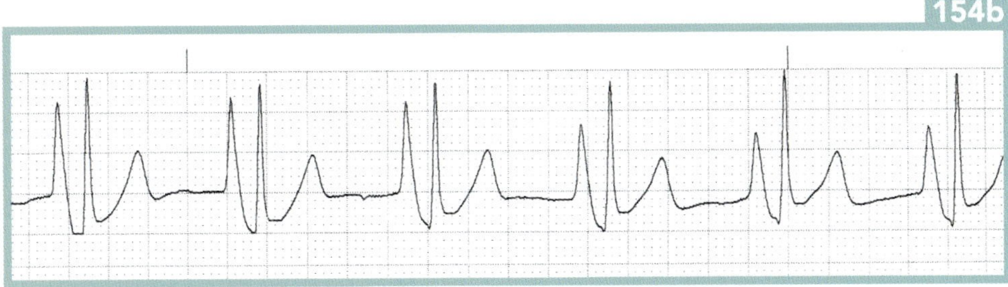

154b

QUESTION 155

155i. Draw the Mapleson classification of anaesthetic flow systems.

ii. List the common names used for these systems and any major limitations they may have.

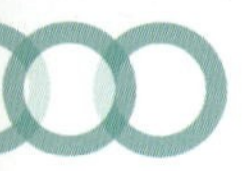

Answer 154

154i. At the start of **154b**, the catheter tip is presumed to be in the middle of the right atrium. The very large, biphasic, sometimes M-shaped P wave indicates that the tip of the CVP catheter is approximately in the middle of the right atrium. (The negative part of the p-wave is seen to be 'cut off' at the bottom of the tracing).

ii. The tracing shows (from beginning to end) a decreasing size of the biphasic p-wave, indicating that the tip of the catheter is moving away from the centre of the right atrium. It has to be advanced to obtain the large biphasic pattern again, which would be correctly placed in the middle of the right atrium to allow attempts to suck out any air, should an air embolism occur.

Answer 155

155i. See **155**.

ii. Mapleson A is the Magill and Lack circuit. Mapleson B and C are often used as portable short-term devices for hand ventilation (e.g. in recovery room/at cardiac arrest). These systems have significant rebreathing of exhaled gases even with very high fresh gas flows. Inspiration is supplied from the same space into which the previous breath was expired. Mapleson D is the modified Bain circuit. Mapleson E is Ayre's T piece and the Bain circuit. 'Mapleson F' was not originally classified by Mapleson but is the Jackson-Rees modification of Ayre's T-piece.

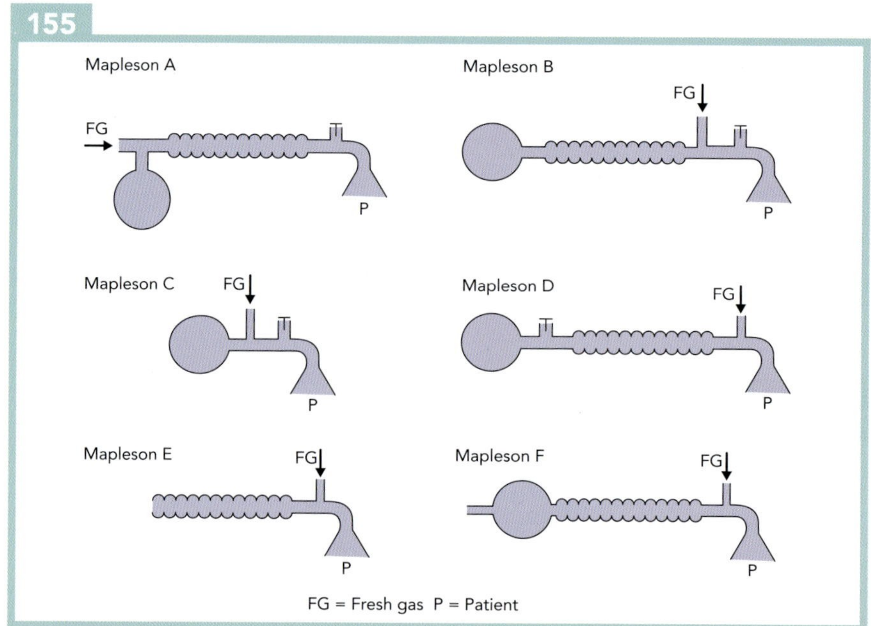

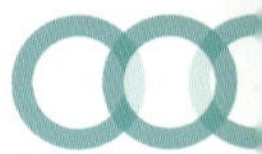

QUESTION 156

156 The postoperative CXR of a female patient who has had a prolonged procedure under GA is shown (**156**). Following the procedure she is unable to move her legs. She has no light touch or pin prick sensation but vibration sense and proprioception are intact.

i. What procedure was performed?

ii. Explain this patient's neurological deficit. Why should the anaesthesiologist be aware of this postoperative complication?

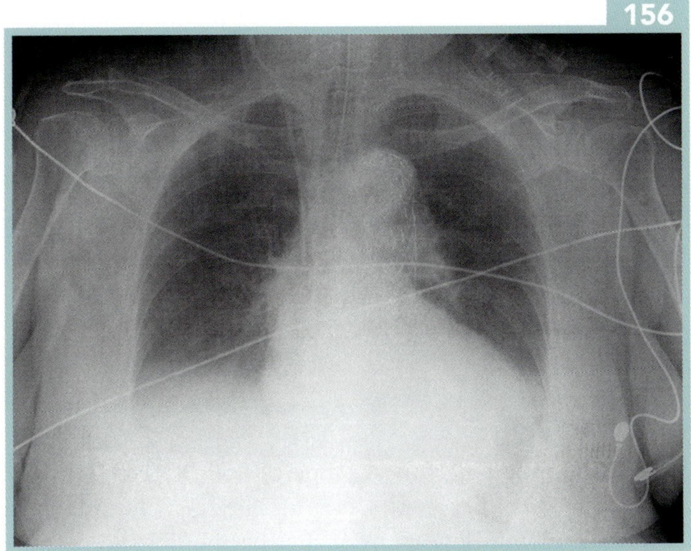

156

QUESTION 157

157i. Arterial waveforms are regularly viewed by anaesthesiologists. Why do they need to understand fast Fourier transform (FFT) and analysis (see also case **229**)?

ii. What is damping, and why does it happen?

iii. What is critical damping?

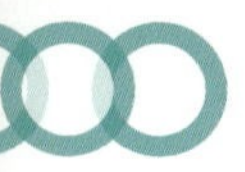

Answer 156

156i. This woman had a dissecting aortic aneurysm and has had an endovascular stent placed in the aorta to repair the lesion. The aortic stent is visible at the start of the descending aorta.

ii. This type of paraplegia, with sparing of the posterior sensory columns, is known as anterior cord syndrome and is due to inadequate anterior spinal artery perfusion. This is supplied rostrally from the vertebral arteries but also has feeder branches from the aorta distally. Patients undergoing prolonged aortic procedures, cardiac surgery or major abdominal surgery are vulnerable to this complication, which is detected postoperatively. Prolonged hypotension may be a contributing factor in some patients. The anaesthesiologist must investigate all complaints of postoperative leg weakness after major surgery or hypotensive episodes.

Answer 157

157a

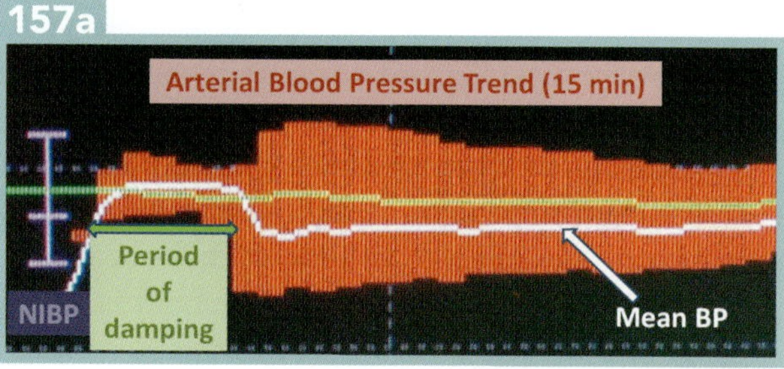

157i. Because their construction (i.e. by Fourier analysis, see case **229**) can be misleading if they become damped (**157a**) or resonate.

ii. Damping occurs when the mechanical properties of the arterial line 'absorb' too many higher waveform harmonics. (**157a**). The trace then shows mainly the fundamental waveform, with few, if any, higher harmonics and minimal oscillation. This 'damped trace' underreads systolic BP and can overread (falsely high) diastolic BP. This can happen if a blood clot, kink or air bubble is introduced accidentally or the 'stiffness' of the line is insufficient. Arterial lines are therefore stiff and inflexible with a relatively narrow bore. It is essential to differentiate this cause of systolic BP hypotension from true hypotension when both systolic and diastolic BP decrease (**157b**).

157b

Arterial Blood Pressure Trend (30 min)

Mean BP

iii. The damping in a system that causes the waveform to return to zero as quickly as possible after the stimulus is finished, without overshooting. The waveform is therefore correctly displayed. This situation exists when the fundamental harmonic is complemented with the optimum number of harmonics and neither overdamping nor hyperresonance occurs.

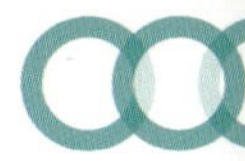

QUESTION 158

158 What is underdamping (see also case **157**)?

QUESTION 159

159 A haemoglobin–oxygen (Hb–O_2) dissociation curve is shown (**159**).

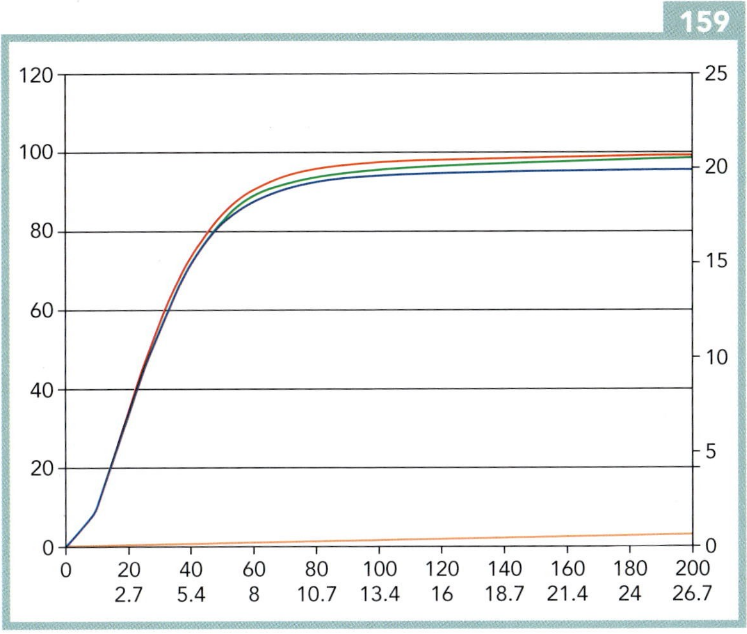

i. What parameter is represented on the x-axis (abscissa)? What are the units and what are the maximum values at sea level?

ii. Name two parameters that can be represented on the y-axis (ordinate) and their units. What are the maximum values at sea level (for a normal Hb concentration)?

iii. A healthy person breathes 100% O_2 and has arterial blood gases measured. Will the value on the x-axis increase? If yes, to what value? If not, explain why not. Will the value on the y-axis increase? If yes, to what value? If not, explain why not.

iv. What is represented by the lower, orange, straight line on the graph?

v. What are the two components of blood O_2 content (i.e. how is O_2 carried in blood)? What are the relative amounts of each of these components? Are both components important under normal conditions?

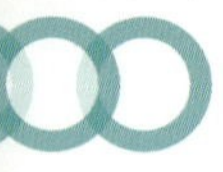

Answer 158

158 Underdamping occurs in an arterial line that is too stiff, too short or has too narrow a gauge. The fluid oscillates and the line overreads the systolic BP because of an exaggerated waveform. Exaggerated underdamping with excessive 'oscillation' makes the BP waveform difficult or impossible to determine accurately.

Answer 159

159i. The parameter represented on the x-axis is the PO_2 of blood. The units are kPa (0–26.7) or mmHg (0–200).

ii. Parameters that could be represented on the y-axis are: (1) saturation (the units are percentage saturation [max. 100% saturated]; (2) oxygen content (the units are ml O_2 per 100 ml blood [max. O_2 content in blood is ± 20 ml O_2 per 100 ml blood]).

iii. The value on the x-axis will increase to a theoretical maximum of 100 kPa (760 mmHg) (actually determined by the alveolar gas equation, which is approximately equal to 100 kPa [760 mmHg] minus the water vapour pressure (6.3 kPa) [47 mmHg] minus the PCO_2 (5.3 kPa) [40 mmHg], so measured oxygen level can never exceed 90 kPa (670 mmHg).

The value on the y-axis will not increase significantly, as Hb cannot take up any more O_2 once it is fully saturated at 100% (i.e. if Hb is fully loaded [20 ml O_2 per 100 ml blood], it cannot take up any more oxygen).

A higher FIO_2 will slightly increase the O_2 content dissolved in the plasma (i.e. from 0.3 ml O_2 per 100 ml blood to a theoretical maximum of 2.1 ml O_2 per 100 ml blood [at 100 kPa (760 mmHg) PO_2]).

iv. It represents O_2 dissolved in the plasma.

v. They are Hb–O_2 (19.7 ml O_2 per 100 ml blood) and O_2 dissolved in plasma (0.3 ml O_2 per 100 ml blood). Dissolved O_2 is not important under normal conditions but becomes relevant when Hb is very low (and the Hb–O_2 content is quite low).

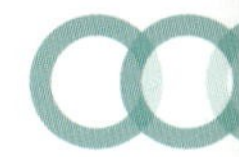

QUESTION 160

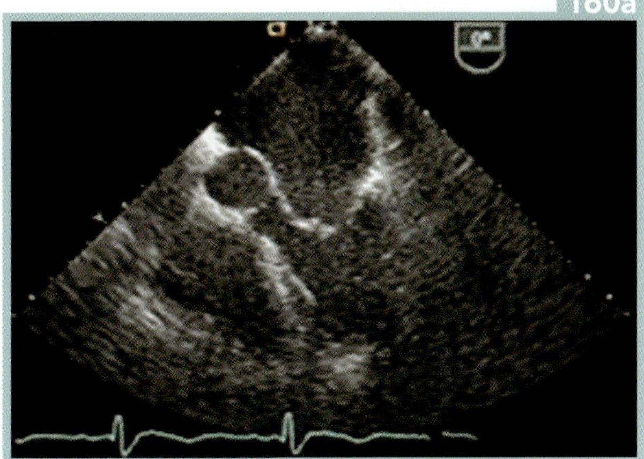
160a

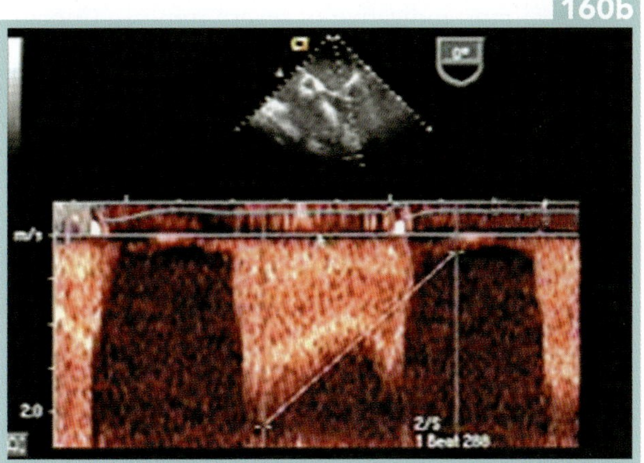

160b

160 A 58-year-old female complains of worsening shortness of breath with exertion but is scheduled for a surgical procedure. Preoperative TOE is performed (**160a, b**).

i. What is the diagnosis?

ii. What can be said about the severity of the problem as shown in **160b**.

QUESTION 161

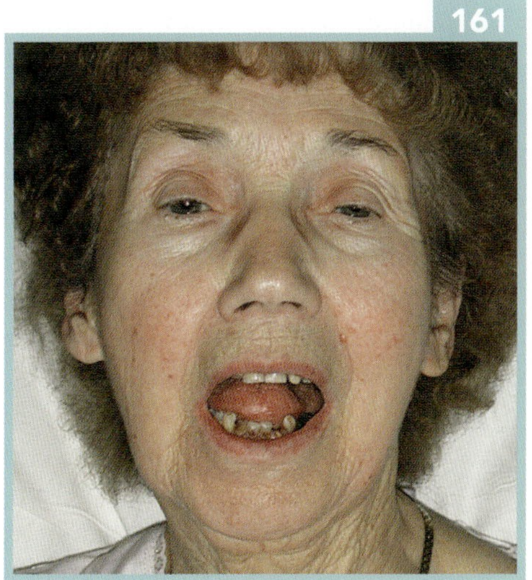
161

161 This patient (**161**) has dry eyes and a dry mouth and has notable dental caries. She presented with rest pain in her left leg due to peripheral vascular disease. The circulation to her fingers is poor and she often gets cold fingers that can be tingly and numb.

i. What is the likely diagnosis that may explain her dry eyes and dry mouth?

ii. What other pathologies may occur associated with this condition?

iii. Why is this a potential problem for the anaesthesiologist?

Answer 160

160i. This four-chamber view shows a stenosed mitral valve (MV) in diastole. The MV leaflets are abnormal; they do not open fully in diastole and exhibit the characteristic 'doming' of stenosis. A continuous wave Doppler from just below the MV in the left ventricle is shown (**160b**). The time for flow across the MV is prolonged.

ii. The area of the MV can be estimated from measurement of the pressure half-time (P1/2 time) using the equation:

$$\text{Valve area (cm}^2\text{)} = 220/\text{P1/2 time (msec)}$$

The slope of the continuous wave Doppler velocity profile is used to determine the P1/2 time. For this patient the P1/2 time is 236 msec, so the MV area is 0.93 cm^2, indicative of severe stenosis. (Normal MV area should be 4–6 cm^2. Below 2 cm^2 is usually symptomatic.)

Answer 161

161i. Sjögren's syndrome (dry eye syndrome or keratoconjunctivitis sicca). Occurring in isolation, this is primary Sjögrens or sicca syndrome, which tends to be severe, including salivary or parotid gland enlargement, dysphagia, dyspareunia and severe dental caries.

ii. Rheumatoid arthritis with dry eyes, mouth, vagina and skin is named secondary Sjögren's. Other connective tissue diseases (e.g. SLE, mixed connective tissue disease, polymyositis, myasthenia gravis, progressive scleroderma, autoimmune liver disease, thyroiditis) can cause secondary Sjögren's. Raynaud's syndrome or vasculitis, lymphadenopathy, leucopenia and hepatosplenomegaly, hyperglobulinaemic purpura, macroglobulinaemia, renal tubular acidosis or glomerulonephritis, pneumonia and diffuse interstitial fibrosis and intrasalivary or lymphomatous malignancies are associated with Sjögren's.

iii. Anaesthetic problems include potential for dental damage, myasthenia, thyroid disease, vasculitis affecting the renal artery, pulmonary complications and difficult intubation owing to thick perioesophageal/oropharyngeal tissues. This patient had a right femoral embolectomy to clear atheromatous plaque. Intubation was difficult because of the dental caries and brittle teeth. Oesophageal and oropharyngeal sclerosis made visualisation of the vocal cords impossible. Intubation was achieved by use of a gum elastic bougie.

Raised immunoglobulin levels, anti-Ro antibodies (present in 70% of cases) and macroglobulinaemia worsened this patient's ischaemic symptoms by increasing blood viscosity. Her cold hands were attributed to Raynaud's phenomenon. After full investigation by rheumatologists, nifedipine was commenced as a vasodilator and her renal function frequently reviewed.

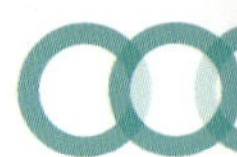

QUESTION 162

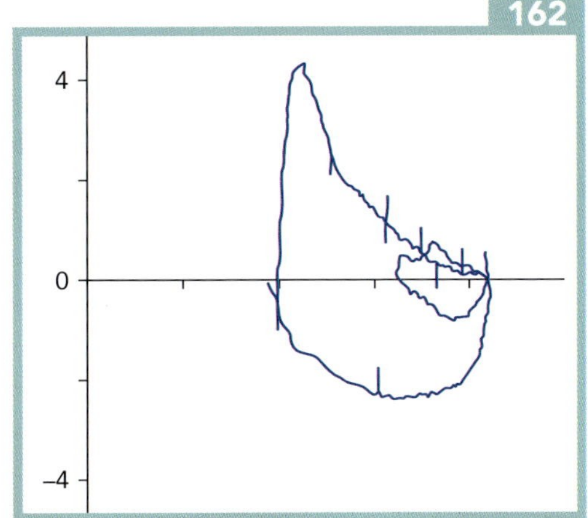

162i. What test is represented by this graphic (**162**)? What do the larger and smaller 'circles' represent?

ii. What parameter (measurement) is depicted on the x-axis (abscissa)? What are the units of the parameter?

iii. What parameter (measurement) is depicted on the y-axis (ordinate)? What are the units of this parameter?

iv. How is FEV_1 (forced expiratory volume in 1 second) determined?

QUESTION 163

163 This ECG tracing (**163**) was recorded during a colonoscopy in a fit, healthy 37-year-old female.

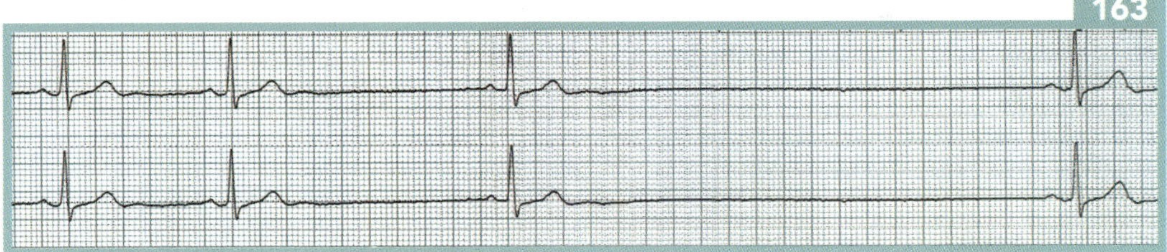

i. What is the starting heart rate?

ii. What is the slowest heart rate demonstrated on this strip?

iii. How can the heart rate be quickly calculated on an ECG strip like this?

iv. Is there a p-wave associated with every QRS complex?

v. What is the diagnosis?

vi. What is the treatment?

vii. List eight other sites where pressure or traction could have similar effects.

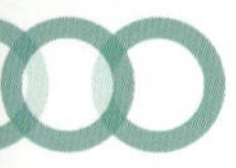

Answer 162

162i. A spirometry trace. The flow–volume loop is depicted, with the larger (outer) circle representing the maximal effort (vital capacity effort) and the smaller (inner) circle representing a tidal volume effort.

ii. Volume. The units are volume units (i.e. litres).

iii. Flow. The units are flow units (i.e. litres per second or litres per minute).

iv. There is no 'time' on either axis (only volume and flow). The measuring instrument indicates upright marks at various time points, one of which indicates when, on the flow signal, 1 second has elapsed.

Answer 163

163i. Approximately 50 bpm.

ii. Approximately 15 bpm.

iii. Count the number of large blocks between two QRS complexes. Divide 300 by the number of large blocks (e.g. for the starting heart rate there are 6 large blocks between the complexes). 300 divided by 6 equals 50. (This works because there are 300 large blocks in a minute at the standard paper speed of 25 mm per second.)

iv. Yes, indicating a sinus rhythm.

v. Bradycardia.

vi. The immediate treatment is to ask the surgeon (proceduralist) to immediately desist with pressure, traction and/or inflation of the bowel or the patient may slow to asystole. Atropine may be required (0.6–1.2 mg IV).

vii. Include: eyes (pressure or traction on eye muscles); traction of intracranial structures; laryngoscopy and intubation; traction on neck structures; traction on intrathoracic structures (e.g. mediastinum); traction on intra-abdominal structures; dilatation of the cervix (e.g. D&C or D&E); stretching of the rectum.

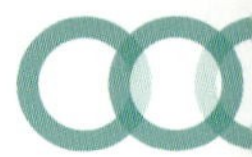

QUESTION 164

164 With regard to this ECG (**164**):

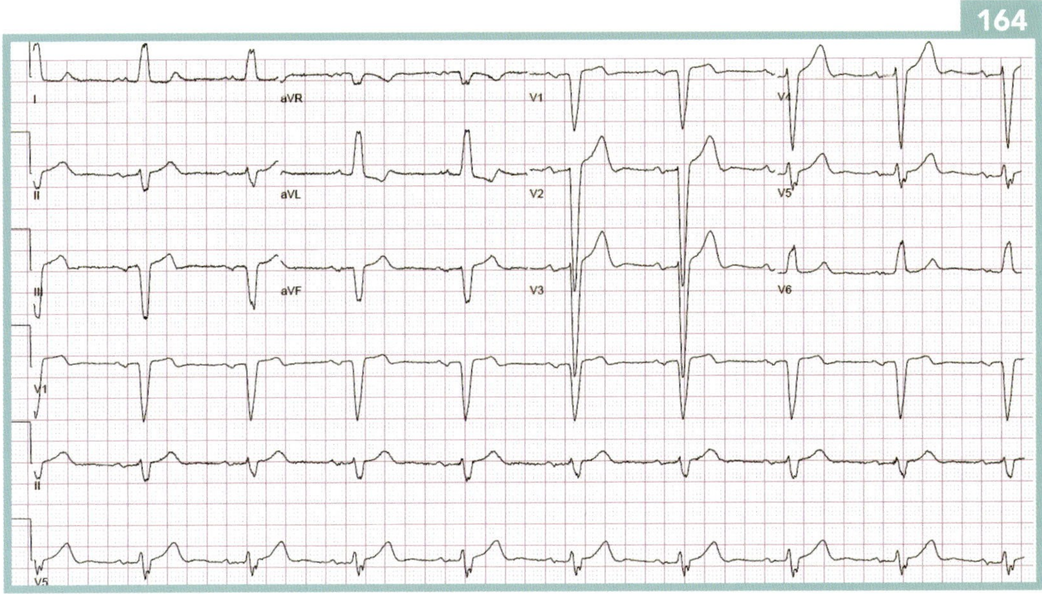

i. What is the rate?

ii. What is the PR interval?

iii. What is the duration of the QRS complex?

iv. Consider lead V6: what is the direction of the terminal voltage of the QRS complex?

v. What is the axis in the peripheral leads?

vi. What are the abnormalities in this ECG?

vii. Is it a trifascicular block?

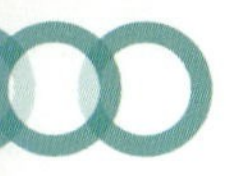

Answer 164

164i. 55 bpm (just over 5 large blocks; 300 divided by the number of large blocks gives the rate).

ii. Approximately 6 mm (6 little blocks, each being 40 msec), with the formal measurement being 228 msec, indicating a first-degree heart block.

iii. Almost 4 mm (the formal measurement being 150 msec), indicating a bundle branch block.

iv. The terminal voltage in V6 is positive, indicating that the slow depolarisation is on the left side of the heart. This implies a left bundle branch block (LBBB).

v. The axis of the peripheral leads is quite negative, with both leads II and III being negative (formal measurement is –44 degrees), supporting a diagnosis of LBBB.

vi. The final interpretation is sinus bradycardia with a first-degree heart block, LBBB and left axis deviation.

vii. It is not a trifascicular block, classically described as prolongation of the PR interval (first degree AV block), right bundle branch block and either left anterior fascicular block or left posterior fascicular block. The former is more common and leads to left axis deviation, the latter to right axis deviation.

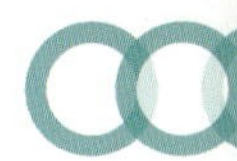

QUESTION 165

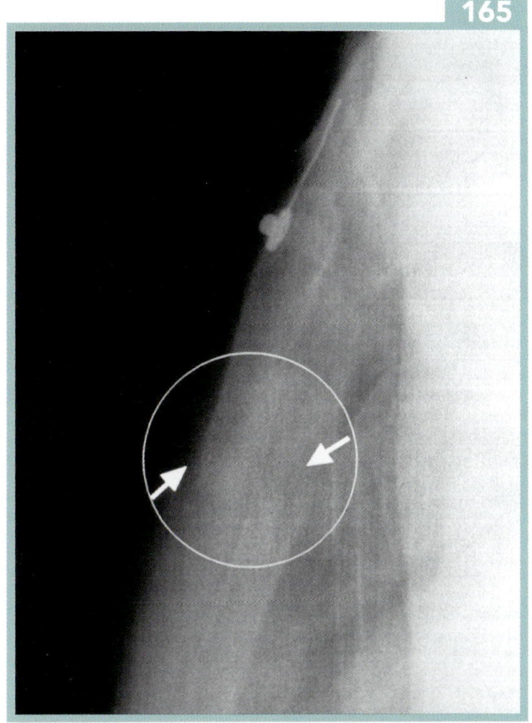

165i. What abnormality can be seen on this lateral sternal (**165**) X-ray taken from a conscious 25-year-old woman involved in a car crash?

ii. Do you think she was wearing a seat belt?

iii. What cardiac complications should be anticipated?

iv. What respiratory complications should be anticipated?

QUESTION 166

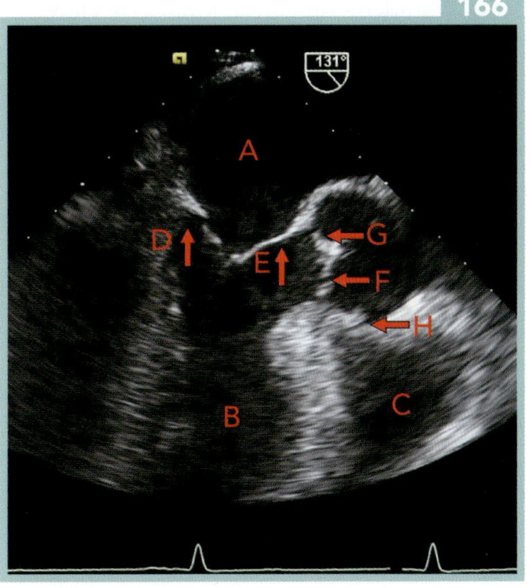

166 A TOE image is shown (**166**).

i. What is this view called?

ii. Which chambers are indicated by A and B?

iii. What area is indicated by C?

iv. What structures are indicated by D and E?

v. What structures are indicated by F and G?

vi. What position is indicated by the arrow at H?

Answer 165

165i. There is a dislocation of the manubrium sterni on the sternal bone, indicating a severe deceleration injury to the chest.

ii. She probably was not wearing a seat belt unless the vehicle was travelling at very high velocity (e.g. over 112 kph [70 mph]). This injury is consistent with hitting the dashboard, which is unlikely if a seat belt is worn.

iii. Cardiac contusions or tamponade are associated with sternal damage. Contusions present as arrythymias or cardiac failure. Tamponade classically presents with low BP, muffled heart sounds, Kussmaul's sign (paradoxical increase in jugular venous pressure with inspiration) and small QRS complexes on the ECG.

iv. Such fracture/dislocations in adults can be associated with thoracic spinal injury and may be accompanied by rib and sternal fractures and damage to underlying soft tissues. Although the patient is neurologically intact, she is at major risk of respiratory failure due to pain from fractured ribs, pulmonary contusions, haemothorax, pneumothorax and flail segments. There is also risk of damage to other mediastinal structures.

Answer 166

166i. A mid-oesophageal, long-axis view.

ii. A is the left atrium, B is the left ventricle.

iii. C indicates the right ventricular outflow tract.

iv. D and E are the posterior leaflet and anterior leaflet of the mitral valve, respectively.

v. F is the right coronary cusp of the aortic valve, G is either the left coronary cusp or the non-coronary cusp of the aortic valve.

vi. H indicates a typical position of the right coronary artery.

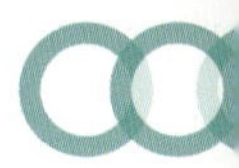

QUESTION 167

167 Blood gas values of four patients are shown in the Table below. Patients 1 and 3 both smoke 20 cigarettes per day.

Values	Patient 1	Patient 2	Patient 3	Patient 4
pH (H^+)	7.37	7.35	7.19	7.48
PO_2 (kPa) (mmHg)	11.7 (88)	8.9 (67)	7.8 (58)	9.2 (69)
PCO_2 (kPa) (mmHg)	5.3 (40)	6.1 (46)	7.6 (57)	4.0 (30)
HCO_3^- (mmol/l)	28	32	32	28
Base excess	0	+4	+4	0

i. Assuming other diagnostic evidence, which patient has the most advanced COPD, patient 1 or patient 3?

ii. Does the blood gas sequence 1 to 3 represent normal clinical progression during a prolonged history of COPD?

iii. Is patient 4 likely to have a diagnosis of COPD?

iv. Could a healthy person visiting Denver (altitude approximately 1,950 metres [6,000 ft] above sea level) have the blood gases of patient 4, and why?

v. Describe the mechanism that enables healthy people to hyperventilate when at higher altitudes.

vi. What medication can be used to modify blood gas altitude effects and how does it work?

Answer 167

167i. Patient 3 has more advanced COPD than patient 1, as patient 3 has hypoxaemia and a high resting CO_2 level.

ii. Yes, these changes can be expected over years. In progressive COPD, hypoxia develops first because ofV/Q mismatch, and in areas of low V/Q ratios (poorly ventilated lung units), shunts develop. As COPD progresses, hypoxic drive fails, PO_2 continues to decrease and PCO_2 rises to above normal. With ongoing progression, PO_2 decreases even further (due to more shunting), the work of breathing increases and the PCO_2 continues to increase above normal values.

iii. No, hyperventilation in the face of COPD and hypoxia is unusual. If patient 4 had COPD, another reason for hyperventilation would be expected (e.g. pneumonia, sepsis).

iv. Yes, a healthy person visiting high altitudes will have a decreased PaO_2 because of the lower partial pressure of oxygen at altitude, so hypoxia develops first and hypoxic drive stimulates respiration, leading to a lower $PaCO_2$.

v. Hypoxia (low PaO_2) at altitude drives the ventilation, leading of hyperventilation with a lowered $PaCO_2$ concentration.

vi. Acetazolamide is a carbonic anhydrase inhibitor and blocks production and reabsorption of bicarbonate by the kidney. This leads to a mild metabolic acidosis, which counteracts the respiratory alkalosis produced by the hypoxic hyperventilation.

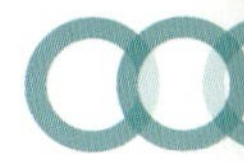

QUESTION 168

168 A normal capnogram with time on the x-axis, CO_2 concentration on the y-axis and several points indicated on the tracing is shown (**168**).

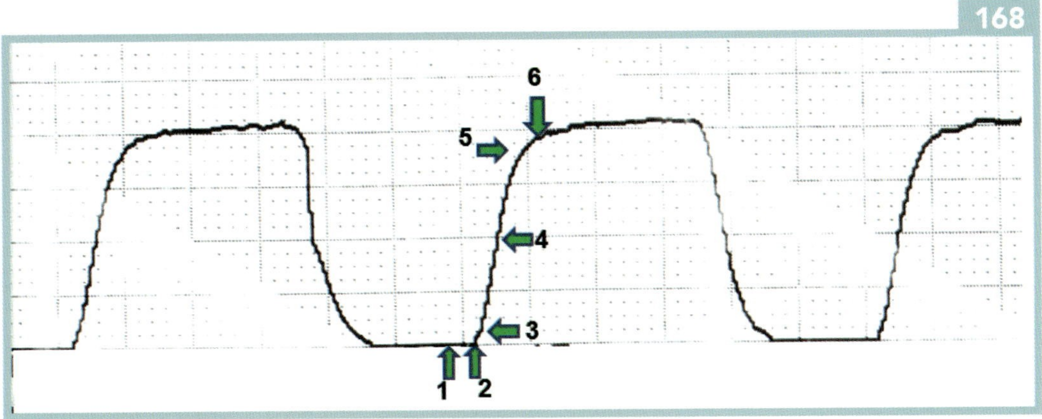

i. When does exhalation start: number 1, 2 or 3?

ii. When has all the anatomical dead space been exhaled: number 3, 4, 5 or 6?

iii. Explain why anatomical dead space is also called 'serial' dead space.

iv. When (which number) does alveolar gas start to reach the sampling point, and when (which number) does alveolar dead space gas start to reach the sampling point?

v. Explain why the alveolar dead space gas is also called 'parallel' dead space.

vi. Does anatomical ('serial') dead space gas affect the end-tidal CO_2 reading? Explain your answer.

vii. Does alveolar ('parallel') dead space gas affect the end-tidal CO_2 reading? Explain your answer.

viii. Does alveolar dead space gas increase or decrease the A-a CO_2 gradient?

ix. What are the constituents of physiological dead space?

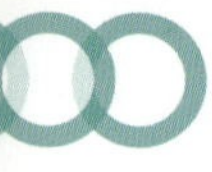

Answer 168

168i. At 1. The first gas to pass by the sampling point is inspired anatomical dead space gas, which is fresh, unused gas – it was not in contact with the alveoli and it did not pick up any CO_2. At the end of inspiration, the fresh, unused gas in the anatomical dead space can be thought of as 'good' gas. This gas would be relevant in mouth-to-mouth ventilation, especially in a child.

ii. Fresh, unused gas in the anatomical dead space dilutes exhaled alveolar gas, and has been exhaled by number 6, when there is no more dilution noted.

iii. Anatomical gas is exhaled first, followed by alveolar gas, hence the nomenclature 'serial dead space'.

iv. Alveolar gas reaches the sampling point at number 2 (i.e. as soon as CO_2 is noted in the exhaled gas, alveolar gas is present).

v. Alveolar dead space gas is exhaled at the same time as alveolar gas, hence the nomenclature 'parallel' dead space.

vi. Anatomical dead space gas is exhaled early in exhalation (in series, prior to the alveolar gas), and therefore does not affect the end-tidal CO_2 reading.

vii. Alveolar dead space gas (containing a lower CO_2 concentration) is exhaled at the same time (in 'parallel') as the alveolar gas and therefore does affect the end-tidal CO_2.

viii. The A-a CO_2 gradient is increased.

ix. The anatomical and alveolar dead spaces. Many discussions on V_a/Q ratios do not differentiate between anatomical and alveolar dead spaces, but only talk about physiological dead space.

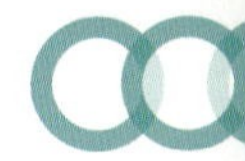

QUESTION 169

169 A 70-year-old man presents for major surgery. He has a history of coronary artery disease and prior myocardial infarction. His ECG is shown (**169**).

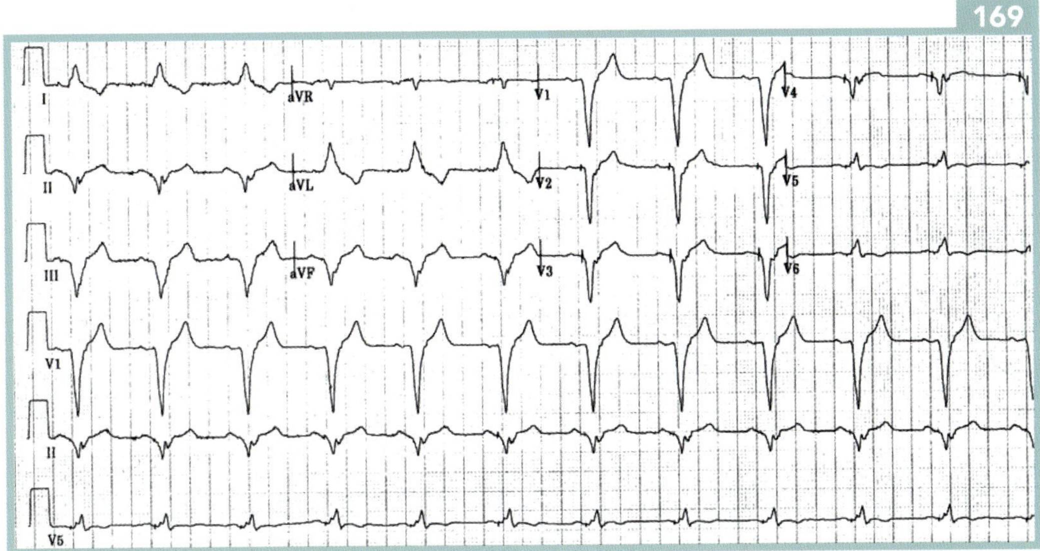

i. What does the ECG show? Look specifically at leads V2, V3 and V4.

ii. Delineate the International Pacemaker Nomenclature (3-letter code).

iii. In what mode (3-letter code) is this pacemaker functioning?

iv. What perioperative management should the patient receive?

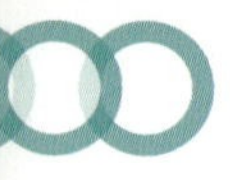

Answer 169

169i. Wide, bizarre QRS complex with a left bundle branch-like pattern. The sharp spikes preceding each QRS complex, most obvious in leads V_2–V_4, reveal a properly functioning ventricular pacemaker positioned in the right ventricle. The QRS configuration is that expected from a pacemaker in this position.

ii. See Table below.

First letter (indicates the chamber paced)	Second letter (indicates the chamber sensed)	Third letter (indicates mode of response to sensed beat)
A (atrium)	A (atrium)	I (inhibited)
V (ventricle)	V (ventricle)	T (triggered)
D (duel-both)	D (dual-both)	D (dual-both)
	O (no sensing function)	O (no sensing function)

iii. The ECG provides information about the pacemaker mode. Each ventricular pacemaker spike is preceded by a normal-appearing p-wave, a constant P-R interval of 0.14 seconds and no apparent atrial pacemaker spike. Using the basic 3-letter designation of pacemaker type, this pacemaker is operating in the VAT mode. The pacer senses the patient's intrinsic p-wave, which then triggers a ventricular-pacing impulse. Since the pacer fires on each beat, this ECG does not provide information regarding whether or not the patient is pacemaker dependent.

iv. This patient may be pacemaker dependent. Pacemaker function must be maintained perioperatively, despite electrical interference from electrocautery. If left operating in its current mode, the pacemaker could sense electrocautery as atrial or ventricular electrical activity. If sensed as rapid atrial activity, the pacemaker may produce a rapid ventricular rate, up to its built-in upper rate limit. If the electrocautery is interpreted as ventricular activity, it may be inhibited or not fire at all, potentially leading to periods of asystole. Therefore:

- The pacemaker should be reprogrammed to a VOO (fixed rate) mode, with the sensing function disabled, during surgery.
- In an emergency, when reprogramming is not possible, placing a magnet over the pacer generator box in the event of pacemaker inhibition during electromagnetic interference should restore pacing at a 'fixed rate' mode. Using the magnet in this way, in the presence of electromagnetic interference, could result in reprogramming the pacer in unpredictable ways.
- If there is a reasonable likelihood of pacemaker failure, percutaneous pacing electrodes could be used as an alternative means of pacing during the surgical procedure.

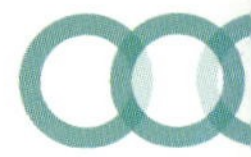

QUESTION 170

170 This patient has a long-standing cervical spine fracture at the C4 level.

i. What is the abnormality on the chest radiograph (**170a**)?

ii. This chest radiograph (**170b**) was performed twenty minutes later. What procedure has been performed?

iii. Why did this happen?

170a

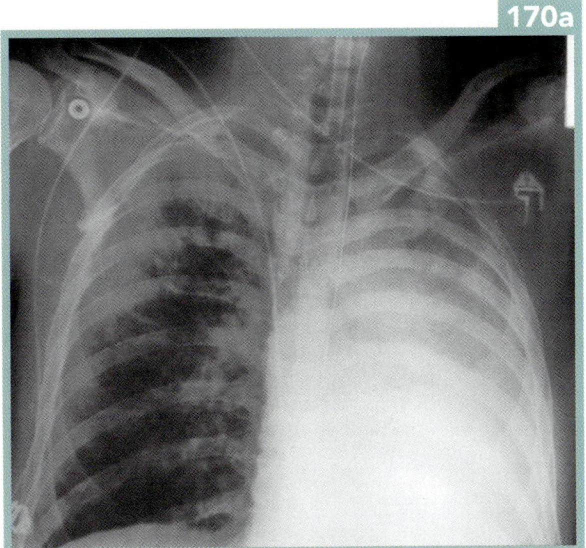

170b

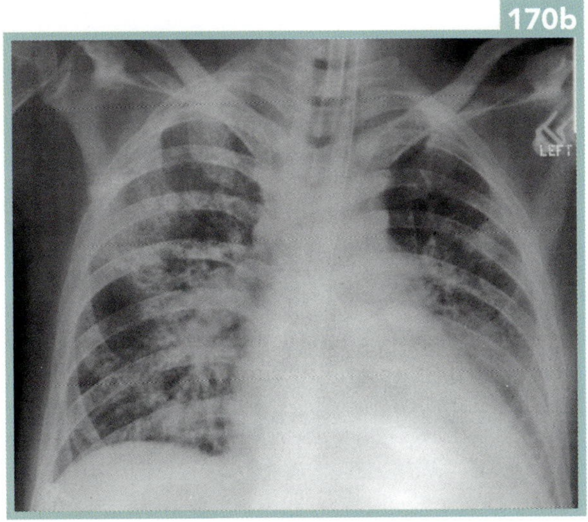

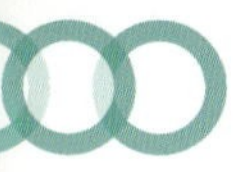

Answer 170

170i. Partial left lower lung collapse with mediastinal shift to the left, the cardiac silhouette is indistinct and the left hemidiaphragm shadow is lost. An ET tube is visible.

ii. At fibreoptic bronchoscopy a plug of mucus was removed from the left main bronchus with resultant partial re-expansion of the left lung.

iii. Acute hypoxia is common in patients with acute tetraplegia. Traumatic tetraplegic patients often have chest injuries or fat emboli, which increase the risk of respiratory failure. Paralysis of the intercostal muscles reduces vital capacity and the patient is reliant on diaphragmatic breathing alone. There is also paralysis of the abdominal muscles, which are essential for effective coughing.

The plug in this patient's bronchus was only pea-sized and would have been easily cleared by a healthy subject. However, this patient aspirated seawater at the time of injury and had signs of pneumonia.

Up to 50% of acute tetraplegics (C3 and below) require ventilatory support, either by non-invasive methods or formal intubation. If a patient is able to breathe spontaneously after the trauma, later weaning from the ventilator is usually possible. High lesions (C2 and above) may have no spontaneous respiration and require long-term ventilation.

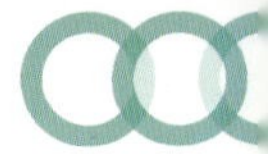

QUESTION 171

171 A 69-year-old female with a history of coronary artery disease and a pelvic fracture after a motor vehicle accident has been in the ICU for 12 hours.

i. What is the yellow catheter contained in a polythene cover and inserted below the green triple lumen CVP line as illustrated (**171a**)?

ii. Why is this device used less frequently than it used to be?

iii. Why is mixed venous oxygen saturation (MVO_2) a useful parameter to measure in a critically ill patient, and what has this measurement been superseded by?

iv. What is the differential diagnosis for the trend over 4 hours in MVO_2 (depicted in **171b**) assuming that arterial oxygenation is adequate?

171a

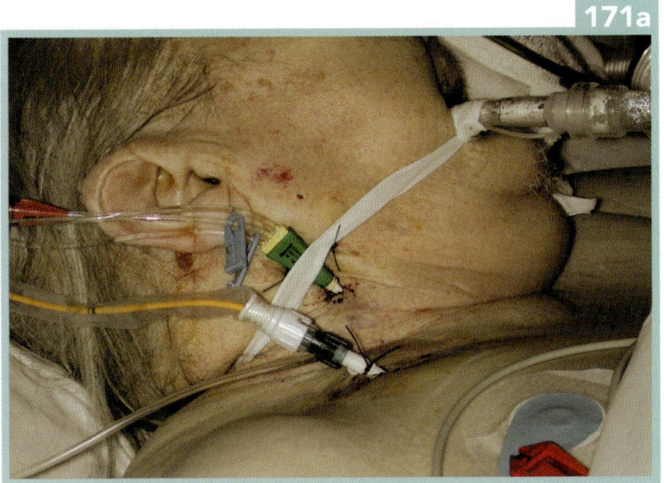

171b

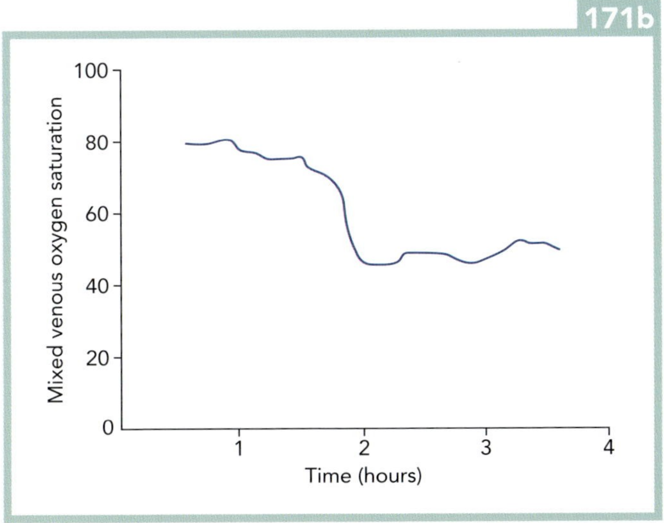

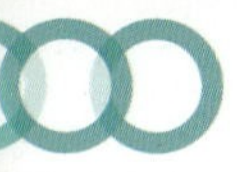

Answer 171

171i. A pulmonary artery (PA) catheter is inserted into the right internal jugular vein. PA catheters were frequently inserted into critically ill patients because by having their tip in the PA they enabled both cardiac output (CO) and MVO_2 to be measured. These two measurements allow calculation of oxygen delivery and consumption.

ii. Other less invasive ways of assessing CO are now available. PA catheter insertion can lead to tricuspid/pulmonary valve damage, arrhythmias and pulmonary infarction. TOE and/or less invasive CO measurement (e.g. Lidco, Picco) have replaced the PA catheter. MVO_2 measurements have been largely superseded by central venous oxygen saturation measurement, which is a close approximation of MVO_2 and only requires sampling from a central venous line. Similar conclusions can be drawn from both saturations measurements.

iii. MVO_2 is the percentage oxygen saturation in venous blood from the body as a whole and is measured accurately from samples taken through the pulmonary artery catheter. MVO_2 is the end result of blood leaving tissues after they have consumed oxygen and represents a balance between arterial oxygen delivery and tissue oxygen consumption.

$$\text{Oxygen delivery} = \text{CO} \times \text{oxygen content (Hb} \times \text{\% saturation} \times 1.34)$$

This is helpful in critically ill patients because if they are shocked or septic, insufficient tissue perfusion is occurring and MVO_2 falls. Measures can then be taken to boost oxygen delivery (e.g. checking arterial oxygen is sufficient, fluid loading to try and increase CO, inotropic support and/or increasing Hb level, so called 'goal-directed therapy', the goal being a MVO_2 of 70% or greater.

iv. If arterial hypoxia is not present, oxygen delivery must be failing due to decreased CO from either hypovolemia or ventricular dysfunction leading to inadequate oxygen delivery to the tissues. Increased oxygen consumption from shivering and/or fever or sepsis can also increase oxygen uptake, causing a reduction in MVO_2.

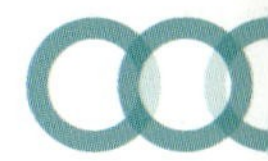

QUESTION 172

172 The ECG and arterial BP traces at a paper speed of 6.25 mm per second (one quarter of the usual paper speed of 25 mm per sec) in a spontaneously breathing patient are shown (**172**). The BP varies (i.e. decreases with inspiration, even though the negative intrathoracic pressure with spontaneous breathing increases the venous return). This phenomenon is called 'pulsus paradoxus'.

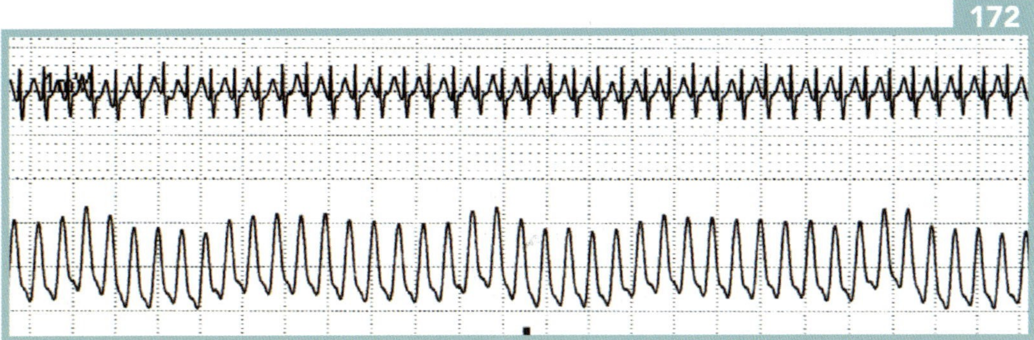

i. Is 'pulsus paradoxus' an abnormal (pathological) phenomenon or an 'accentuation of normal'?

ii. List four reasons why the negative inspiratory pressure with spontaneous breathing would decrease the BP (during the inspiratory phase of spontaneous breathing).

iii. Explain why BP increases during exhalation (with spontaneous breathing).

iv. Is it acceptable to use pulse pressure variation with spontaneous breathing to gauge volume status? Explain your answer.

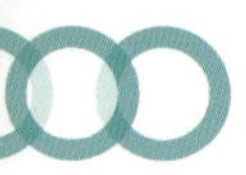

Answer 172

172i. An accentuation of a normal phenomenon.

ii. Inspiration (spontaneous) causes a decreased BP in normal subjects. The reasons for this are: (1) inspiration (spontaneous) decreases intrathoracic pressure, which increases venous return to the right heart; (2) increased right heart filling causes a septal shift to the left side, thereby decreasing the compliance of the left ventricle ("stiffer") and, therefore, decreased left ventricular filling for a given filling pressure (left ventricular end diastolic pressure), leading to a smaller stroke volume; (3) inspiration (spontaneous breathing) increases the volume of the pulmonary vascular bed, with less venous return to the left heart (leading to a smaller stroke volume); (4) inspiration (spontaneous) decreases pulmonary venous pressure, leading to less pressure to fill the left heart (smaller stroke volume).

iii. Exhalation (spontaneous breathing) increases pulse pressure in normal subjects. This happens when each of the four causes listed above is reversed.

iv. It is not acceptable: (1) the pressure fluctuations in the chest with spontaneous breathing are not constant; (2) the physiology underlying the pulse pressure variations as an indicator of volume status is based on positive pressure in the chest (Valsalva manoeuvre) and not on negative pressure variations (pulsus paradoxus physiology).

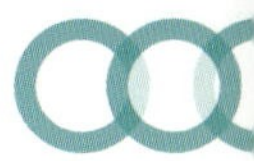

QUESTION 173

173 ECG and pulse oximeter traces are shown (**173**). The ECG rate is recorded as 123 bpm by the electronic monitor.

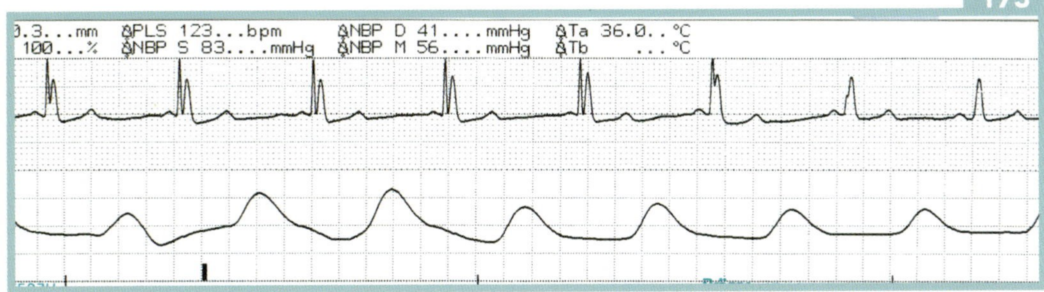

i. Describe and analyse the ECG rhythm. Why does the monitor record a rate of 123 bpm?

ii. What is the rate demonstrated by the pulse oximeter? The electronic monitor reports heart rate and pulse rate separately. Why this distinction?

iii. How does the very last ECG complex differ from the earlier complexes?

QUESTION 174

174 With regard to the four lung volumes: inspiratory reserve volume, tidal volume, expiratory reserve volume and residual volume:

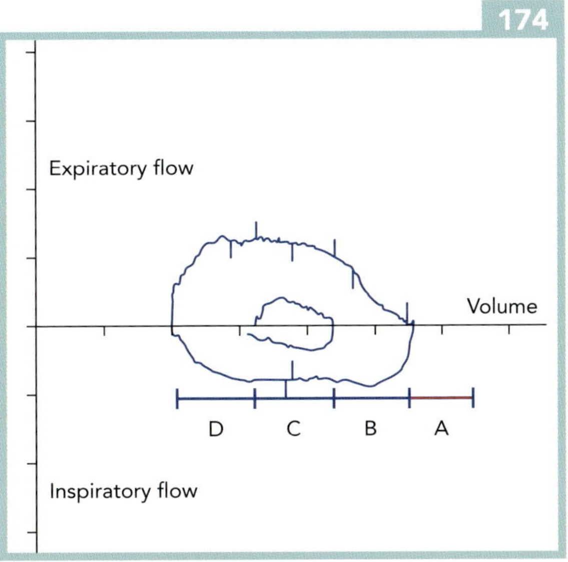

i. Match these four lung volumes with the volumes (areas) noted as A, B, C, and D on the x-axis of the flow–volume loop (**174**).

ii. Is the lung volume indicated by A actually measured with the flow–volume loop?

iii. Mention three techniques to measure the lung volume indicated by A.

iv. Is this a normal flow–volume loop? Explain your answer.

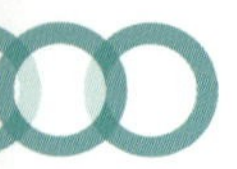

Answer 173

173i. This is normal sinus rhythm as indicated by the very last beat of the tracing. The ECG monitor is 'counting' two electric pulses for every one ECG complex. The interference is being caused by the nerve stimulator, which is continuously stimulating at 1 Hz (mimicking another 60 bpm), which is very close to the patient's true heart rate, and the two electrical impulses are almost in-phase and overlapping.

ii. The pulse oximeter is demonstrating a pulse rate of around 60 bpm. A quick check is to count the large blocks on the ECG trace (five blocks from a peak to another peak in this case). Then divide 300 by the number of large blocks, which gives a pulse rate of 60 bpm. The heart rate reported by the monitor is the rate of the ECG (electrical impulses). The pulse rate is the rate of the pulsatile (mechanical) activity, which may be the pulse oximeter or the arterial blood pressure.

iii. The very last ECG complex was recorded after the nerve stimulator was switched off, and demonstrates a normal sinus rhythm.

Answer 174

174i. A = residual volume; B = expiratory reserve volume; C = tidal volume; D = inspiratory reserve volume.

ii. The residual volume (A) is not measured with a flow–volume loop.

iii. The residual volume can be measured using (1) a helium dilution technique, (2) a whole body plethysmography box or (3) a nitrogen wash-out test after inhalation of a single breath of a tracer gas (typically oxygen).

iv. The flow–volume loop in **174** is an example of a fixed airway obstruction (specifically, tracheal stenosis after several weeks of ventilation including a tracheostomy).

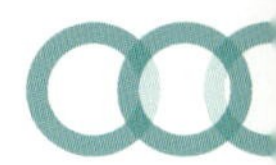

QUESTION 175

175 The devices indicated by A and B on this patient (**175**) are used for monitoring patients with brain injury.

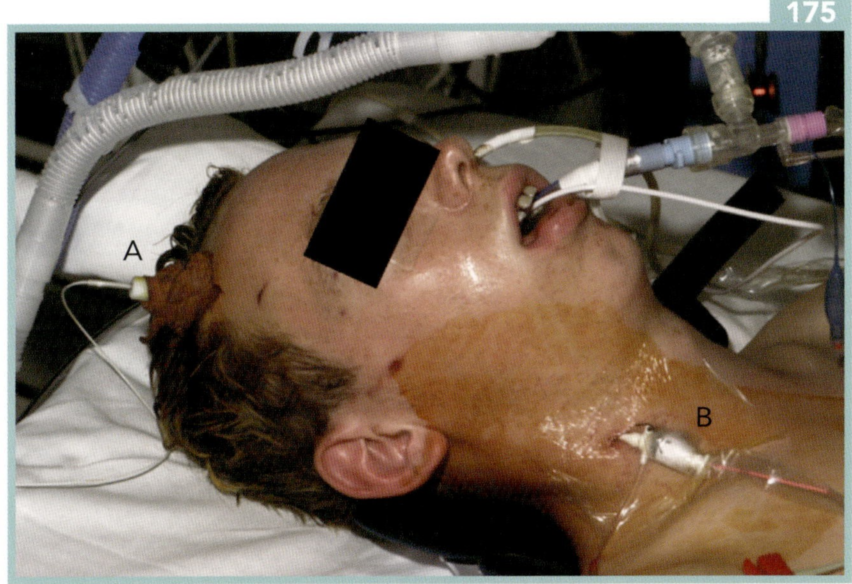

i. What are they?

ii. What are the risks associated with their use?

iii. Discuss their clinical usefulness.

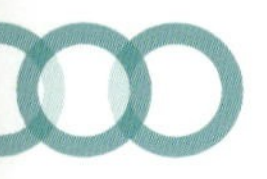

Answer 175

175i. A is an intracranial pressure (ICP) monitor, also known as an ICP bolt. The illustration shows an intraparenchymal fibreoptic transducer. Other types are available. B is a jugular bulb catheter.

ii. The risks of both devices are infection and haemorrhage. Experienced personnel should insert these devices under full sterile technique.

iii. In head injury, ICP monitoring is important for both recognition of a sudden increase in ICP secondary to an acute bleed and also for calculation of cerebral perfusion pressure (CPP). CPP is compromised secondary to any intracranial mass within the vault of the skull (e.g. a haematoma, a cerebral contusion or generalised cerebral oedema secondary to a diffuse brain injury). A CPP above 70 mmHg is a goal of head injury management and is calculated thus:

$$\text{CPP} = \text{MAP (mean arterial pressure)} - \text{ICP}$$

CPP guides the neurosurgeon/intensivist as to when to manipulate MAP with fluids and vasopressors.

A jugular vein catheter measures oxygenation in venous blood leaving the brain by a fibreoptic transducer connected to a light emitting diode and works by the same principles as a pulse oximeter. It is placed within the jugular sinus by being passed retrogradely up the internal jugular vein. Normal saturation of jugular venous blood ($SjVO_2$) is 55–75%.

Low $SjVO_2$ implies excessive O_2 extraction by brain tissue and a sluggish cerebral blood flow (CBF). Therapeutic manoeuvres include checking for good oxygenation and correct positioning of the patient's head to assist adequate arterial flow and venous drainage. Echocardiography, a pulmonary artery catheter or at least a CVP line should be used to ensure adequate fluid loading and allow safe use of vasopressors (e.g. noradrenaline) to elevate MAP to optimise cerebral perfusion.

A high $SjVO_2$ may be due to either excess CBF (luxury perfusion) or a lack of metabolic activity within cerebral tissue because of cell death. CT can distinguish between these two situations. With 'luxury perfusion', high ICP and high $SjVO_2$ may require mild hyperventilation to a pCO_2 of 4–4.5 kPa (30–35 mmHg) to reduce CBF by vasoconstriction. Once PCO_2 is optimised, if $SjVO_2$ remains high, sedatives can be added to suppress metabolic activity.

Although the catheter picks up global cerebral ischaemia, focal ischaemia may not be detected and caution should be taken not to overinterpret a normal or high jugular venous oxygen level.

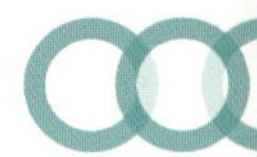

QUESTION 176

176 List 17 reasons why 'normal saline' (**176**) is neither normal nor physiological.

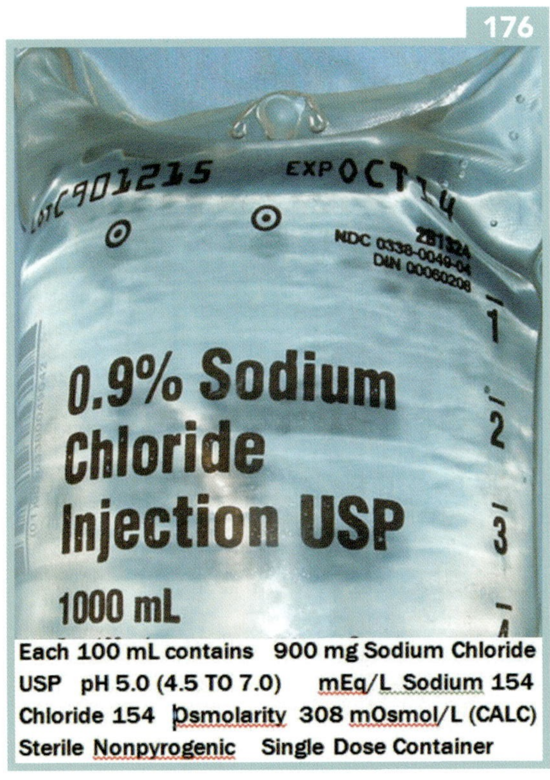

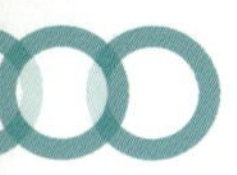

Answer 176

176 • A 'normal' solution contains 1 mole of substance per litre. In chemistry, a one normal solution of NaCl is 0.5 molar Na(Cl) assuming complete dissociation. Physiological dissociation is approximately 1.7 ions per mole, so one normal of NaCl is 1/1.7 = 0.588 molar. This is roughly four times more concentrated than medical 'normal saline' of 0.154 molar (or 154 mmol [mEq]/l). The unit symbol 'N' is used to denote 'mol/l' when referring to normality. Alternatively, the symbol 'Eq/l' is sometimes used. Although losing favour, medical reporting of serum concentrations in 'mEq/l' (= 0.001 N) still occurs.

- It contains 0.9 % NaCl, which is hypertonic. A NaCl solution of 0.83 % would be isotonic.
- 'Normal saline" (at 20°C) has an osmolality and osmolarity of 308 mOsmol/l, which is hypertonic compared with the normal physiological osmolarity of 285 mOsmol/l.
- It does not have a physiological colloid osmotic pressure.
- The Na^+ concentration is 154 mEq/l, which is higher than physiological concentrations.
- The Cl^- concentration is 154 mEq/l.
- 'Normal saline' leads to a hyperchloremic acidosis as it leads to a decrease in H^+ ion excretion by the kidney.
- The pH of 'normal saline' in the container is 6.5–7.0. This does not cause acidosis as 'normal saline' does not contain any H^+ ions.
- 'Normal saline' does not have any buffering capacity.
- It is said to have 'negative free water', which means that water has to be added to the hypertonic solution to make it isotonic.
- 'Normal saline' causes a retention of H^+ ions. As an example, it is used to treat the alkalosis of pyloric stenosis with its attendant projectile vomiting.
- 'Normal saline' leads to a retention of K^+ ions; therefore, it is used to treat hypokalemia (especially when in concert with hyponatremia).
- 'Normal saline' produces an osmotic gradient; for instance, across the blood–brain barrier.
- Normal saline (in the bag) is fully ionized, while it is only partially ionized in the blood.
- It does not contain any Ca^+.
- 'Normal saline' does not contain any K^+.
- It would be possible to generate any number of examples of constituents not present in 'normal, physiological saline'.

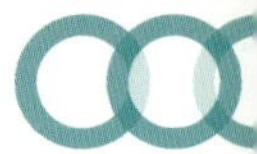

QUESTION 177

177 A pressure trace of an arterial BP wave form is shown (**177**). The subject is blowing against a pressure gauge (e.g. a mercury sphygmomanometer). The four phases are marked as 1, 2, 3 and 4.

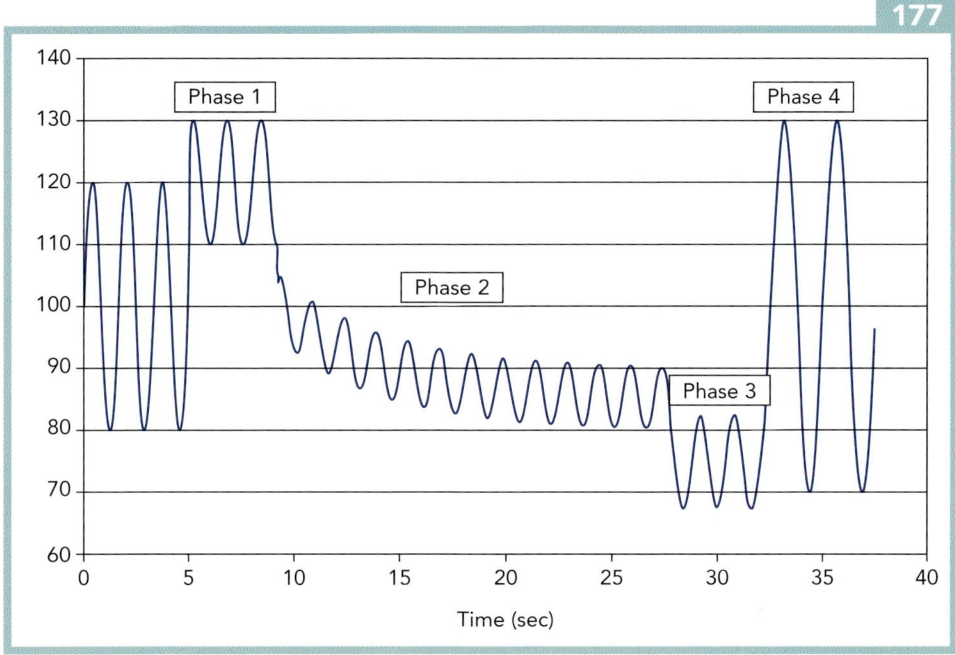

i. What is the manoeuvre called?

ii. What pressure is typically generated during this manoeuvre?

iii. What are the physiological causes of each phase of the manoeuvre? Specifically, explain why the blood pressure initially increases, even though the increased intrathoracic pressure decreases the venous return.

iv. What is the manoeuvre called when the patient generates a negative pressure?

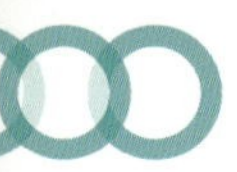

Answer 177

177i. Valsalva manoeuvre.

ii. Classically, the subject blows against a resistance maintaining a pressure of 40 mmHg for 30 seconds.

iii.
- Phase 1 is caused by the increased intrathoracic pressure, which increases the pressure inside the left ventricle. This leads to an increased BP and a larger stroke volume. The heart also works effectively works against ('sees' or encounters) a lower output impedance (lower 'resistance').
- Phase 2 is caused by the decreasing venous return (preload) due to the increased intrathoracic pressure. Peripheral venous constriction occurs to improve venous return in the later periods (stages, parts, phases) of phase II. Arterial vasoconstriction (afterload) also increases in an attempt to maintain the BP.
- Phase 3 is caused by the reverse phenomenon of phase I: the additional advantage of the higher intrathoracic pressure is removed from the left ventricle, which works against ('sees') an effective increase in output impedance ('resistance') and the BP decreases, while also resulting in a decreased stroke volume.
- Phase 4 is caused by the enhanced venous return due to venoconstriction. The BP oscillates up and down while the compensatory mechanisms find a new balance.

iv. Mueller manoeuvre.

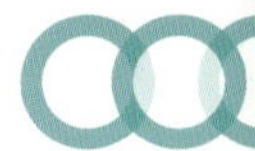

QUESTION 178

178i. What disease is demonstrated in these two images (**178a, b**)?

ii. What are these skin lesions called?

iii. What tissues are affected by this condition?

iv. What are the anaesthetic implications of this disease?

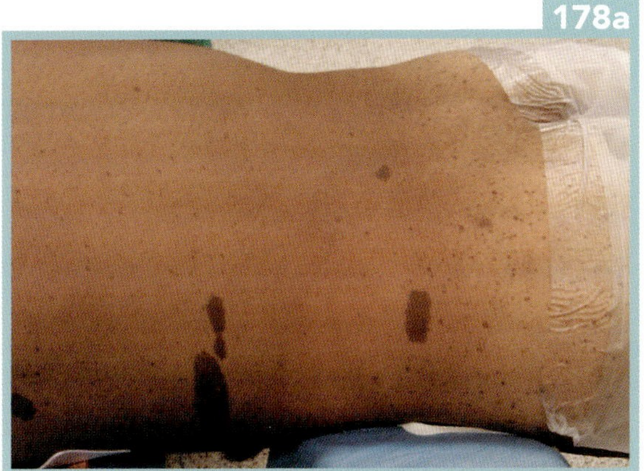

178a

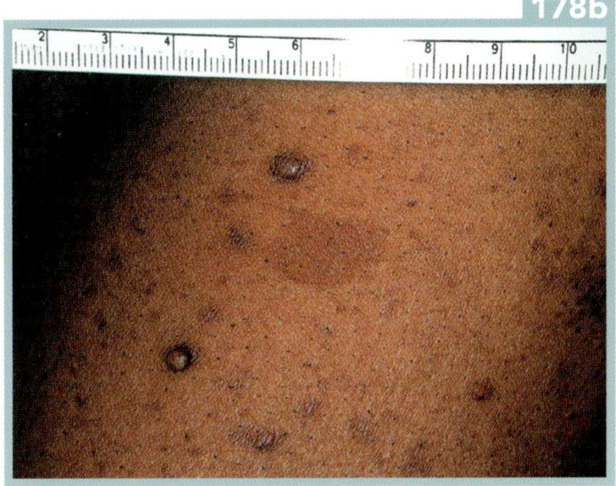

178b

QUESTION 179

179i. Write down the concentrations of all the positive ions and all the negative ions in lactated Ringer's solution (LRS).

ii. Do the same for Hartmann's solution.

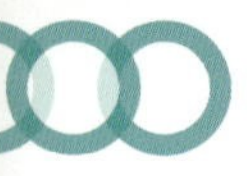

Answer 178

178i. This patient has Von Recklinghausen's neurofibromatosis (neurofibromatosis 1).

ii. Image **178a** shows flat uniformly pale brown macules, known as Café-au-lait spots, which vary in size from 0.5 to 20 cm and can be found on any cutaneous surface. Six or more spots greater than 1.5 cm in diameter are presumptive evidence of neurofibromatosis in children over 6 years of age and adults. The raised lesions in **178b** are neurofibromas.

iii. The lesions in neurofibromatosis affect tissues derived from neuroectoderm. These include neurofibromas, plexiform neurofibromas, optic nerve gliomas and astrocytomas of the brain and spinal cord. Hamartomas and meningiomas may also develop. The disease is genetic and autosomal dominant, although manifestations may not occur until early childhood or adulthood.

iv. The anaesthesiologist may encounter these tumours as an incidental finding in a patient presenting for other reasons, or because surgery is planned for excision of painful lumps from the skin or excision of intraspinal or intracranial tumours. These tumours may occur intracranially or along nerves, with possible intracranial mass effects and/or intraspinal lesions/tumours. Practitioners should be wary of performing spinals and epidurals. Associated abnormalities are scoliosis, phaeochromocytoma, renal artery stenosis, pulmonary fibrosis, obstructive cardiomyopathy or fibrous dysplasia of bone.

Answer 179

179i. SI units: sodium 130 mmol/l; potassium 4 mmol/l; chloride 109 mmol/l, calcium 1.5 mmol/l; lactate 28 mmol/l; osmolarity 273 mOsmol/l. (US units: sodium 130 mEq/l; potassium 4 mEq/l; calcium 2.7 mEq/l; lactate 28 mEq/l; osmolarity 273 mOsmol/l.)

ii. Hartmann's solution is very subtly different. SI units: sodium 131 mmol/l; potassium 5 mmol/l; chloride 111 mmol/l, calcium 2 mmol/l; lactate 29 mmol/l; osmolarity 273 mOsmol/l. (US units: sodium 131 mEq/l; potassium 5 mEq/l; chloride 111 mEq/l; calcium 4 mEq/l; lactate 29 mEq/l; osmolarity 273 mOsmol/l.)

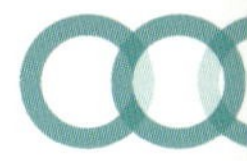

QUESTION 180

180 Give 17 reasons why lactated Ringer's solution (LRS) is neither normal nor physiological. (**Note:** There are many more than 17. These reasons also apply to Hartmann's solution, which is only marginally different.)

QUESTION 181

181 What common pathology can cause these two varying CT scan appearances (**181a, b**)?

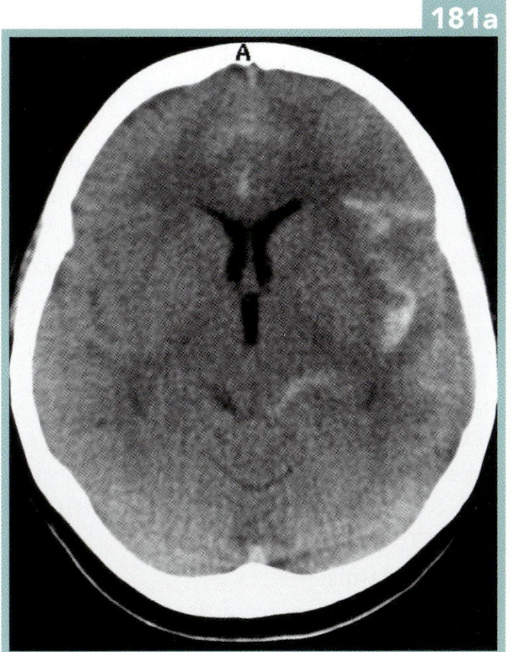

181a

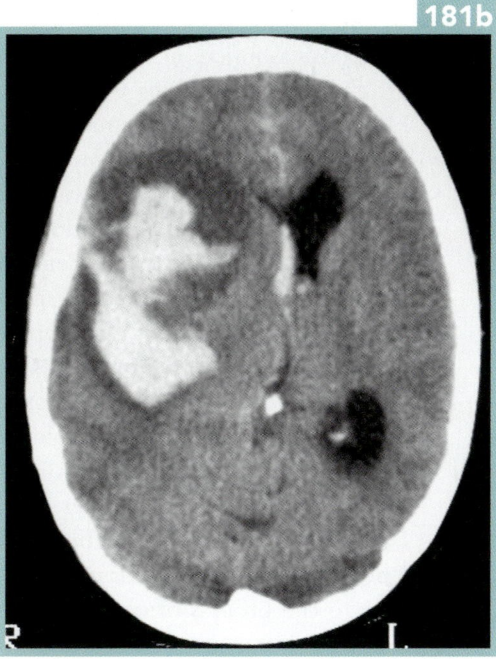

181b

Answer 180

180 • A normal solution would contain 1 mole of substance per litre of solution (i.e. contain a much higher concentration of solutes).

- LRS contains 25 mmol (mEq)/l of lactate. The upper limit of normal is 2 mmol (mEq)/l.
- The osmolarity (mOsmol/l at 20°C – temperature dependent) is lower.
- The osmolality (mOsmol/kg – temperature independent) is lower.
- No colloid osmotic pressure constituents.
- The Na^+ concentration is lower than physiological concentrations at 130 mmol (mEq)/l.
- The Cl^- concentration is high but within the physiological range.
- LRS contains sodium lactate, which leads to an alkalosis after the lactate is metabolized in the liver after 3–4 hours (with normal liver perfusion and normal temperature).
- The pH of the solution in the bag is 6.5. However, LRS does not cause (nor aggravate) an acidosis as it does not contain any H^+ ions. The term 'lactic acidosis' is, in reality, a 'hydrogen lactate acidosis' with the hydrogen ion increase causing the acidosis.
- LRS does not have any significant buffering capacity.
- LRS is hypotonic and contains positive 'free water' (a little less than 100 ml/l of LRS). The concept of 'free water' indicates that water needs to be removed to produce an iso-osmolar solution.
- LRS contains Ca^{2+} in a concentration that differs (higher) from that in blood. Before the advent red cell storage with saline-adenine-glucose-mannitol (SAGM) solutions, citrate was an anticoagulant which could 'clump' red cells if mixed with the calcium in LRS. Citrate can be used for donor whole blood collection prior to packed cell processing but citrate residues are tiny after processing so LRS is compatible with blood transfusion.
- LRS produces an osmotic gradient. For example, free water will tend to move across the blood–brain barrier, thereby increasing the intracranial pressure (ICP).
- LRS does not contain any bicarbonate (HCO_3^-).
- The viscosity of LRS is lower than blood and plasma.
- Due to the process of osmosis of free water, LRS will increase the ICP due to the lower-than-physiological osmolality. This might be clinically relevant with the infusion of large volumes and/or raised ICP.

Answer 181

181i. Subarachnoid haemorrhage has occurred in both cases. A generalised subarachnoid bleed is shown in **181a**, and this can be secondary to one or more of the following: a hypertensive crisis, an aneurysmal rupture or the rupture of an arteriovenous malformation. A massive bleed within the territory supplied by the middle cerebral artery after trauma is shown in **181b**. There is also hydrocephalus and a notable midline shift.

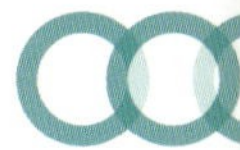

QUESTION 182

182i. How would each of the patients in case **181** be likely to present?

ii. What are the complications of these conditions?

QUESTION 183

183 A 56-year-old woman has had an uneventful laparoscopic cholesystectomy. Six hours later she looks pale, her peripheries are cool, her BP is 75/45, her pulse is 90 and her oxygen saturation on air is 92%. She is complaining of severe chest pain, nausea and abdominal discomfort. She has been started on high-flow oxygen and her saturations are now 100%. Fluid resuscitation using 500 ml of Ringer's lactate solution has been started. Her ECG is shown (**183**).

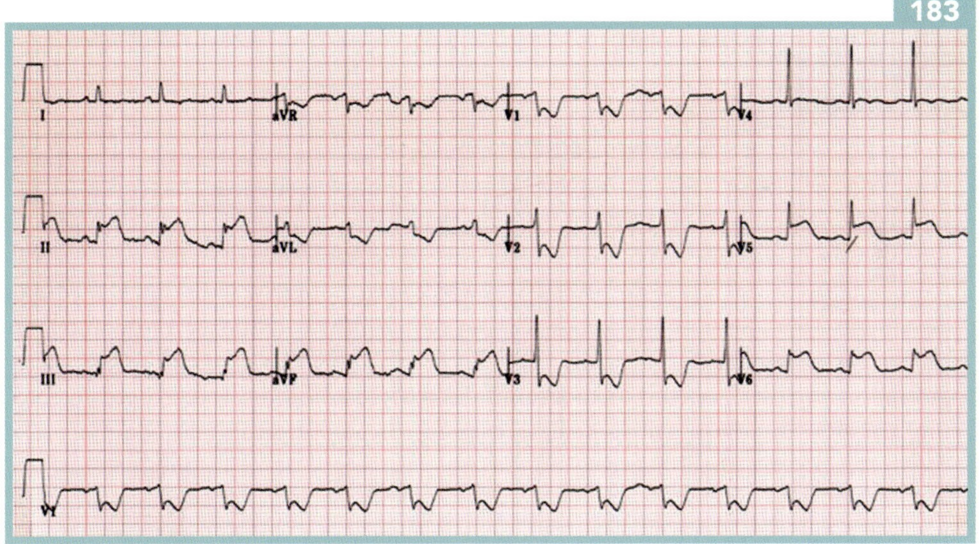

i. What is likely to have happened?

ii. Is the use of oxygen correct? Justify your answer.

iii. How should the clinical problem be managed?

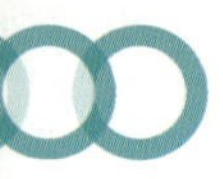

Answer 182

182i. Both of these patients would usually present with a sudden onset, severe headache. The patient in **181a** is likely to have signs of meningism and may have seizures, as this CT scan does not show signs of raised intracranial pressure (ICP) and the patient's symptoms are more likely to result from the irritant effect of subarachnoid blood. The patient in **181b** will show signs of raised ICP, focal neurological deficit and an altered conscious level.

ii. The immediate complications resulting from both of these cases are serious, with an expected 10% mortality, and include: (1) raised ICP from the intracerebral haematoma; (2) hydrocephalus causing a raised ICP; (3) re-bleed; (4) seizures; (5) neurogenic pulmonary oedema; (6) myocardial infarct/ischaemia; (7) arrhythmia; (8) hypertension or hypotension. Factors 5–8 result from the huge sympathetic discharge at the time of the bleed.

Later complications include: re-bleed; vasospasm, which can cause severe neurological damage (typically 4–10 days post subarachnoid haemorrhage); cerebral infarct; cerebral oedema; chest infection; electrolyte abnormalities (cerebral salt-wasting syndrome or, less commonly, syndrome of inappropriate antidiuretic hormone, or diabetes insipidus).

Answer 183

183i. The ECG shows an early, inferolateral, acute myocardial infarction (AMI) (i.e. ST segment elevation in leads II, III, aVF, V5 and V6 with ST depression in aVL and V1–3).

ii. Supplemental oxygen is appropriate (as initial O_2 saturations <94%) but the patient is now hyperoxic. Theoretically, hyperoxia can be harmful as coronary vasoconstriction can occur, extending the ischaemic area. Hyperoxia may also generate oxygen-free radicals in partially perfused areas around the AMI, causing tissue damage. Ninety-four to 98% saturations are optimal, so oxygen concentration should be reduced and the reason for the initial hypoxia sought (e.g. pulmonary oedema/pneumonia).

iii. Immediate management includes IV opiate analgesia and aspirin (300 mg chewable). An ECG is vital for correct diagnosis. Urgent cardiological consultation is required as angiography and percutaneous intervention may be needed. Additional antiplatelet therapy may also be suggested by the cardiologist (clopidogrel, 600mg). Fluid resuscitation should be stopped. Baseline troponin should be measured and repeated at 6 hours. Baseline raised troponin above the upper reference limit (URL), with a 20% rise at 6 hours and with a positive ECG, is diagnostic for AMI. If baseline troponin is below the URL, a rise of >50% from baseline confirms AMI. This patient is unstable and needs urgent cardiological intervention. Thrombolytic therapy is contraindicated by the recent surgery. Angioplasty, only available in hospitals with an angiography suite and trained personnel, may prevent permanent cardiac damage. Inotropic support for short-term cardiovascular support may be harmful by increasing cardiac work in an already compromised heart.

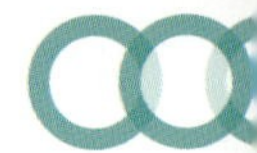

QUESTION 184

184 A magnetic resonance imaging (MRI) scan of a 56-year-old woman presenting with sudden onset deafness in her left ear is shown (**184**). She is otherwise healthy.

i. What abnormality does this MRI scan show as indicated by the red arrow?

ii. What intraoperative anaesthetic considerations must be taken into account for an open removal of this lesion?

iii. How would you manage this patient postoperatively?

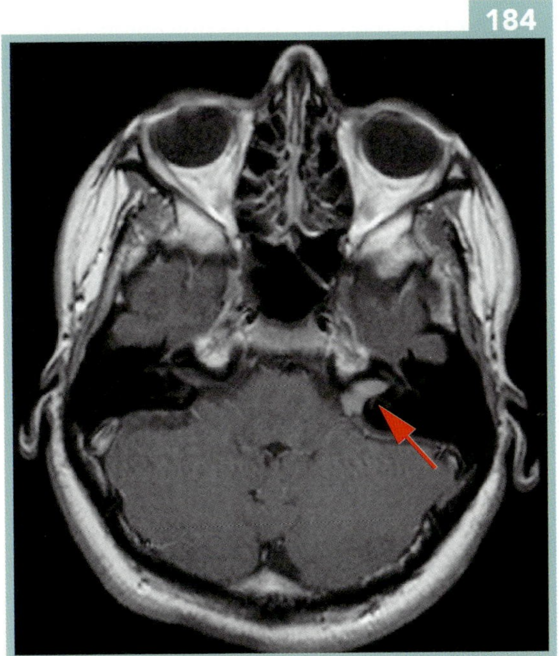

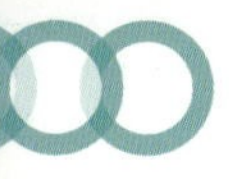

Answer 184

184i. A vestibular schwannoma (previously known as an acoustic neuroma).

ii. The following considerations must be taken into account:

- Prolonged surgery with the risks of hypothermia and pressure sores.
- Kinking of the ET tube with neck flexion and rotation. Downward migration of the tube can occur when the neck is flexed during positioning of the patient.
- Peripheral nerve palsies, particularly sciatic nerve and brachial plexus.
- Patient positioning may be prone, park bench or sitting. The sitting position allows better surgical access and improved drainage of blood from the operative field, but increases the potential for venous air embolus and postural hypotension. Postural hypotension can be prevented by adequate intravascular volume loading prior to patient positioning.
- There is a requirement for intraoperative facial nerve stimulation to assist the surgical technique, so no neuromuscular blockade should be administered after the initial dose for tracheal intubation.
- Arrythmias may occur, particularly severe bradycardia or asystole due to brainstem retraction. The use of atropine may remove signs of impending damage to the brainstem. Bulbar palsy may be present preoperatively.
- Smooth awakening from anaesthesia.

iii. Good postoperative management involves:

- Extubating the patient when the end-tidal arterial CO_2 difference is normalised, the patient has been rewarmed and bulbar palsy excluded.
- Close monitoring of respiratory, cardiovascular and neurological systems of the patient in a critical care area.
- Hypertension should be avoided postoperatively as this may increase the likelihood of posterior fossa haematoma developing.
- Large doses of anti-emetics are required.

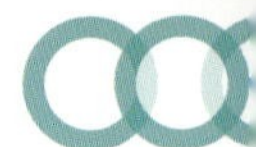

QUESTION 185

185i. What does this graph show (**185**)?

ii. What do VO_2 and VCO_2 mean?

iii. What is the significance of the crossing lines?

iv. Is it pathological for a 70 kg 49-year-old man?

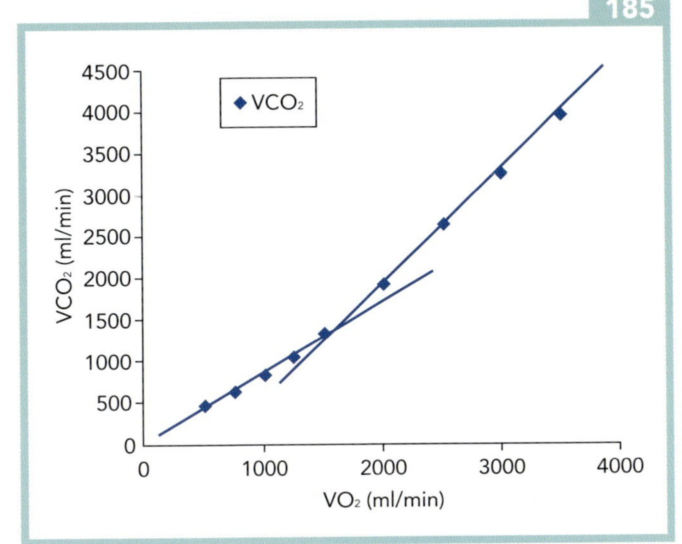

QUESTION 186

186 Two standard ET tubes (7.5 and 8.0 mm) as well as a left-sided double lumen ET tube (39 FG) are shown (**186a**). For an adult male, an 8 mm ET tube would typically be selected for intubation for abdominal surgery, while a 39 FG double lumen tube might be selected for one-lung ventilation for lung surgery (e.g. pneumonectomy).

i. What actual measurement does the size 8 mm indicate (i.e. from where to where is the distance of 8 mm measured)?

ii. What does the unit 'FG' (also known as 'F') indicate? Specify the abbreviation and specify the measurement and units (i.e. from where to where is the measurement 39FG made).

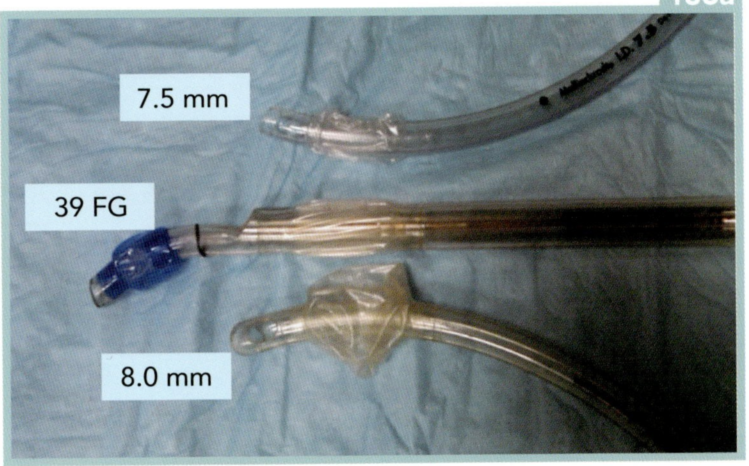

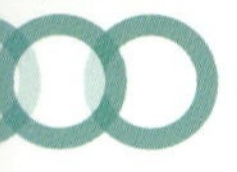

Answer 185

185i. This graph is derived from cardiopulmonary exercise testing (CPET). The uptake of oxygen and the production of carbon dioxide are measured by this technique.

ii. VO_2 stands for oxygen uptake; VCO_2 stands for carbon dioxide production.

iii. The lines cross at the point where the relative rate of increase in VCO_2 changes compared with the VO_2. This indicates carbon dioxide production increasing relative to oxygen consumption because significant anaerobic metabolism is starting. This normally occurs at >40% of maximum oxygen consumption. In this patient it occurred at 1.5 l/min (49% of maximal oxygen consumption).

iv. This patient weighed 70 kg, so this represents an anaerobic threshold of 21.4 ml/kg/minute, which is normal. Patients up to 80 years of age with an anaerobic threshold below 11 ml/kg/minute are at high risk of cardiovascular complications after major surgery, especially if it is associated with ischaemic heart disease. Patients over 80 may have lower anaerobic thresholds and their results are therefore more difficult to interpret.

Answer 186

186i. The 8 mm ET tube has an inner diameter (ID) of 8 mm. The measurement is from the inner wall on the one side to the inner wall on the other side (**186b**).

ii. FG is an abbreviation for French gauge. The FG is the outer circumference in mm. A 39 FG tube therefore has an outer diameter of 13 mm. To calculate the diameter, divide the circumference by Pi (π), or for an approximation, divide by 3.

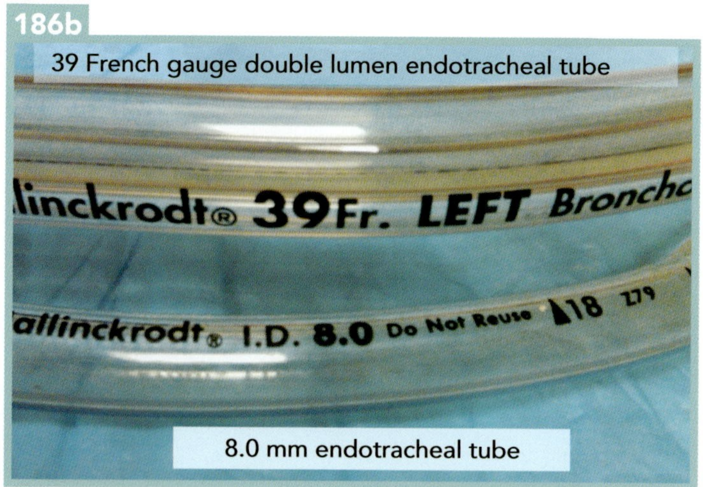

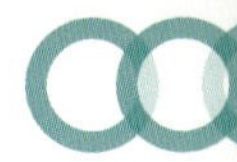

QUESTION 187

187 Draw a conventional anaesthetic circle breathing system ('circle system') and indicate the placement (position) of each of the following items (constituents).

a. Fresh gas flow inlet position.
b. One-way valve in the inspiratory limb.
c. One-way valve in the expiratory limb.
d. Y-connector to the patient.
e. Connector to the limb that leads to: e1 – anaesthesia reservoir bag and pop-off valve (APLV = adjustable pressure limiting valve); e2 – ventilator.
f. Soda lime absorber.
g. Selector switch to select between manual ventilation and controlled ventilation.
h. Pop-off valve (APLV).
i. Anaesthesia reservoir bag.
j. Ventilator.

Check your drawing by looking at **187a** before looking at the answer.

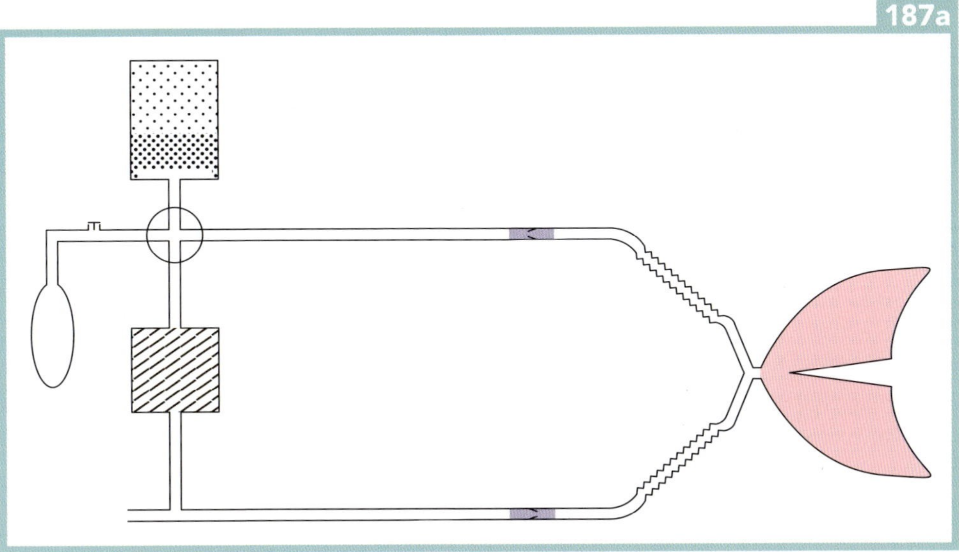

Answer 187

187 The items a-j are shown in **187b**.

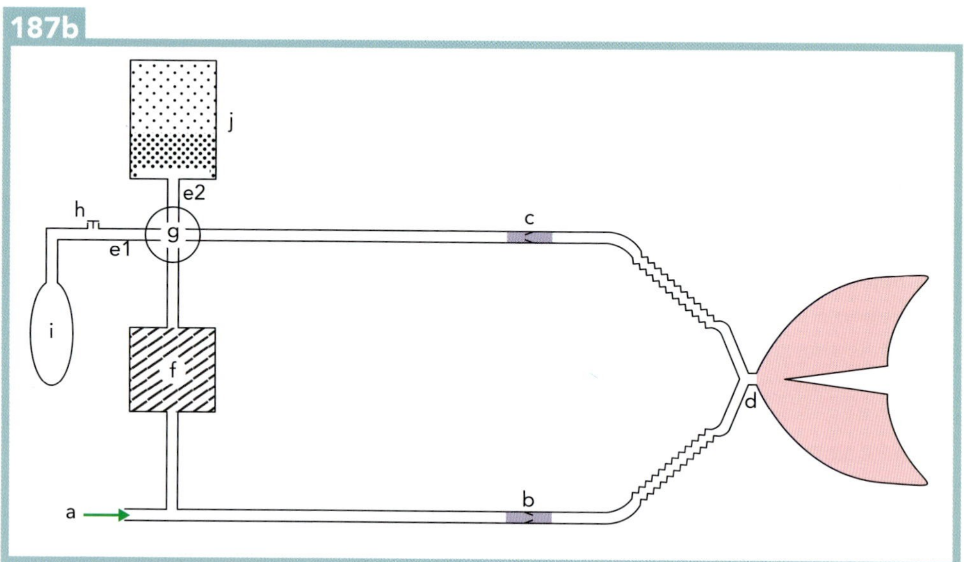

a. Fresh gas flow inlet position.
b. One-way valve in the inspiratory limb.
c. One-way valve in the expiratory limb.
d. Y-connector to the patient.
e. Connector to the limb that leads to: e1 – anaesthesia reservoir bag and pop-off valve (APLV = adjustable pressure limiting valve); e2 – ventilator.
f. Soda lime absorber.
g. Selector switch to select between manual ventilation and controlled ventilation.
h. Pop-off valve (APLV).
i. Anaesthesia reservoir bag.
j. Ventilator.

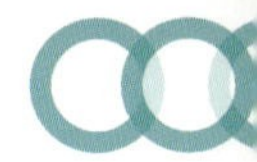

QUESTION 188

188 An ECG (top trace) and an arterial line with a low arterial BP are shown (**188a**). A single period of high pressure is noted, with a sudden decrease in the high pressure state. An arterial line is shown (**188b**) where the arterial catheter was kinked ('period of damping'), then unkinked and then gradually became kinked again. An episode of hypotension is shown (**188c**).

i. If an arterial line demonstrates a very low systolic BP, as in the 'period of damping' in **188b**, how can the pop-test (flush-test) differentiate between a true low BP and an overdamped arterial line, and how can the trend of the diastolic and mean BPs help to differentiate between a truly low systolic BP and a damped trace with a false-low systolic BP?

ii. Describe the interpretation of the pop-test (flush-test) as demonstrated in **188a**.

iii. Describe the concept of 'damping' as related to overdamped arterial lines.

iv. List some causes of overdamped arterial lines.

v. Given an extreme/excessive amount of damping, what BP value will be approximated?

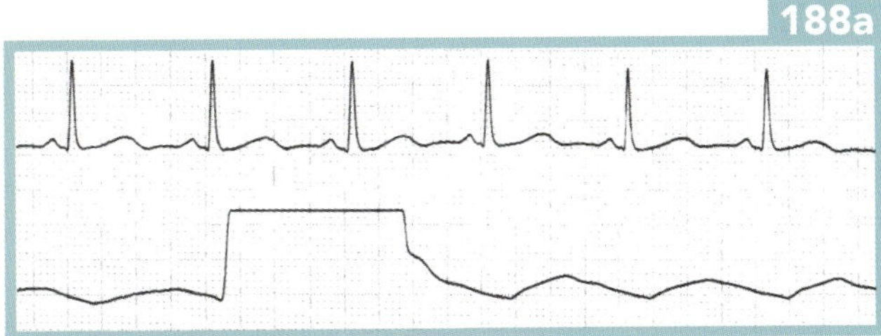

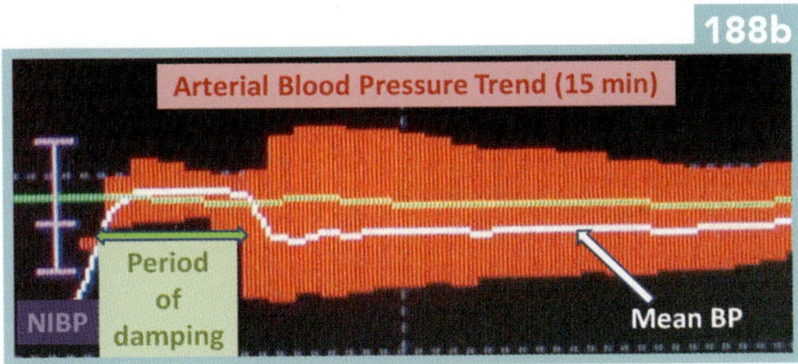

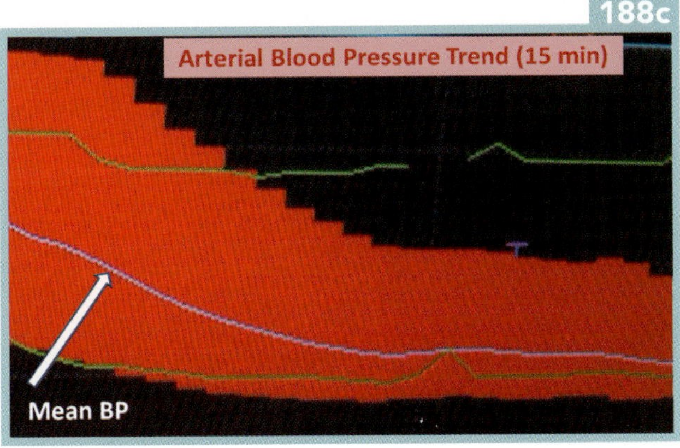

Answer 188

188i. The pop-test (flush-test) can be used to check if the arterial line is overdamped by noticing a slow return to baseline. The trend of the diastolic BP will demonstrate an increase in diastolic BP while the systolic BP is decreasing (**188b**, arrow). The trend of the mean BP will not show a decrease, as would be expected with a true hypotension. With a true episode of hypotension, all three measures of BP (systolic, diastolic and mean) will be decreasing (**188c**).

ii. It demonstrates a very slow return to the physiological BP tracing and values, with no oscillations. This is indicative of an overdamped arterial line.

iii. Damping occurs in an overdamped arterial line and is diagnosed by a slow return of the pressure trace to the BP values, with an absence of oscillating waves.

iv. An overdamped arterial line is mostly caused by a large air bubble in the line, which leads to a very low natural frequency response. Other common causes are an increased resistance in the arterial line, such as a kink, and/or a partially obstructed line due to blood clots.

v. When the arterial line is damped, the systolic excursion is decreased, leading to a falsely-low systolic BP and the diastolic excursion is also decreased, but this leads to a falsely-high diastolic BP. Both these phenomena are seen in **188b** (Period of damping) and the pulse pressure appears narrow. Given 'extreme' damping, the mean BP would be approximated and this is actually how the mean BP is determined by the equipment: the BP voltage is passed through a filter that 'dampens' and removes any excursion, thus only the mean BP remains.

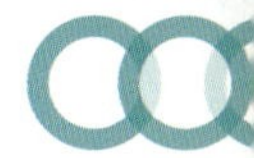

QUESTION 189

189 A patient is undergoing surgery in the sitting position. A change in the precordial Doppler sound monitor is noted associated with lower end-tidal CO_2 ($ETCO_2$) (**189a**) and decreased oxygen saturation (**189b**). The arterial line (initially damped) shows a normal BP (**189b**).

i. What do these changes indicate?

ii. Why does the $ETCO_2$ concentration decrease with this event? Explain the underlying physiology.

iii. In this scenario, could significant air be sucked out from the right atrium? What Doppler sound would be associated with significant amounts of right ventricular air?

iv. List the monitors that can detect gas (air) embolism. Rank from most to least sensitive.

v. List some anatomical sites (and/or surgeries) associated with air (room air) embolism. Embolism from pressurised infusion of air/CO_2 for procedures such as laparoscopy should not be included.

vi. Explain why gas embolism on the venous system can cause a stroke on the arterial system.

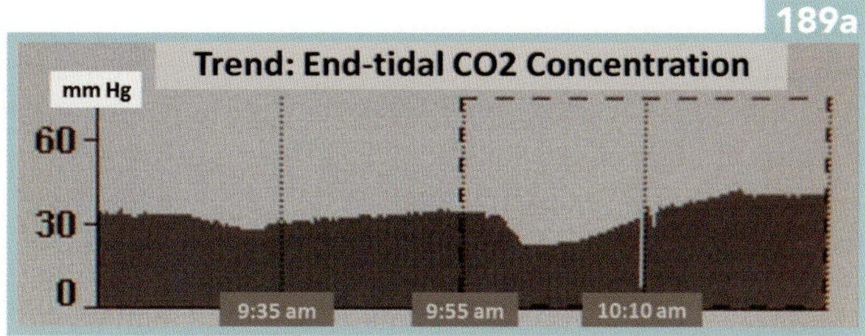

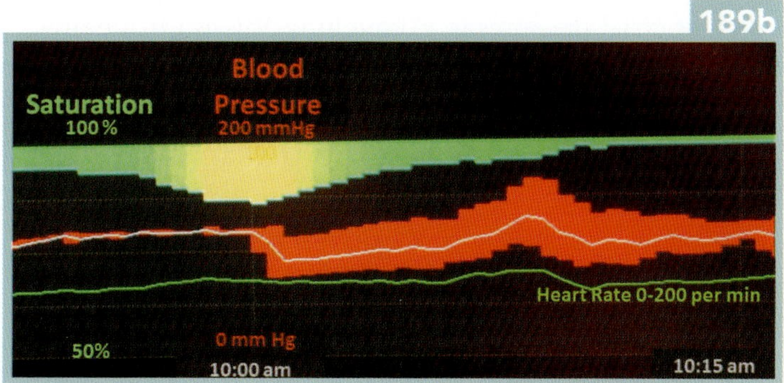

Answer 189

189i. An air embolus has occurred causing muffled heart sounds and a huge reduction in cardiac output, hence no $ETCO_2$.

ii. When limited gas (air and/or CO_2) enters the vasculature, gas bubbles break up and obstruct smaller branches of the pulmonary artery and the precapillary sphincters. Capillary blood flow to downstream alveoli is obstructed, leading to alveolar (aka 'parallel') dead space. Gas from this type of dead space is exhaled in parallel with alveolar gas, dilutes the alveolar gas plateau and increases the end-tidal to arterial CO_2 gradient.

iii. There are signs of air embolism but arterial BP is still normal, so an 'air lock' has not developed, therefore a significant amount of air in the right atrium is unlikely. The typical 'mill wheel murmur' of an air lock was not heard.

iv. (1) Transoesophageal Doppler; (2) precordial Doppler; (3) end-tidal nitrogen pressure (ETN_2 – requires the patient to be inhaling only oxygen to notice the small increase in nitrogen tension on a mass spectrometer).

Pulmonary artery pressure, capnography ($ETCO_2$), cardiac output, CVP, saturation, BP and right ventricular strain on ECG are not sensitive enough to be sole monitors for air embolism.

v. Craniotomy (sitting, prone and supine); shunt placement (e.g. ventriculoperitoneal shunt); central line (e.g. CVP) placement; cervical spine surgery (sitting and prone); thoracic and lumbar spine surgery (prone); uterus (hysterectomy and caesarean section); liver surgery; orthopaedic surgery (joint replacement, stemmed prosthesis insertion); otolaryngological procedures (sitting, head-up and supine).

vi. Two possible mechanisms are:

- Postmortem studies of victims of fatal car crashes showed that 28% had a 'probe patent foramen ovale' (i.e. the foramen ovale was not anatomically closed ['fused'], but 'physiologically' closed by the higher pressure in the left atrium). Increased right atrial pressures (e.g. coughing, Valsalva manoeuvre, pulmonary hypertension such as repeated gas emboli) can lead to right atrial pressure exceeding left atrial pressure and a paradoxical gas embolism developing.
- Gas emboli may also pass through pulmonary anatomical shunts.

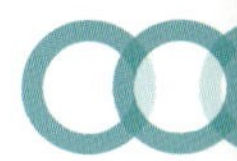

QUESTION 190

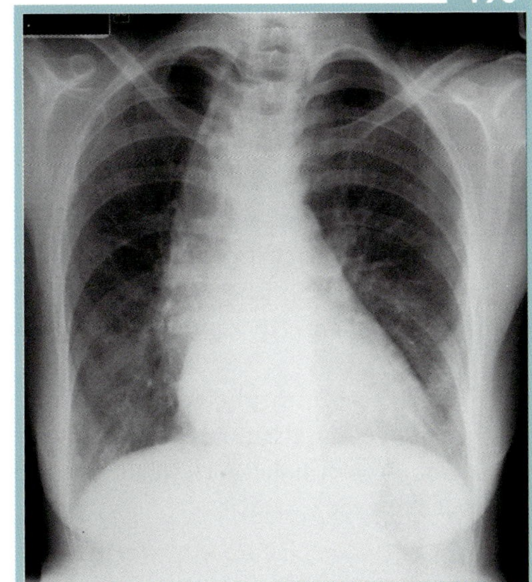
190

190 This CXR (**190**) was a routine film for a woman presenting for cholecystectomy. On direct questioning the patient mentions pain radiating to her back, which is associated with difficulty swallowing. Occasionally, food material regurgitates into her throat. Her family has ignored her complaints and insists that she has gallstones because of a positive abdominal ultrasound.

i. What condition does this patient have?

ii. What other conditions could mimic this condition?

iii. Why is this X-ray and history a source of concern for the anaesthesiologist?

iv. Are the gallstones pathological?

QUESTION 191

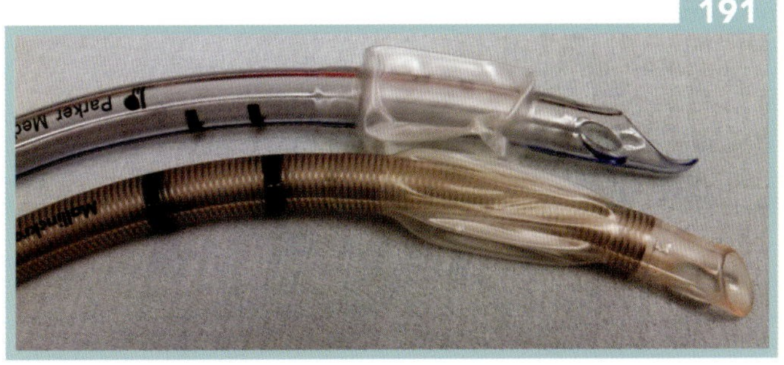

191

191i. What is the distance from the vocal cords to the carina in the normal adult patient?

ii. In which direction does the bevel point on a standard ET tube (lower tube, **191**)?

iii. Why might this be a problem during the management of a difficult intubation using a gum-elastic-bougie or an ET exchanger?

iv. Why does the 'Parker' ET tube (upper tube, **191**) have a curved tip with the bevel pointing posteriorly?

v. Why do some ET tubes have two lines on them near the cuff?

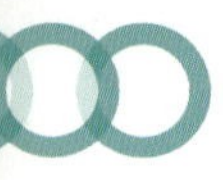

Answer 190

190i. Achalasia of the cardia.

ii. Although the symptoms this patient complains of are classical for achalasia, it can mimic gastritis, cholecystitis or an oesophageal tumour.

iii. The danger, shown clearly by the dilatation of the oesophagus on CXR, is that upper oesophageal contents (secretions or unswallowed food) can be aspirated and severely soil the lungs on induction of anaesthesia. A rapid sequence induction is needed to prevent aspiration of oesophageal contents.

iv. Thirty percent of the adult population over age 40 have gallstones. This may be a purely circumstantial finding and not necessarily pathological without classical symptoms of colicky right subcostal pain radiating to the ipsilateral shoulder or between the scapulae.

Answer 191

191i. The typical distance from the vocal cords to the carina is said to be 4 inches (10 cm).

ii. The bevel ('flat side') points to the left, implying that the 'sharp point' is pointing to the right side.

iii. The 'sharp point' on the right side might 'hang up' on the right vocal cord when advancing the tube ('rail-roading') over the bougie or the tube exchanger.

iv. The 'Parker' ET tube has the bevel ('flat side') pointing towards the posterior side, also with the tip curved posteriorly. This causes the tip of the tube to 'ride on' the anterior side of the introducer, gum-elastic-bougie or tube exchanger without encountering ('hanging up on') the right vocal cord.

v. The two lines indicate the manufacturers' suggestions as to the position of the vocal cords after intubation.

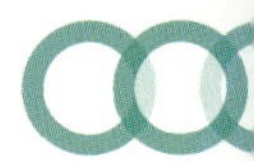

QUESTION 192

192 A researcher measures the time (in minutes) for soda lime to become exhausted on a human patient simulator using standardised conditions of CO_2 production. The data sets in the Table below are collected after the researcher has performed five runs with each type of soda lime.

Company	Duration of soda lime activity in minutes					Mean	Median	Mode
A	478	504	504	513	516			
B	491	492	505	505	512			
C	484	485	490	508	508			

Company A claims the means as measured prove that their soda lime lasts the longest.

Company B calculates the medians (middle values) for the three groups and claims their product lasts the longest.

Company C calculates the modes (most frequently occurring) for each type of soda lime and claims their product lasts the longest.

i. Calculate the mean, medians and modes for each data set.

ii. Which company's claim is correct?

iii. What should the researcher have done prior to the study to avoid such 'searching or fishing' for the best statistical test for their data?

iv. Are the differences in duration clinically relevant?

v. What should the researcher have done prior to the study in terms of clinically relevant differences?

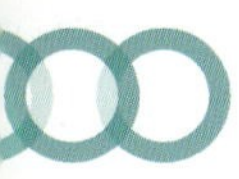

Answer 192

192i. See below:

Company	Duration of soda lime activity in minutes					Mean	Median	Mode
A	478	504	504	513	516	503	504	504
B	491	492	505	505	512	501	505	505
C	484	485	490	508	508	495	490	508

ii. Theoretically, each company's claim of 'best' is correct: given the measurement quoted by each company, that specific product is the 'best' and lasts the longest.

iii. The researcher should ideally have performed a pilot study, examined the distribution of the data (normally distributed or not) and decided on an appropriate statistical test prior to performing the study.

iv. The differences seem quite small when related to total duration (e.g. expressed as a percentage, or fraction, of duration).

v. Ideally, the researcher should have established what would be considered a clinically relevant difference in duration of action prior to performing the study. Such a clinically relevant difference might be arbitrary or be based on the literature (if such exists). **Note:** Even though a difference might be 'statistically significant', the difference might not necessarily be 'clinically relevant' or 'clinically important'.

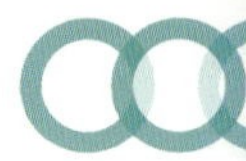

QUESTION 193

193 A medical researcher thinks that most patients with arm and leg fractures are much shorter than patients with gunshot wounds and wishes to test this hypothesis. The height distribution of patients presenting to a small hospital with arm fractures and gunshot wounds is shown (**193**).

i. Are the data normally distributed?

ii. Is there possibly a selection bias in the data if the hospital is located between an equestrian race track and the police barracks.

iii. The data are on an interval scale and a Student's t-test was used to test for differences in the heights of patients with fractures and gunshot wounds. No statistically significant difference was found. Is a Student's t-test appropriate for this data set? Explain your answer. Give three requirements necessary before a Student's t-test may be used.

iv. Would a Mann-Whitney U test (or another non-parametric test) be appropriate for this data set? Explain your answer.

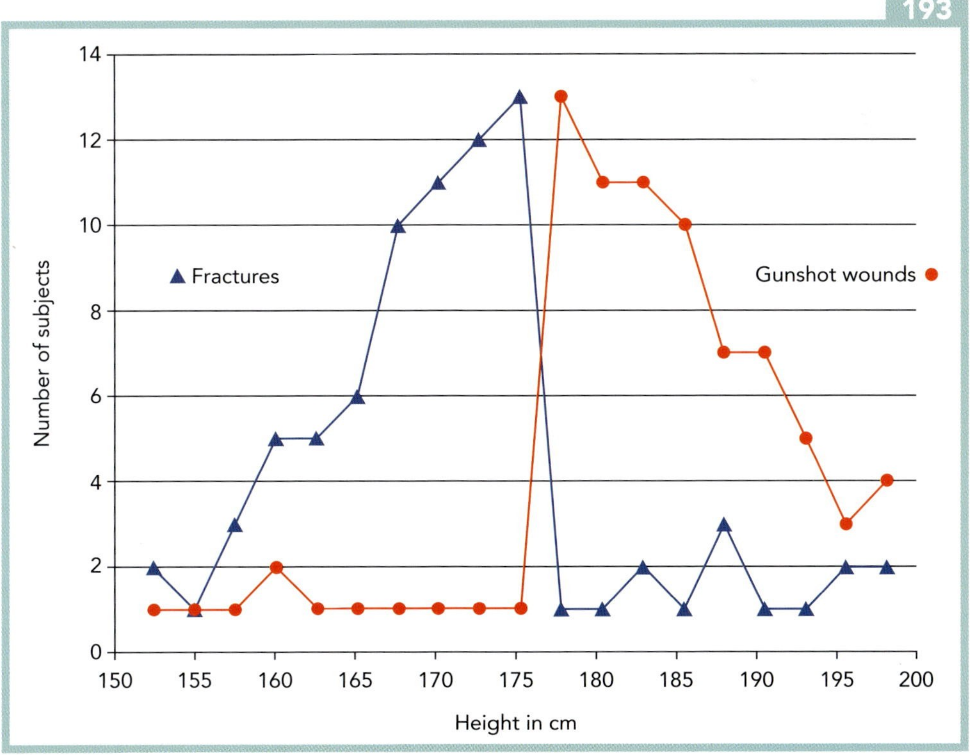

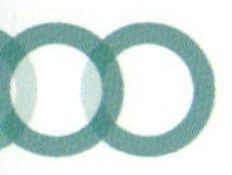

Answer 193

193i. The graph shows the heights of patients with fractures to have a peak at 175 cm (70 in) and very few taller subjects. The graph also shows the heights of patients with gunshot wounds to be mainly above 178 cm (71 in) and only a few shorter subjects. The data are not normally distributed, but are skewed (left and right).

ii. Yes, there is most likely a selection bias. Jockeys from the race track would tend to be smaller and have more fractures, while the policemen from the barracks would tend to be taller and have more gunshot wounds. It is possible for jockeys to occasionally have gunshot wounds and for policemen to have fractures.

iii. A Student's t-test is not appropriate because the data are not being normally distributed. Provisions/requirements necessary before a Student's t-test may be used include normal distribution, interval data, similar variances (distributions) of the data, independent variables (except for paired t-test).

iv. A Mann-Whitney test is a so-called 'distribution free' test (i.e. it does not matter if the data are not normally distributed). The test ranks the groups from small to large (or large to small) and tests for the number of occurrences of one condition (fractures) before occurrences of the second condition (gunshot wounds). From the data distribution, it is clear that a statistically significant majority of fractures do occur in patients shorter than the subjects with gunshot wounds. The Student's t-test was not the correct test to select, and therefore it did not identify the statistically significant difference between the groups.

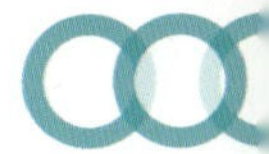

QUESTION 194

194 The kidney shown (**194**) has been removed from a 54-year-old male donor and is about to be transplanted into a suitably matched recipient. The forceps are holding the renal artery and vein. In addition to providing safe and effective GA for both patients:

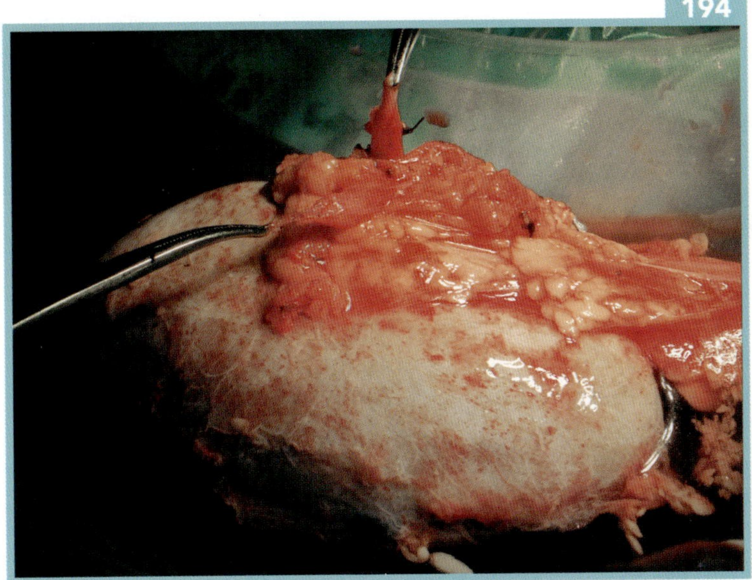

194

i. What specific intraoperative management is relevant to the donor to maximise the chances of successful transplantation?

ii. How is the recipient managed intraoperatively to maximise the chances of successful receipt of the transplanted organ?

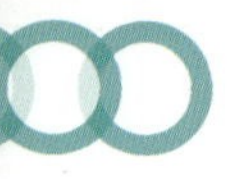

Answer 194

194i. The donor should be healthy with normal renal function. Management can be divided into:

- Fluids. Preoperatively at least 1 litre of IV fluid should be given to boost urine output and additional IV crystalloid (usually Hartmann's solution) should be given to achieve a positive fluid balance of approximately 3–4 litres during surgery. Oesophageal Doppler may also be useful in optimising perfusion. When the kidney has been removed, this fluid loading ceases in order to prevent overloading the donor once the kidney has been removed.
- Maintenance of good perfusion pressure to the donated kidney. Arterial line monitoring should be established to ensure that arterial BP does not fall below a mean arterial pressure of 70–80 mmHg, as below this level renal perfusion can be adversely affected.

ii. Management of the recipient should concentrate on:

- Fluids. A CVP line is essential and, arbitrarily, a CVP level of 7–10 mmHg should be attempted to ensure optimal fluid loading for the transplanted kidney. Use of transoesophageal Doppler can also further aid fluid management to optimise the cardiovascular conditions for the implanted kidney. Large volumes of normal saline (2–3 litres) may be required if the patient appears preoperatively dry. Hartmann's solution should not be used as it contains potassium, which may be elevated postoperatively until the new kidney establishes itself.
- Renal tubular assistance. Mannitol (12.5–25g [125–250 ml of 10% solution]) aids renal perfusion, promotes free radical scavenging and encourages a diuresis in the transplanted kidney.
- Immunosuppression. Should be commenced as soon as possible after implantation of the donor kidney. The drugs likely to be administered intraoperatively are the calcineurin inhibitors basiliximab or daclizumab (for induction immunosuppression) and supplemental immunosuppressive steroids (e.g. methylpredisolone).
- Lines. Arterial lines are discouraged as the patient's arterial tree should be maintained as intact as possible. Arteriovenous shunts will be needed for dialysis if the transplant fails. Peripheral venous lines or BP cuffs should not be sited on the side of an established fistula.

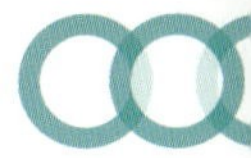

QUESTION 195

195i. Describe the basic physiological reasons for myasthenia gravis (MG) (**195**, from *Browse's Introduction to the Symptoms & Signs of Surgical Disease*, Fifth Edition, 2014, with permission).

ii. Why is this important to understand in anaesthesia?

iii. What are the symptoms of MG?

iv. What drug treatments are available?

v. What tests can be employed to aid diagnosis?

195

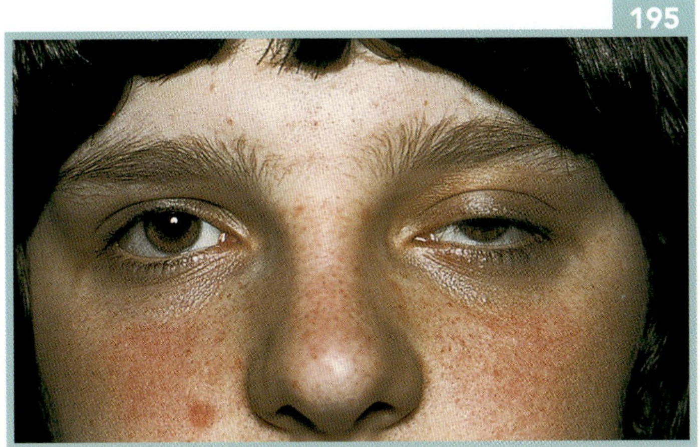

Answer 195

195i. MG is a disorder of neuromuscular transmission caused by either genetic anatomical or acquired immunological abnormalities of the neuromuscular junction (NMJ). Anatomical distortion of the postsynaptic muscle membrane, or its disruption by antibodies, reduces the effect of acetylcholine (ACh) and decreases nerve impulses.

ii. Muscle relaxants (and reversal agents) affect ACh levels at the NMJ and should be avoided in a myasthenic patient to prevent very prolonged/dangerous paralysis. Regional or local anaesthesia should be used when possible. 'Deep' inhalational anaesthesia without relaxants can be used but this leads to cardiovascular depression at muscle relaxing doses. If relaxants are essential, perioperative neuromuscular transmission must be monitored by a nerve stimulator. Reversal agents should not be used as they unpredictably disturb ACh levels at the muscle end-plate. Prolonged postoperative ventilation should be expected for myasthenic patients.

iii. MG is often picked up by ocular signs (ptosis or diplopia – often unilateral) (66% of cases) or oropharyngeal muscle weakness (difficulty chewing, swallowing or talking) (16%), but limb weakness is rare. Symptoms worsen as the day progresses or with fatigue, emotional upset, systemic illness (especially viral infections), hypothyroidism or hyperthyroidism, pregnancy, the menstrual cycle, drugs affecting neuromuscular transmission and increases in body temperature. After 15–20 years the weakness may become fixed, with atrophic muscles.

iv. There is no complete treatment for MG. Cholinesterase inhibitors (e.g. pyridostigmine/neostigmine) retard enzymatic hydrolysis of ACh at cholinergic synapses, allowing ACh accumulation at the NMJ and prolonging its effect. Marked improvement can occur with steroids. Azothiaprine, cyclosporine or cyclophosphamide are second-line treatments but may cause immunosuppression. Plasma exchange and IV immunoglobulin can alleviate symptoms for short-term benefit prior to surgery.

v. The Tensilon® test assists diagnosis. Weakness improves after IV edrophonium chloride. IM neostigmine, which has a longer duration of action, may work better in some patients and is particularly useful in children, whose response to IV edrophonium chloride may be too brief to observe. Electromyography and repetitive nerve stimulation (RNS) are useful for diagnosis. A significant decrement to RNS in either a hand or shoulder muscle is found in most (60%) patients with MG.

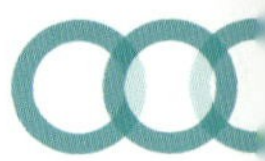

QUESTION 196

196 Consider a classic anaesthetic machine that does not have fresh gas flow compensation:

i. What does it mean when an anaesthetic machine is not 'fresh gas flow compensated'? Use the drawing shown (**196**) to explain your answer.

ii. List three possible changes in ventilator settings and one other setting that could affect the contribution of the fresh gas flow to the tidal volume.

iii. Does lack of fresh gas flow compensation affect the tidal volume in 'volume mode settings' on the ventilator?

iv. Does lack of fresh gas flow compensation affect the tidal volume in a 'pressure mode' of ventilation?

v. Does fresh gas flow compensation influence the tidal volume in manual mode (i.e. with 'hand ventilation')?

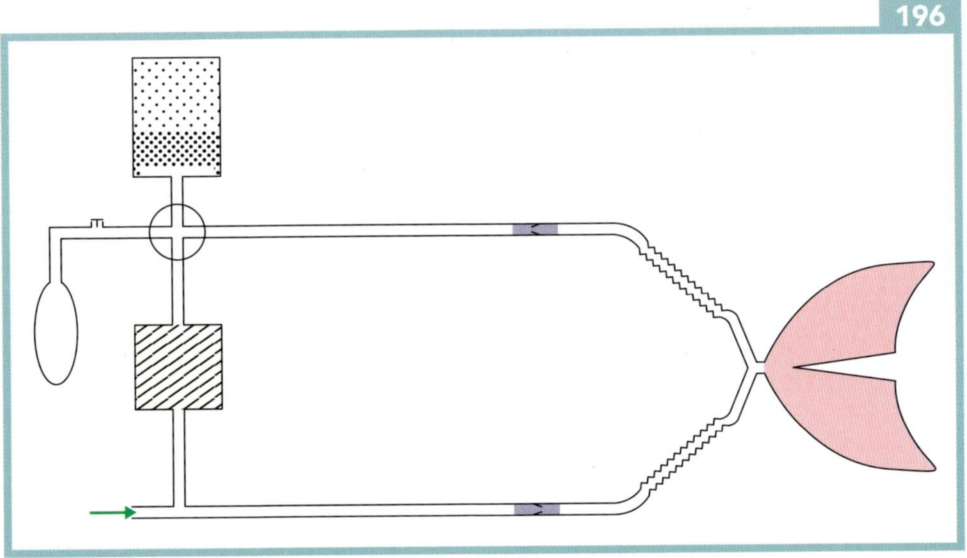

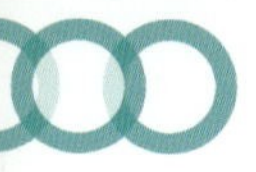

Answer 196

196i. Fresh gas flow, in older anaesthetic machines, continues to flow into the circle system throughout all phases of ventilation. The volume of fresh gas flow that flows during the period of inspiration is in addition to the tidal volume provided by the ventilator (with volume mode settings). The tidal volume delivered to the patient therefore varies with the settings (inspiratory duration) of the ventilator as well as with the amount of the fresh gas flow during the inspiratory period. The phenomenon of fresh gas flow affecting the tidal volume delivered to the patient is called 'not fresh gas flow compensated'.

ii. Any change in ventilator settings that alters the duration of inspiration would alter the contribution of the fresh gas flow to the tidal volume delivered by the ventilator. For instance: respiratory rate; I:E ratio; inspiratory duration (on anaesthetic machines with this setting); the fresh gas flow rate as set on the flow meters affects the tidal volume.

iii. During the inspiratory phase with a volume mode setting on the ventilator, no gas escapes from the breathing system and the tidal volume is affected.

iv. In the pressure mode of ventilation, the tidal volume is dependent on the maximum pressure (peak inspiratory pressure) in the breathing system, and any extra gas from the flow meters will not have any effect on the tidal volume.

v. During manual ventilation, the tidal volume is limited by the pop-off pressure, and extra fresh gas flow does not affect the tidal volume.

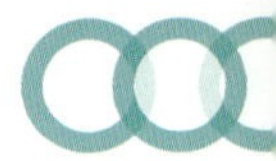

QUESTION 197

197 A soda lime absorber is shown (**197a**). The inspired CO_2 is noted to be increasing on the capnogram.

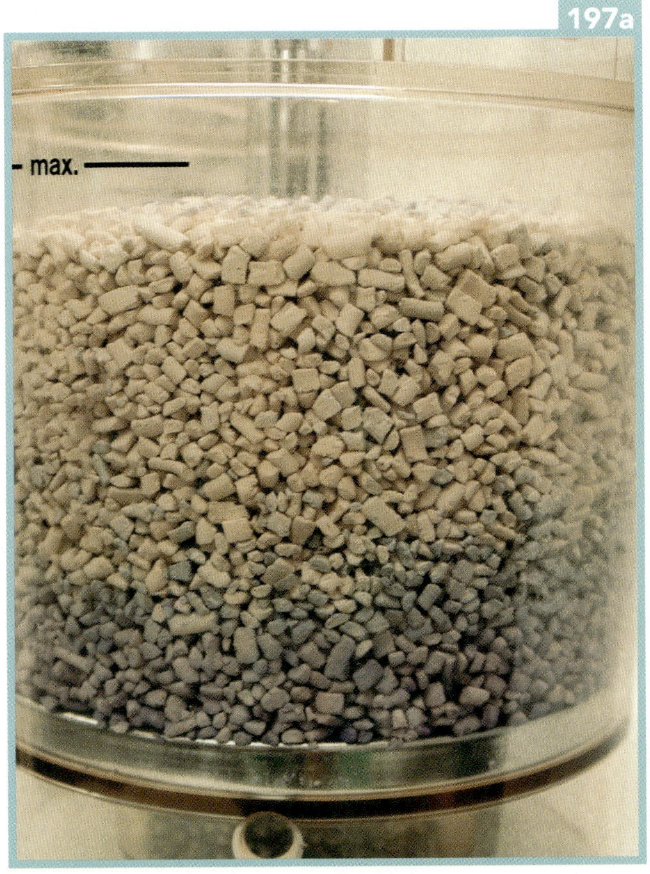

197a

i. Could the soda lime be exhausted even though the colour change has not yet reached the top of the canister?

ii. If this does happen, what mechanisms might cause this?

iii. Does 'channelling' occur in an upright soda lime canister?

iv. Describe a second mechanism that might lead to CO_2 breakthrough without a colour change.

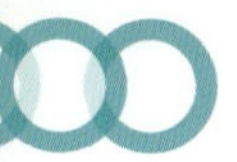

Answer 197

197i. Yes, CO_2 breakthrough can occur even though the soda lime does not appear to be exhausted (see **197b**).

ii. 'Channelling' can occur when exhaled gas passes through an area of the canister that is not filled with soda lime. It is much commoner in canisters that are horizontal.

iii. Channelling can occur in an upright canister, as indicated in **197b**.

iv. CO_2 breakthrough can occur by 'reactivation'. Over time, the colour change can be reversed as the slow reaction catches up. However, the colour change to blue with a second exposure is not reliable.

197b

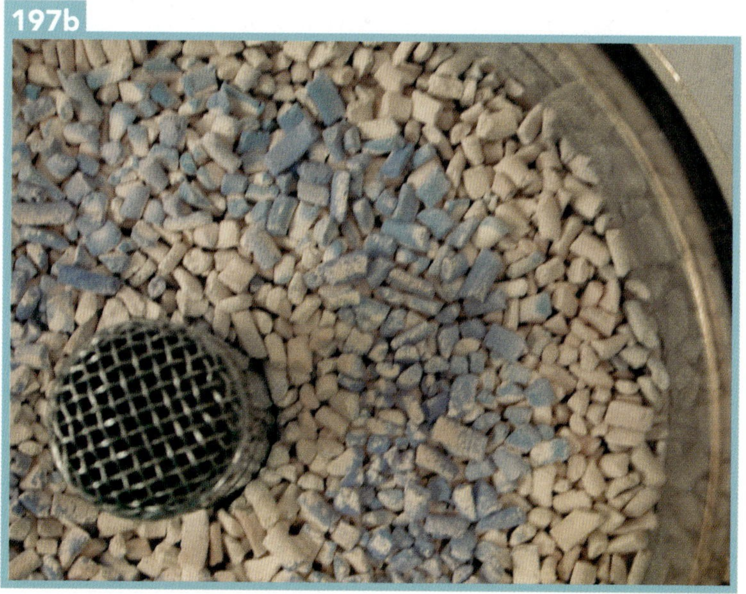

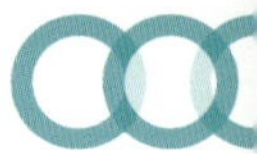

QUESTION 198

198 During the preanaesthesia check, the internal compliance of an anaesthetic machine is reported as 2.8 ml per cmH_2O (**198**). If a normal patient is ventilated with a tidal volume of 700 ml, and the resulting plateau pressure is 20 cmH_2O (assume that the measurements are accurate):

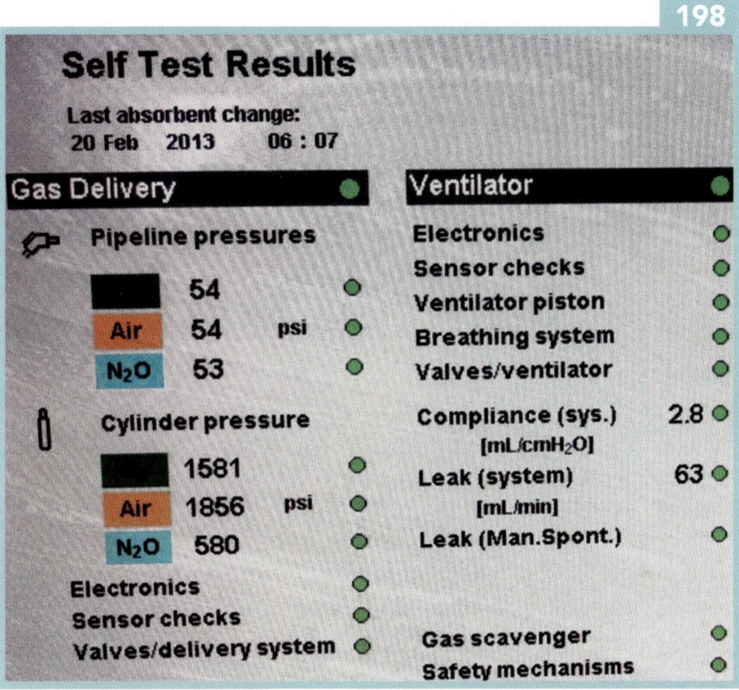

i. Explain what you understand by the concept 'internal compliance of an anaesthetic machine'.

ii. What factors affect this measurement?

iii. Given a basic (non-computerised) anaesthetic machine: (1) what volume of gas will be pumped out of the ventilator bellows (or piston); and (2) will the volume of gas pumped into the patient's lungs be more, equal to, or less than 700 ml?

iv. At a plateau pressure of 20 cmH_2O, calculate the volume of gas involved in question (ii) (i.e. any difference between ventilator output and volume received into the lungs).

v. Which gas law is applicable?

vi. Given a computerised anaesthetic machine (with 'compliance compensation'), what tidal volume will the ventilator put out to the patient's lungs?

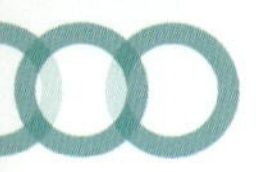

Answer 198

198i. 'Internal compliance of an anaesthetic machine' describes the compressibility of gas inside the machine (i.e. for every 1 cmH_2O pressure increase in the system, a certain amount of gas will be compressed inside the piping, ventilator and breathing system).

ii. A major factor is the internal volume of the breathing system (hence thinner tubes for use in paediatrics). Another factor is the volume in the ventilator at the end of the inspiratory stroke (bag-in-the-box or piston design).

iii. (1) The volume exiting the bellows might be 700 ml; (2) because some of the gas will be compressed inside the anaesthetic machine and breathing system, the gas entering the patient's lungs will be less than 700 ml.

iv. Given a compliance of 2.8 ml per cmH_2O and a plateau pressure of 20 cmH_2O, the amount of gas compressed inside the anaesthetic machine and breathing system will be 56 ml of gas (20 cm H_2O times 2.8 ml per cm H_2O).

v. Boyle's Law ($P1 \times V1 = P2 \times V2$).

vi. Modern, computerised anaesthetic ventilators often compensate for internal compliance by adding an extra amount of gas, over the set tidal volume, to compensate for the 'loss' due to compressibility (internal compliance) inside the anaesthetic machine and breathing system. In this case, the anaesthetic machine will put out a tidal volume of 756 ml. There is a design limit for such compensation; for example, the engineers might elect to provide a maximum compensation of 50% of the set tidal volume.

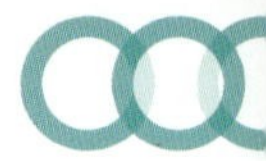

QUESTION 199

199 A 10 kg (22 lb) child is being ventilated with a set tidal volume of 100 ml and a plateau pressure of 20 cmH_2O. The anaesthetic is continued in the magnetic resonance imaging (MRI) suite for a postoperative MRI scan. A non-MRI compatible anaesthetic machine is available outside the MRI suite and a very long set of corrugated tubing as part of a circle system is used (**199**).

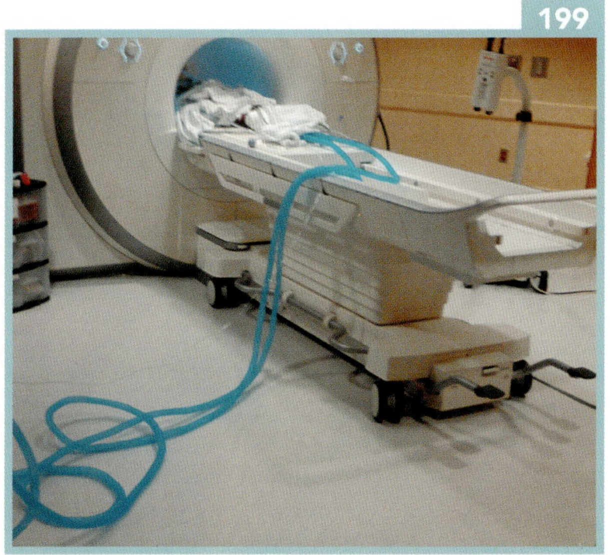

199

i. What is the (approximate) compliance of the child's lungs?

ii. How can you determine the internal compliance of an anaesthetic machine with lengthy corrugated tubing?

iii. Given an internal compliance of 5 ml per cmH_2O for the anaesthetic machine and long breathing tubes, what volume of gas is compressed inside the machine and breathing tubes (i.e. what is the internal compliance of the anaesthetic machine and breathing system)?

iv. If a tidal volume of 100 ml is set on the anaesthetic machine, what tidal volume can we expect the child's lungs to receive?

v. Would it be acceptable and/or advantageous to use a pressure controlled rather than a volume controlled ventilation mode under these circumstances? Explain your answer.

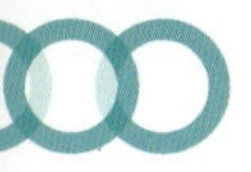

Answer 199

199i. The compliance of the child's lungs is calculated from the change in volume (delta V) divided by the change in pressure (delta P). In this case, 100 ml divided by 20 cmH_2O, giving a compliance of 5 ml per cmH_2O.

ii. One method to determine the internal compliance of a system with very long tubes is as follows: the outflow of the circle system (outlet of the Y-connector) is totally occluded, a smallish tidal volume (e.g. 50–100 ml) is set on the machine so that the pressure developed will be in the range of the plateau pressure of the prospective patient. In this case a tidal volume of 50 ml was used and the pressure was found to be 10 cmH_2O, giving a compliance of 5 ml per cmH_2O (i.e. 50 ml divided by 10 cm H_2O).

iii. At a plateau pressure of 20 cmH_2O and a compliance of 5 ml per cmH_2O, the amount of gas compressed in the anaesthetic machine and breathing tubes is 100 ml.

iv. Given that the compliance of the child's lungs and the compliance of the anaesthetic machine are equal, the set tidal volume will be distributed equally between the two compliances, and the child's lungs will only receive a tidal volume of 50 ml (with a ventilator setting of 100 ml tidal volume).

v. Using a pressure controlled ventilation mode would cause the ventilator to continue to increase the outflow from the ventilator until the pressure reaches the desired level (in this case, 20 cm H_2O). This would overcome the increased compliance due to the long corrugated tubing and ensure that the tidal volume into the child's lung would be sufficient.

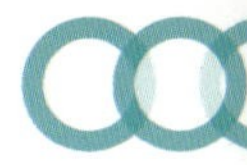

QUESTION 200

200 An 18 g needle has a greater diameter (is 'thicker') than a 22 g needle (**200**).

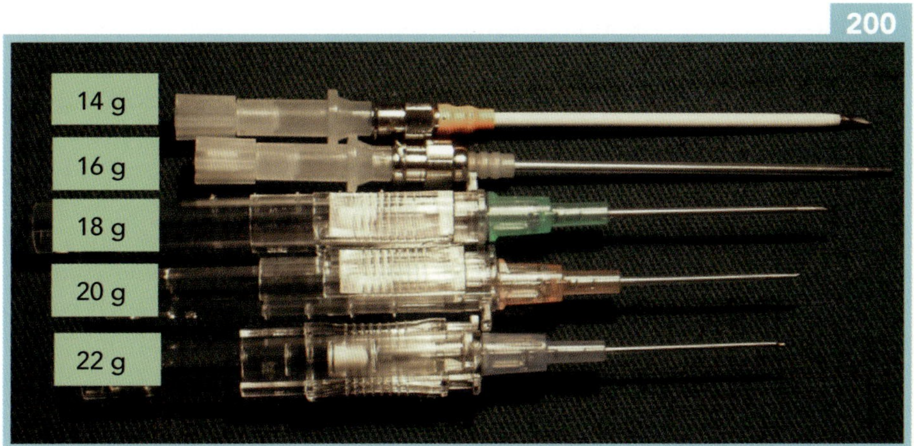

i. What does the abbreviation 'g' indicate?

ii. What does the abbreviation 'SWG' indicate?

iii. Why does a higher number (e.g. 22 g) indicate a smaller diameter than 14 g?

iv. Does 18 g indicate inner diameter or outer diameter?

v. How long does it take to infuse 1 litre of crystalloid solution through each of the cannulae below, and what is their maximum flow per minute?
   - a, 14 g (orange).
   - b, 16 g (grey).
   - c, 18 g★ (green).
   - d, 20 g★ (pink).
   - e, 22 g★ (blue).

   ★ = not considered suitable for emergency resuscitation in adults.

Answer 200

200i. The abbreviation 'g' indicates gauge (i.e. the diameter of the needle).

ii. It indicates Standard Wire Gauge. Earlier names associated with this form of gauge are, in the UK, Holtzapffel and Stubs Wire Gauge. In the USA the terms US Birmingham Wire Gage and British Standard Wire Gauge were used.

iii. Historically, during the wire making process, a rod of metal is heated and 'pulled' (stretched) through a specific sized hole in a draw plate. With each additional pull through the next smaller hole in the draw plate, the wire is stretched to a thinner gauge. The SWG indicates the number of pulls through the machine. Hence, a 22 SWG has been pulled through a smaller hole than a 16 gauge. Each pull (and decrement in size) had to be within specific tolerances, so that the wire would not break during the pulling process.

iv. It indicates the outer diameter.

v. Minimum times for 1 litre infusion and maximum flow rates in ml/minute are:
a = 3.7 minutes (270 ml/minute);
b = 4.2 minutes (236 ml/minute);
c = 10 minutes (103 ml/minute);
d = 15 minutes (67 ml/minute);
e = 32 minutes (31 ml/minute).

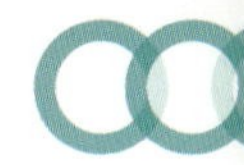

QUESTION 201

201 A cardiopulmonary exercise test (CPET) result from a patient with an oesophageal cancer with a poor prognosis is shown (**201**). The graph shows how the ventilatory anaerobic threshold (VAT) is determined by the V-slope method.

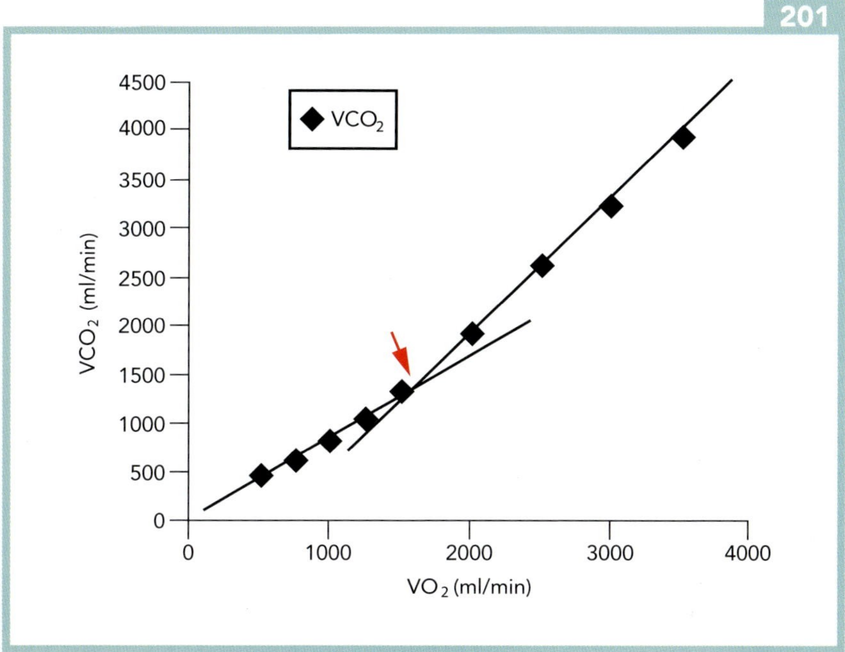

i. What two things need to be known before this test can be interpreted correctly, and what three calculations constitute the CPET?

ii. What physiological principle needs to be known to understand CPET.

iii. Define PVO_2. What is normal in a resting state and at peak exercise?

iv. What does the arrow indicate?

v. Is this test result acceptable to allow oesophageal resection for carcinoma?

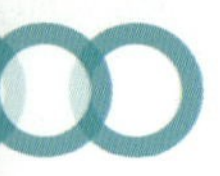

Answer 201

201i. The patient's weight has to be known so that the oxygen uptake can be normalised for body weight. The exercise protocol also needs to be known in order to judge whether the patient has been correctly exercised and a true result is shown. The patient is usually placed on an exercise bike and VO_{2max}, VAT and maximal heart rate are recorded.

ii. The Fick equation (uptake of oxygen by the tissues equals cardiac output times the arterial mixed venous oxygen content) is essential to understanding CPET:

$$VO_{2max} = (SVmax \times \text{ Heart rate max}) \times (CaO_{2max} - CvO_{2max})$$

The maximum rate at which a person can take in and utilise oxygen defines the functional aerobic capacity. If this capacity is likely to be exceeded during surgery, there is a high chance of detrimental cardiovascular events associated with surgery.

iii. PVO_2 (l/minute) is the peak oxygen uptake achievable by the patient and is the point at which a plateau occurs on a graph of VO_2 and work rate. In a resting subject it is usually about 3.5 ml/kg/minute or 250 ml. This rises to about 15 times more in extreme exercise (30–50 ml/kg/minute). Athletes can achieve up to 80 ml/kg/minute.

iv. The arrow shows the VAT. Patients with a high operative adverse cardiovascular event rate have a VAT of <10 ml/kg/minute; those with a good cardiovascular prognosis have a VAT of >18 ml/kg/minute.

v. The VAT is the point at which the slope of the relative rate of increase in VCO_2 relative to VO_2 changes, illustrated by the point at which the two lines superimposed on the patient's readings cross. In this patient, it occurred at a VO_2 of 1.5 l/minute, or 50% of PVO_2 and at 1,750 ml/minute oxygen uptake. As a VAT greater than 40% is normal, and this patient's peak oxygen content is satisfactory, it seems that these measures of physiological reserve suggest that he will survive the immediate surgical period. However, because of the nature of oespohageal cancer, overall survival is difficult to predict.

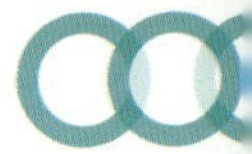

QUESTION 202

202 A 21-year-old male weighing 60 kg (132 lb) is anaesthetised for incision and drainage of a perianal abscess with the following drugs: propofol 180mg, fentanyl 100μg and amoxicillin/clavulinic acid 1.2 g. A laryngeal mask is inserted. His BP is found to be 60/20 mmHg immediately after induction and he develops bronchospasm and marked erythema of his entire body. There is marked 'tracking' along the vein where the antibiotic was injected.

i. What is your differential diagnosis?

ii. Describe the clinical features of the most likely diagnosis in detail.

iii. Outline the correct treatment.

iv. How is the pathology further quantified?

QUESTION 203

203i. How would you interpret this ECG (**203**)?

ii. What are the advantages of the type of device demonstrated by this ECG?

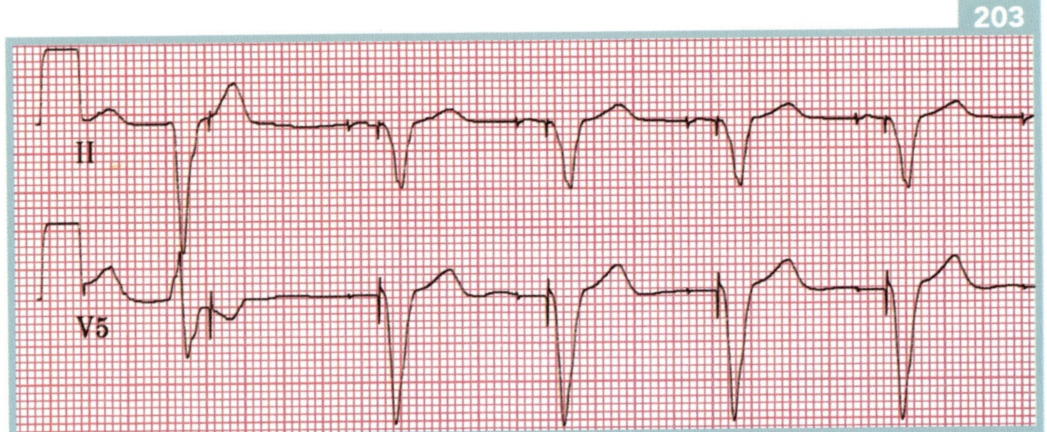

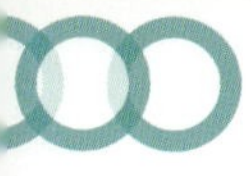

Answer 202

202i. The BP drop alone may be anaesthesia overdose or unmasked severe sepsis (the patient is very slight), but bronchospasm and erythema mean that anaphylaxis is the most likely diagnosis.

ii. All these features are not necessarily present (incidence in brackets): cardiovascular collapse (88%); erythema (45%); bronchospasm (36%); angioedema (24%); cutaneous signs/rash (13%); urticaria (8.5%); generalised oedema (7%).

iii. Emergency treatment (the 'anaphylaxis drill'). Stop administering the suspected drug and terminate any surgical procedure as soon as possible. Maintain the airway and give 100% oxygen. Lay the patient flat with the feet elevated. Give adrenaline. In cardiovascular collapse, up to 0.5 to 1 mg (5–10 ml of 1:10,000) should be given IV by titration at a rate of 0.1 mg/min. This is potentially dangerous and should only be performed by experienced personnel. The minimum dose should be given and stopped when BP is restored. For milder reactions, 0.5 mg adrenaline may be given IM. Rapid fluid loading with crystalloid or colloid solution must be undertaken, with possibly litres of fluid required to counter the extravasation of fluid into the tissues. A continuing adrenaline infusion may be necessary, commencing at 4–8 μg/min (0.05–0.1 μg/kg/min). 5 mg adrenaline should be diluted with 50 ml normal saline and run by controlled infusion at 5 ml per hour. This gives 8.3 μg/min and the effect can be titrated to BP.

Adjunct therapy. Antihistamines counter histamine release caused by anaphylaxis (e.g. chlorpheniramine, 10–20 mg by slow IV infusion). Steroids are helpful but may take 6 hours to be effective (100–300 mg hydrocortisone by IV bolus). Bronchodilators (salbutamol/albuterol) may ease bronchospasm.

iv. Follow up identification of allergen. 5–10 ml of blood should be taken in a plain blood tube for antigen testing to help determine the cause of the anaphylaxis. Repeat samples should be taken 12 and 24 hours after the reaction. Samples are analysed for tryptase (a mast cell enzyme) and IgE. IgE may be 'typed' (for suxamethonium, penicillin, ampicillin and latex) to show the exact cause of the reaction. Tryptase is high soon after a true anaphylactic reaction, falling to normal limits within 24 hours.

Answer 203

203i. The ECG demonstrates the presence of, and regular capture by, an antrioventricular sequential pacemaker.

ii. The atrial 'kick' provided by the atrial pacemaker helps to improve ventricular filling and cardiac output.

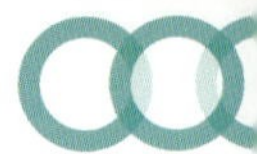

QUESTION 204

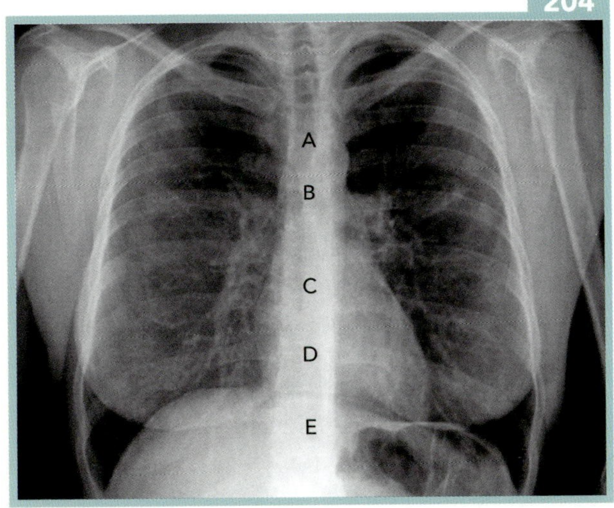

204 With regard to the positions marked A, B, C, D and E on the CXR shown (**204**):

i. At which position(s) would it be appropriate to place the tip of an oesophageal temperature probe? The temperature probe might be incorporated into an oesophageal stethoscope.

ii. Would A or B be ideal (appropriate) positions?

iii. Why would E not be an appropriate position during abdominal surgery?

iv. Which diseases are considered relative or absolute contraindications to the use of oesophageal devices such as a temperature probe or a TOE probe.

QUESTION 205

205 An intra-aortic balloon pump trace of a patient brought to the operating room for cardiac surgery is shown (**205a**).

i. Comment on the arterial wave form.

ii. What action should be taken?

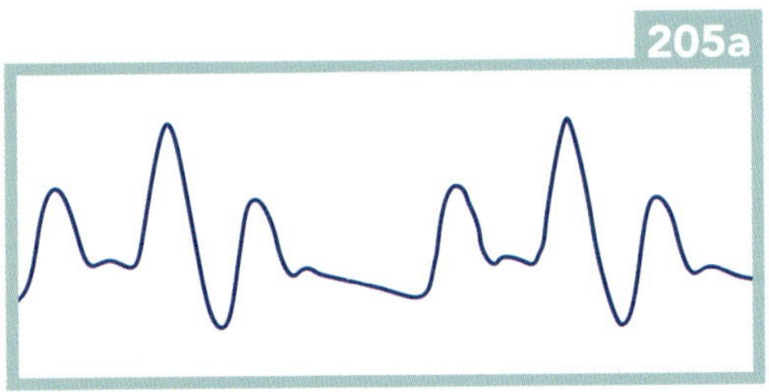

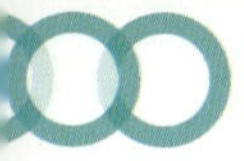

Answer 204

204i. The lower third of the oesophagus, situated behind the heart, is the ideal position for an oesophageal temperature probe (positions C and D).

ii. Position A (behind the trachea) and position B (behind the carina) might be affected by the temperature in the airway (usually colder than core body temperature).

iii. Position E (inside the stomach) might be affected by the temperature surrounding the stomach, such as a saline wash-out of the abdomen. Brief periods (2–3 minutes) of temperature alterations indicate such errors. The gas flow during a laparoscopy might also affect the reading (also usually a false-low temperature).

iv. Oesophageal varices, foreign body in the oesophagus, oesophageal diverticula and oesophageal rupture are contraindications to placement of an oesophageal temperature probe or TOE probe.

Answer 205

205i. The arterial wave form demonstrates intra-aortic balloon pumping in a 1:2 assist ratio. This setting allows identification of landmarks on the patient's arterial trace to guide timing settings. The patient's trace demonstrates late inflation of the balloon. The goal of balloon inflation is to produce a rapid rise in aortic diastolic pressure, thereby increasing oxygen supply to coronary circulation.

ii. Balloon inflation should occur just prior to the dicrotic notch (DN) of the arterial wave. Properly timed inflation will result in a peak diastolic pressure (PDP) greater than peak systolic pressure (PSP). Late balloon inflation results in a PDP that is less than optimal. This reduces aortic perfusion pressure and volume to the coronary arteries. The appropriate action is to make inflation occur earlier, just prior to the DN, as shown in **205b**.

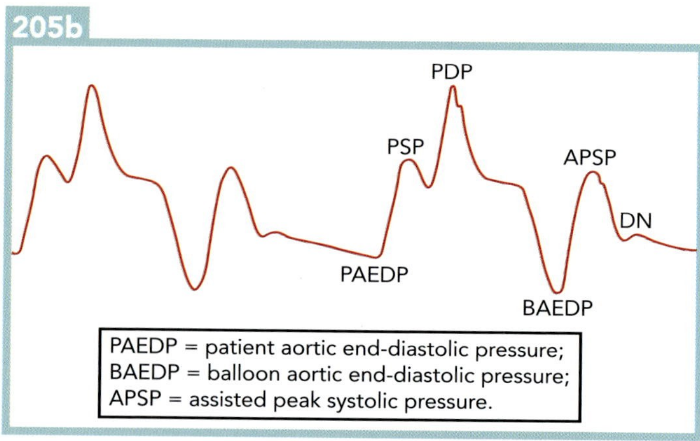

PAEDP = patient aortic end-diastolic pressure; BAEDP = balloon aortic end-diastolic pressure; APSP = assisted peak systolic pressure.

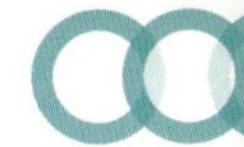

QUESTION 206

206 A CT scan is shown (**206**). The residual volume (RV) in this patient, as measured with a helium dilution rebreathing technique and a nitrogen wash-out technique, is found to be 1.5 litres less than the RV determined with a 'body box' (plethysmographic box).

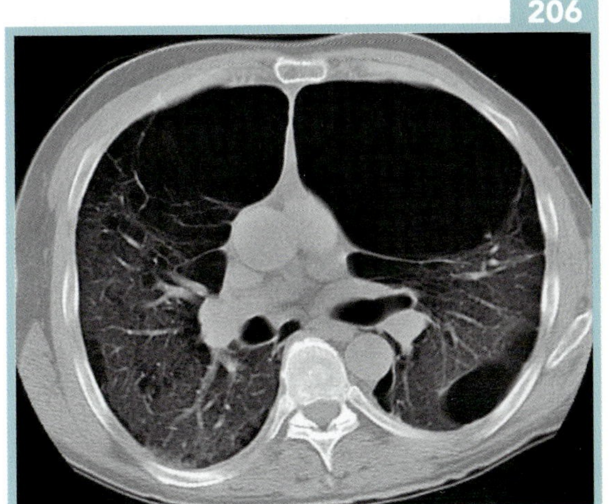

206

i. What characteristic of the bullae would lead to such a discrepancy?

ii. Explain why the volume of some types of bullae should not be measured with a helium dilution or nitrogen wash-out technique.

iii. Would the gas in the intestines be measured as RV with a body box technique?

QUESTION 207

207 A CT scan is shown (**207**).

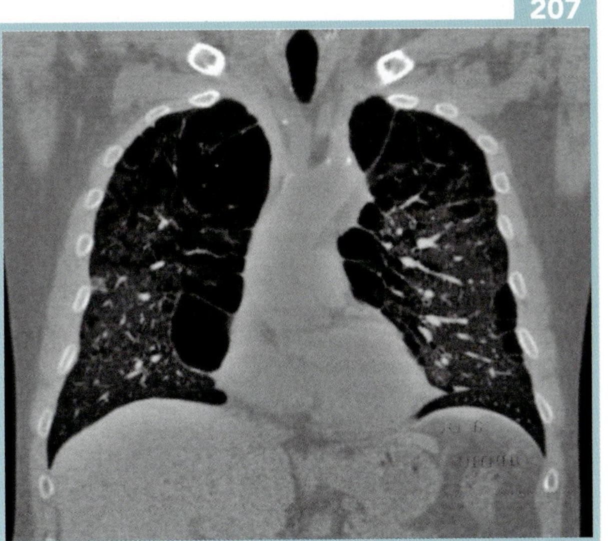

207

i. Would you use nitrous oxide (N_2O) in this patient? Explain your answer.

ii. Are there some patients with lung cavities where it is theoretically safe to use N_2O?

iii. What two tests would you request to compare to determine if N_2O would be safe?

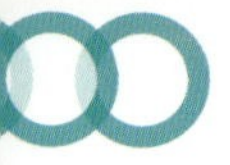

Answer 206

206i. The discrepancy in RV measurements results from whether the bullae are connected to the airways or not connected (i.e. isolated).

ii. Bullae that are open and connected to the airways participate in the mixing of inhaled gases. Such connecting bullae will therefore be measured with a helium dilution and a nitrogen wash-out technique. Isolated bullae, by not being connected to the airways, will not be measured by dilution and inhalation techniques but can be measured by a body box technique, which measures all bullae.

iii. Any gas inside the body (including gas in the intestines) would be measured by a body box technique. It will be compressed by increased pressures in the body box, and the total volume of gas in the body (e.g. lungs, connected bullae, non-connected bullae, intestines) can therefore be calculated using Boyle's Law.

Answer 207

207i. The scan shows multiple large, medium and small bullae throughout both lungs. The use of N_2O would be unwise. Thin-walled bullae such as these would be unlikely to communicate with the airways and are therefore considered 'isolated'. N_2O diffuses rapidly into such bullae by virtue of its low blood solubility and would expand these structures, potentially rupturing them. Pneumothorax, arterial or venous gas embolism and/or intrapulmonary and mediastinal gas are all possible results.

ii. Thick-walled lung abscesses with sputum production communicate with the airways and are less likely to expand, as the N_2O would not be trapped within them.

iii. Two methods of measuring residual volume (RV) can be compared to determine if the bullae are communicating with the airways. A large discrepancy between RV as measured by a helium dilution or nitrogen wash-out technique compared with a body box (plethysmographic) technique would show whether bullae are communicating with the airways or not.

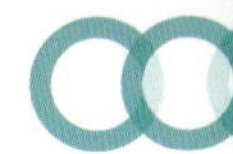

QUESTION 208

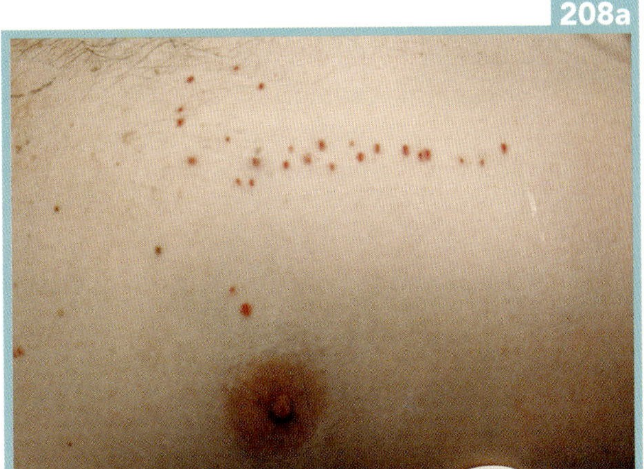
208a

208 An 18-year-old male patient crashed his car. He is behaving inappropriately saying that the car crash was "amazing" and is seemingly oblivious to pain. He has a closed fracture of his right arm and an open fracture of his distal tibia but otherwise appears uninjured.

i. List the differential diagnoses that may explain his mental state.

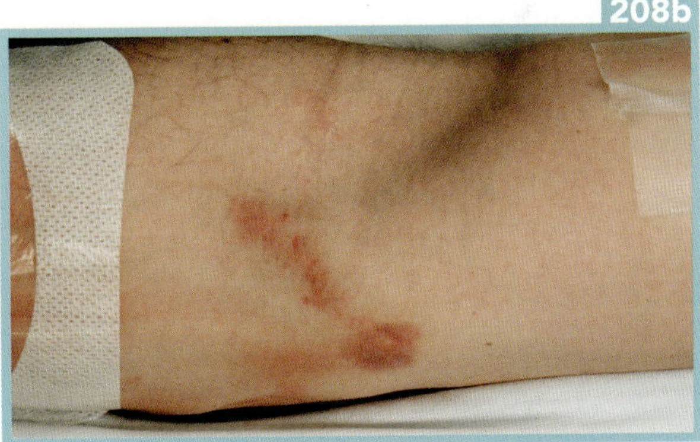
208b

ii. Skin lesions noted on his chest (**208a**) and his left antecubital fossa (**208b**) are shown. Do these images help to explain his condition?

iii. The orthopaedic surgeon wants to take him to the operating room as soon as possible to prevent vascular compromise and tibial sepsis. Is this patient fit for surgery in his current state? Justify your answer.

QUESTION 209

209 A 64-year-old, 80 kg (176 lb) male with benign prostatic hypertrophy had a transurethral resection of the prostate (TURP). He was hypertensive, controlled with a diuretic. Surgery was performed with glycine irrigant and under spinal anaesthesia. The procedure lasted 110 minutes with no adverse events. Minimal sedation was required and the patient was alert and conversant throughout. He was taken to the post-anaesthesia care unit (PACU) in a stable condition with a T10 spinal level. Thirty minutes later the patient became confused and agitated with a mild resting tremor.

i. What should the anaesthesiologist consider as a differential diagnosis?

ii. What should be done in the immediate management of this patient?

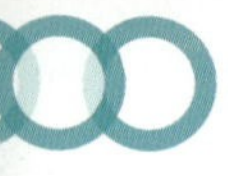

Answer 208

208i. The patient has mania, which can result from a number of causes namely: bipolar disorder; stimulant drug abuse (e.g. cocaine, amphetamines); medications (e.g. steroids or selective serotonin reuptake inhibitors); non-compliance with medications for bipolar or psychotic disorders; thyrotoxicosis; intracranial malignancy.

ii. The lesions on the chest are known as skin popping lesions and are caused by injecting drugs intradermally. In this case the patient had injected cocaine into his chest skin. The lesion in his antecubital fossa shows where he has attempted to inject into his brachial vein. These two signs indicate that substance abuse is highly likely to be the cause for his mania.

iii. Surgery for a compound fracture is urgent but the effects of cocaine should wear off within 15 minutes if the drug was injected or within an hour if there are still intradermal deposits. Cocaine can cause severe hyperthermia, hypertension, arrhythmias and convulsions, especially in overdose, so it is worth waiting for the acute effects to wear off. A history should then be taken to establish an alternative diagnosis as listed above. Assuming the mania was simply due to the cocaine, surgery can then proceed. If mania recurs in the postoperative period, an extended recovery with sedation, ventilation and ICU admission may be needed.

Answer 209

209i. Because of the prolonged resection time (>60 minutes), TURP syndrome is the most likely diagnosis. Massive uptake of hypotonic glycine solution is likely. Serum sodium should determine if dilutional hyponatraemia has caused his change in mental status. Severe hyponatraemia may lead to seizures or cerebral oedema. Other reasons why a postoperative patient may become confused are: uncontrolled pain; early sepsis, in this case catheterisation of the bladder may lead to bacteraemia; a cerebrovascular event (transient ischaemic attack, stroke, hypoperfusion may all lead to confusion; a neurological examination should be carried out looking for signs of facial or limb weakness); disorientation due to medication, particularly benzodiazepines and opiates.

ii. Adequate oxygen saturation should be ensured and respiratory depression excluded. Agitation related to ischaemia of the brainstem from hypoperfusion should be excluded. If the patient remains alert, conversant and other reasons for confusion are excluded, treatment should be conservative. Diuresis with furosemide, fluid restriction and slow administration of normal saline should suffice. Sodium levels must be repeated frequently (every 30 minutes) until the levels begin to increase.

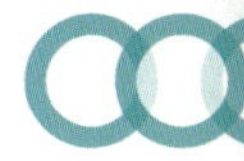

QUESTION 210

210 With regard to the 64-year-old, 80 kg (176 lb) male with benign prostatic hypertrophy who had a transurethral resection of the prostate (TURP) (see case **209**), how should serious consequences of TURP syndrome be managed.

QUESTION 211

211 The supine CXR of a man who crashed his motorbike at high speed is shown (**211**). He is conscious with a GCS of 15 and is complaining of severe shortness of breath and pain in his right neck and shoulder. He has a respiratory rate of 35 and oxygen saturations of 88% on a trauma mask receiving 15 litres/minute oxygen. He has a small right pupil with a possible ptosis. He has no power or sensation in the right upper limb.

i. What are the chest radiograph abnormalities?

ii. Why is this patient tachypnoeic?

iii. Why does he have a small pupil and ptosis?

iv. Should he be intubated immediately?

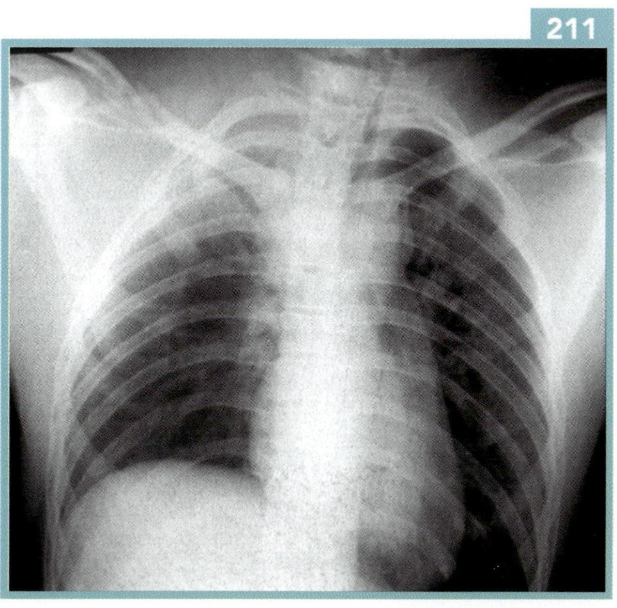

211

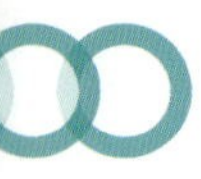

Answer 210

210 Slow correction of the sodium (<10–15 mmol/day) is important for chronic hyponatraemia, but here the recommended correction rate can be exceeded as the hyponatraemia occurred very quickly. Normal levels should be achieved within 12 hours.

This patient's sodium level of 120 mmol/l (mEq/dl) confirms TURP syndrome, so a repeat assessment of mental status is required. If further deterioration has occurred, subsequent intervention should be more aggressive. The huge amount of free water that causes TURP syndrome can cause cerebral oedema with increased intracranial pressure; intubation and ventilation might be required if conscious level decreases by >2 GCS points or seizures occur. CT of the head is needed if intubation has occurred for low conscious level or seizures. If the hyponatraemia is worsening or if seizure activity appears likely by rapidly changing conscious level, aggressive therapy with hypertonic (3%) saline can be initiated. This must be done cautiously because of the potential for (1) CNS injury from hypertonic saline (central pontine myelinolysis) or (2) exacerbation of fluid overload with a hyperosmolar solution. Intubation may also be required because of pulmonary oedema from fluid overload causing respiratory difficulty.

Answer 211

211i. There are fractures of the right clavicle and the 1st, 2nd and 3rd ribs. The right transverse process of the first thoracic vertebra has been avulsed. The right hemidiaphragm is elevated. There is shadowing over the right lung field. There is also has a large pneumothorax on the left chest anteriorly.

ii. He is tachypnoeic because of the severe nature of his chest trauma. He had a phrenic nerve paralysis, left-sided pneumothorax and bilateral lung contusions.

iii. This man has a right brachial plexus injury involving the cervical sympathetic plexus, thus his stellate ganglion and sympathetic chain. This is also known as Horner's syndrome. His phrenic nerve was also damaged.

iv. It takes a large amount of energy to break the first three ribs and clavicle. Damage to underlying tissue, in this case nerve and lung, has occurred. Such patients require intensive care until it is clear that there are no major vascular or cardiorespiratory problems. It would be safer to intubate this patient early as his injuries are severe and his pulmonary contusions will worsen before they improve.

QUESTION 212

212 Compare and contrast the two graphics showing the plasma ('blood') concentrations of propofol (**212a, b**). Graph **212a** shows the plasma concentration of propofol using a constant infusion rate irrespective of accumulating drug plasma levels. Note that the plasma concentration continuously increases and, even after 36 hours of infusion, has not yet reached a steady state. Graph **212b** shows the plasma concentrations of propofol using a variable infusion rate as delivered by a computer controlled infusion (also called target controlled infusion [TCI]). The computer produces an initial rapid rate of infusion to achieve the desired target concentration and, thereafter, gradually decreases the infusion rate as the peripheral compartments 'fill up'.

i. Give a reason why it would be advantageous to 'know' the plasma concentration during the maintenance phase.

ii. Considering the context-sensitive half-time, give a reason why it would be advantageous to 'know' the plasma concentration during the wake up phase.

iii. How can one mimic the variable (decreasing) infusion rate to attain an approximate constant plasma concentration of propofol?

212a

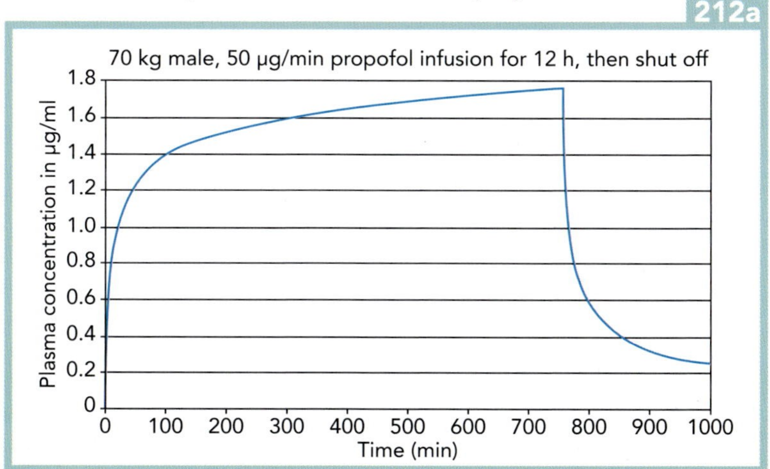

212b

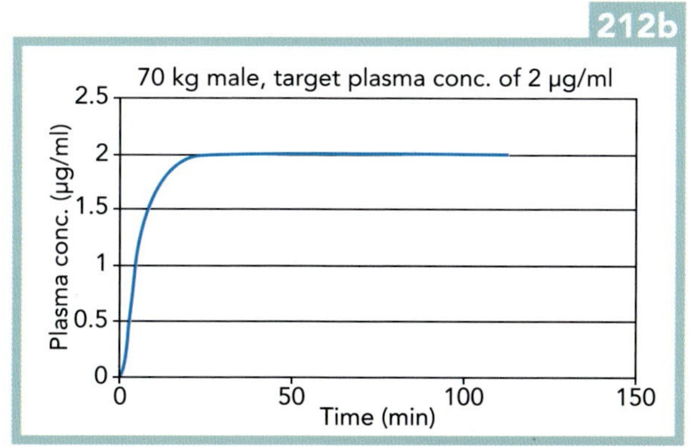

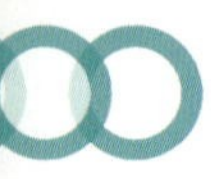

Answer 212

212i. TCI uses a real time pharmacokinetic model to calculate the infusion rate to achieve a desired or 'target' blood concentration at any point. It is advantageous to know what plasma concentration is needed for more painful periods of the surgery, and quickly attain (or target) that specific concentration again. Another advantage is that the plasma concentration remains at the selected concentration, as the computer continuously 'dials back' the infusion rate.

ii. The context-sensitive half-time means that it takes longer to wake up after an infusion than after a bolus of the same drug, even though the peak concentration attained by each may be the same. This happens because it takes longer for the infused drug to decrease in concentration. Knowing this means that it is easier to predict when the patient will wake up after an infusion. This is achieved by the computer continuously calculating what would happen to the plasma concentration if the infusion were to be discontinued at this point, and calculating how long it would take to reach the wake up concentration of propofol.

iii. Graph **212c** shows the bolus, excretion, transfer (BET) technique of attaining a relatively constant plasma concentration by administering a bolus of propofol, followed by an infusion rate of 200 μg/kg/minute (12 mg/kg/hour) for 10 minutes, followed by an infusion rate of 166 μg/kg/minute (10 mg/kg/hour) for 10 minutes, followed by an infusion rate of 133 μg/kg/minute (8 mg/kg/hour) for 10 minutes. (See: www.LearningTIVA.com)

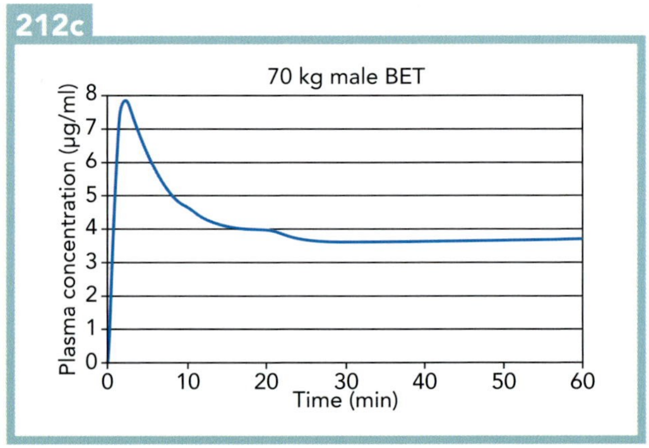

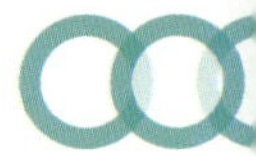

QUESTION 213

213 A 3-year-old male child has blue sclerae and suffered a femur fracture after a minor trauma.

i. What orthopaedic procedure is shown (**213**)? Why is this procedure an anaesthetic challenge?

ii. What are the long-term cardiopulmonary effects of this condition should the patient survive to adulthood?

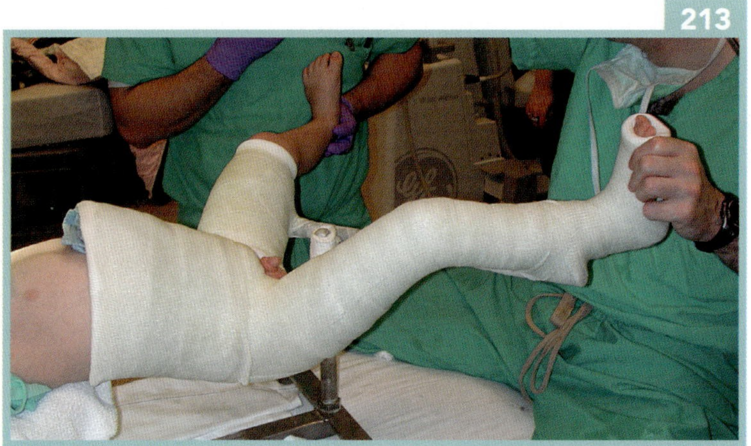

213

QUESTION 214

214 Metabolic processes, for example metabolism of drugs by liver cells, are usually divided into two types.

i. What are phase 1 drug reactions?

ii. What are phase 2 drug reactions?

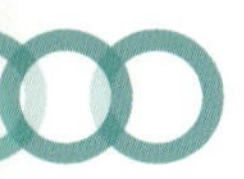

Answer 213

213i. This is a child with osteogenesis imperfecta after suffering a femoral fracture. He is too young for an internal fixation, therefore a 'spica cast' is being placed. The cast reaches from the xiphisternum over the pelvis down to below the knee of the affected limb. The anaesthetic challenges include:

- Positioning. Having the child's hips on a 'frame' so that the plaster of Paris (in this case - heat-sensitive, washable cast) can be wrapped around the whole child. The child could fall from the frame or the operating table.
- Losing the airway.
- Temperature problems. The child can become hypothermic from exposure or too hot (after the plaster cast had been placed in hot water to soften it, the cast gives off heat which can overheat and/or burn the child).
- Scoliosis-related cardiopulmonary morbidity can cause marked chest wall deformity with restrictive lung defects. Full pulmonary function testing is required prior to anaesthesia as either sudden intraoperative respiratory decompensation or difficult postoperative weaning can occur.

ii. Older patients (age range 19 to 61) may present with osteogenesis imperfecta tarda (OIT), a less severe form of osteogenesis imperfecta. Myxomatous degeneration of heart valves occurs, similar to that seen in Marfan's syndrome. The aortic, mitral and right-sided valves may be affected in descending order of frequency. Aneurysms of the sinuses of Valsalva or ascending aorta have also been described. In one study all adult patients with OIT had a history of multiple fractures, but only some had blue sclerae, deafness and/or 'elfin'/triangular facies. Cardiac surgery has a mortality of almost 50% in these patients.

Answer 214

214i. Phase 1 reactions result in drug oxidation, reduction or hydrolysis. The enzyme responsible for most of these reactions lies in the endoplasmic reticulum. It is known as the 'non-specific cytochrome P-450' or mixed-function oxidase system. Cytochrome P-450 consists of a variety of forms of a superfamily of genetically related haemoproteins, which are the terminal oxidases of the mixed-function oxidase system. Some hydrolytic reactions occur in plasma by cholinesterase, at the neuromuscular junction by acetylcholinesterase or in the cytoplasm of the liver cell by amidases.

ii. Phase 2 reactions involve conjugation of the products of phase 1 reactions with glucuronide, sulphate, acetate, glycine or methyl groups. Some drugs may only be metabolised by phase 2 reactions. Glucuronide conjugation takes place in the hepatic endoplasmic reticulum and enhances the water solubility of drug metabolites. In the liver, Kupffer cells are responsible for drug acetylation. The rate and extent of this reaction in humans are under genetic control. Conjugation with glycine, sulphate and methyl groups occurs in the cytoplasm of the liver cell.

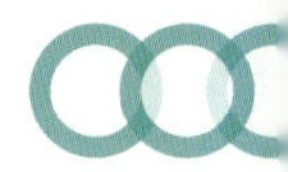

QUESTION 215

215 This ECG (**215**) is of a patient who has had a cardiac transplant.

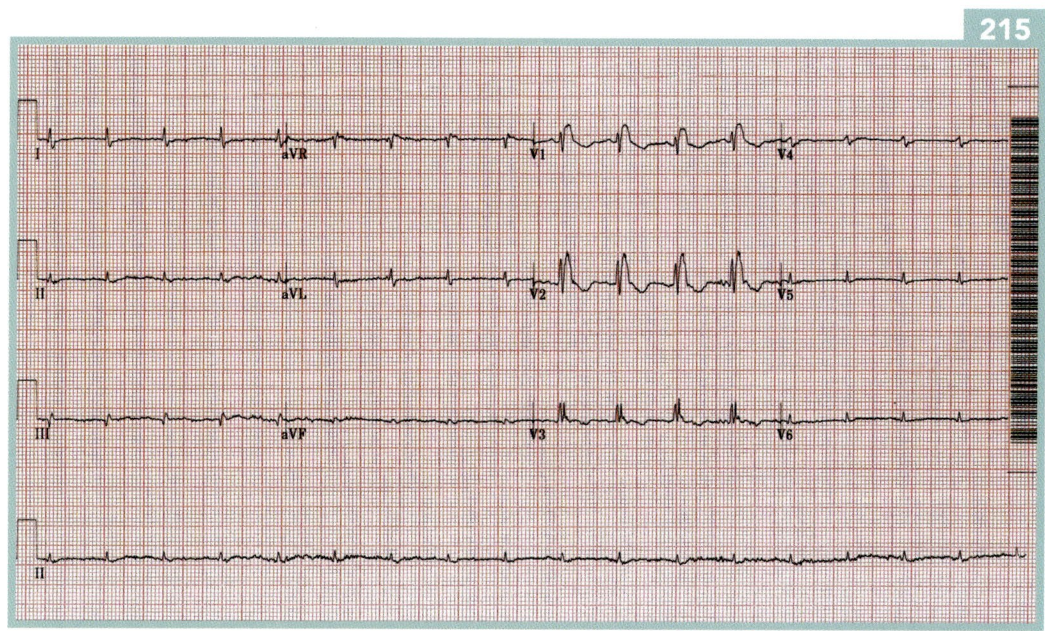

i. What features of the ECG suggest this?

ii. What are the principles of perioperative management of a patient with a cardiac transplant?

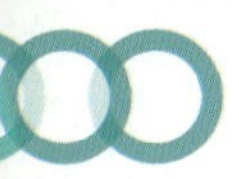

Answer 215

215i. The ECG shows sinus rhythm at a rate of approximately 100 bpm. The axis is normal at +41°. There is a marked right bundle branch block and the QTc interval is prolonged at 478 milliseconds. Any QTc above 450 msec can be associated with arrhythmias. Occasionally, additional P waves may be seen as there may be a residual atrial remnant present.

ii. The donor heart rate is dependent on donor sinus node activity. The transplanted heart has no autonomic innervation and the resting heart rate is typically 90–100 bpm. Ten percent of recipients require a permanent pacemaker. Heart rate cannot adjust to sudden changes of systemic vascular resistance occurring during anaesthesia, so hypotension should be corrected rapidly with adequate preload and the use of vasoconstrictors such as phenylephrine or metaraminol.

Depth of anaesthesia cannot be judged by heart rate. Cardiac vagolytic effects of atropine and glycopyrrolate do not occur and digoxin ceases to be an effective antiarrhythmic due to the inability to increase vagal tone. Direct acting chronotropic agents such as ephedrine and isoprenaline may be necessary to speed up heart rate, but marked sensitivity to adenosine, adrenaline and noradrenaline can be seen. Angiotensin converting enzyme inhibitors, which are used to treat hypertension, can cause intraoperative hypotension.

Immunologically mediated coronary heart disease of the donor heart is common. Attention should be paid to associated diseases such as epilepsy and hypertension.

Long-term treatment with immunosuppressant drugs such as azathioprine, cyclosporine and prednisolone mean infection, malignancy, osteoporosis and renal impairment are more likely. Cyclosporin can be given by IV infusion (one-third of the oral dose) in the perioperative period. IV hydrocortisone, at higher doses than equivalent prednisolone maintenance, can be used instead of prednisolone and azathioprine. There is no contraindication to regional anaesthesia but scrupulous asepsis should be used for all invasive procedures.

Cytomegalovirus (CMV) seronegative patients should receive blood from seronegative donors to prevent CMV infection, which can result in serious disease and even death.

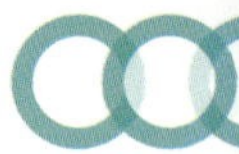

QUESTION 216

216 Capnograph tracings of a spontaneously breathing subject on a Mapleson D, E or F breathing system are shown (**216a–c**). A normal expiratory CO_2 pattern is seen, but a lower CO_2 concentration is also noted during the inspiratory phase.

With regard to **216a**:

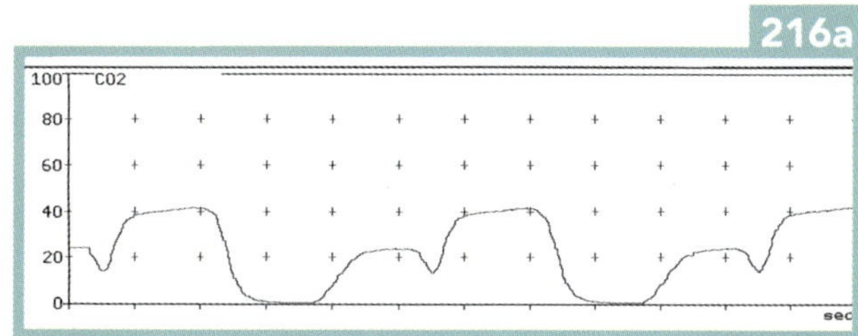

216a

i. Where does the CO_2 during the inspiratory phase come from?

ii. Is the fresh gas flow (FGF) sufficient?

iii. Why is there no CO_2 early in inspiration?

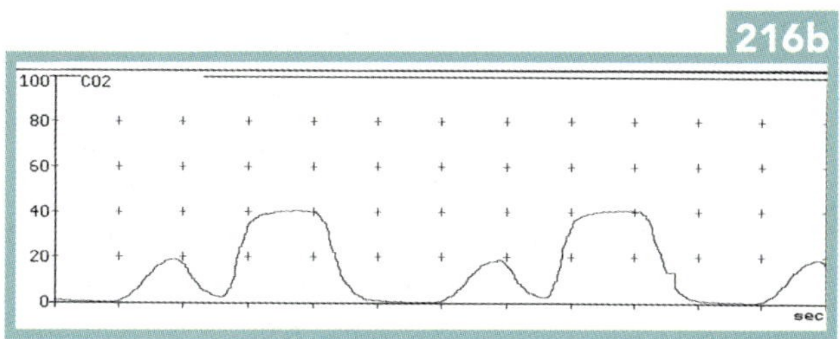

216b

iv. With regard to **216b**, explain why, with increased FGF, the inspiratory CO_2 concentration has decreased.

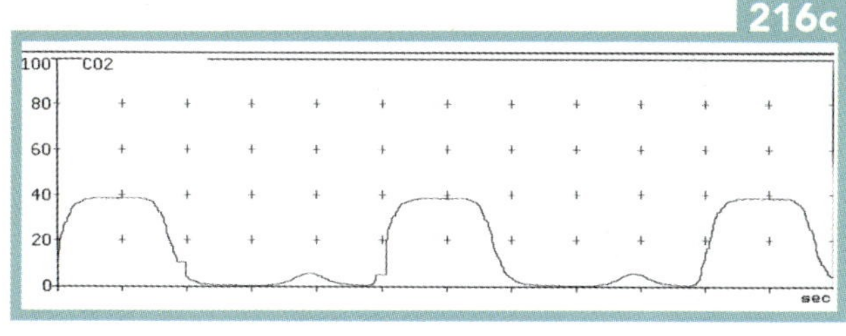

216c

v. A further increase in FGF leads to the inspiratory CO_2 concentration decreasing even more (**216c**). How much FGF should be given to totally eliminate rebreathing? Give the answer as: (a) FGF to minute volume ratio; (b) ml per kg per minute.

vi. How does the peak inspiratory flow rate influence rebreathing of CO_2?

vii. Would a similar pattern of rebreathing be seen when using a Bain breathing system?

QUESTION 217

217i. What is Stewart's physical chemical approach to acid–base analysis?

ii. What is a strong ion in normal blood?

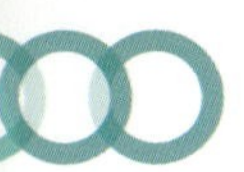

Answer 216

216i. When the instantaneous inspiratory flow rate exceeds the FGF rate, gas is taken from the expiratory limb. The gas in the expiratory limb is previously exhaled gas and contains CO_2, which has been diluted with the constant FGF that was flowing throughout exhalation.

ii. The FGF is still insufficient to prevent rebreathing.

iii. During any expiratory pause, the fresh gas continues to flow and pushes the CO_2-containing gas further down the expiratory limb. So the first gas to be taken from the expiratory limb does not contain any CO_2.

iv. With a higher FGF, less CO_2-containing gas is taken from the expiratory limb. The constant higher FGF also dilutes exhaled gas more.

v. The FGF required to totally eliminate the rebreathing of gas from the expiratory limb is: (a) 3 times the minute ventilation (MV), which is typically 5 litres/minute; (b) 220 ml/kg/minute (5 litres/minute for a 70 kg [154 lb] person is approx. 70 ml/kg/minute).

vi. The peak inspiratory flow rate is three times MV (actually pi [π] $\times$ MV).

vii. The Bain system functions as a Mapleson D system, so the rebreathing characteristics are similar.

Answer 217

217i. Arterial acid–base balance calculation conventionally uses arterial CO_2 tension ($PaCO_2$) and pH (or H^+). This distinguishes respiratory from metabolic acid–base disturbance by considering changes in bicarbonate (HCO_3^-) concentration. In respiratory acidosis a simple relationship between $PaCO_2$ and pH/H^+ exists. The higher the CO_2, the lower the pH (or higher the H^+). Metabolic disturbances are traditionally explained by decreases in HCO_3^- level; however, this may be too simplistic. Stewart's physicochemical approach to acid–base balance provides a more detailed explanation and also explains the development of metabolic acidoses when excess normal saline is administered to a patient.

In Stewart's analysis, HCO_3^- and pH are both determined by three independent variables: pCO_2, strong ion difference and total concentration of weak acids (A_{TOT}). A_{TOT} consists primarily of albumin and haemoglobin. These proteins act as buffers in the whole blood. (See also case **218**.)

ii. Strong ions are those that are fully dissociated in the plasma of normal blood.

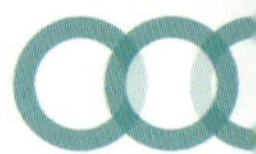

QUESTION 218

218 The balance of cations and anions found in normal blood and the buffer bases that maintain electroneutrality are shown (**218**) (SID = strong ion difference). Why does this explain Stewart's theory?

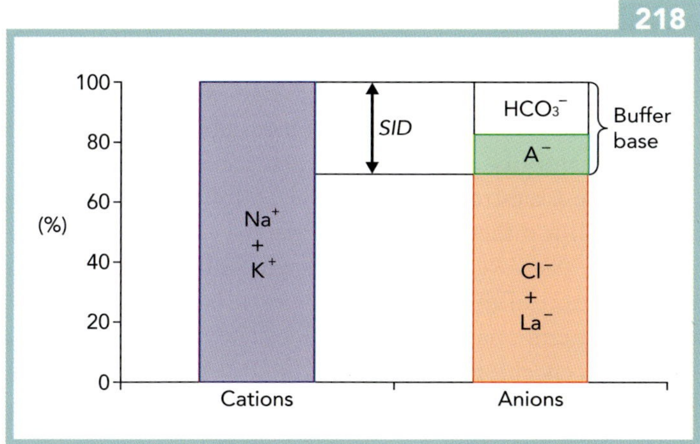

QUESTION 219

219 A 50-year-old, 1.79 m (6 feet), 80 kg (176 lb) male with aseptic necrosis of the right femoral head is pre-assessed for elective femoral hemiarthroplasty. He has chronic fatigue and autoimmune hepatitis (the latter managed by oral steroids).

i. Why does this man have aseptic necrosis?

ii. How would you assess his liver disease?

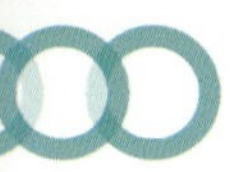

Answer 218

218 SID results from the observation that Na^+, K^+, Cl^- and lactate (La^-) are fully ionised under all physiological conditions and do not bind to albumin or haemoglobin. Stewart's analysis states that only an alteration in one or both of SID and $A_{(TOT)}$ can lead to a change in metabolic acid–base balance.

Buffer base anions ([A] + [HCO_3^-]) interact with SID ions to maintain electroneutrality. With excess saline infusion, excess sodium and a large excess of chloride administered, this disrupts the balance of strong ions, with too many negatively charged chloride ions resulting. Electrochemical neutrality must be maintained so there must be an alteration in the buffer base to counter this effect. HCO_3^- is the easiest molecule for the body to shed renally (compared with chloride, which is difficult for the kidney to excrete, and negatively charged proteins, which take days/weeks to modify). The subsequent loss of HCO_3^- leads to an acidification of the blood and hyperchloraemic metabolic acidosis results. Additionally, temporary excess crystalloid solution dilutes blood proteins, exacerbating the excess chloride ions. This can also be seen during prolonged ICU stays when protein dilution and synthesis can deplete protein levels.

The balance of ions in the blood is illustrated in **218**. With excessive chloride administration, it can be seen that the only ion that can easily be lost is HCO_3^-, thus leading to acidosis.

Answer 219

219i. Chronic steroid use for liver disease is serious because of the associated risks, and his aseptic necrosis may be a consequence of steroid use. Evaluation of the severity of his liver disease is based on risk assessment. Anaesthetic technique selection will also be influenced by hepatic function.

ii. Liver disease is associated with coagulopathy. Questions about easy bruising, duration of bleeding from simple skin cuts and blood with cough, sneeze or tooth brushing can characterise potential coagulopathy. Fatigue is universally reported with liver disease and is more serious if associated with ascites. Laboratory tests are very important for assessing the severity of liver disease. Liver enzymes, proteins and coagulation studies must be done and enzyme elevation is assumed. Trends assess severity, with progression associated with increased enzyme levels. Below normal levels of serum proteins indicate serious liver disease and impaired synthetic function. Elevation of PT and/or APTT reflect significant impairment of synthetic function and would be the most serious finding if abnormal.

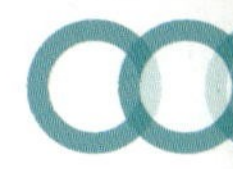

QUESTION 220

220 The severity of liver disease is classified using Child's criteria. Describe in tabular form how the Child's score is calculated. What are the survival rates for the different classes?

QUESTION 221

221 The formula below applies to fluid resuscitation in the first 24 hours after a thermal injury:

Fluid replacement in ml = 4 ml/kg/body surface area (BSA) in the first 24 hours

i. What is this commonly used formula known as?

ii. Does this formula include maintenance fluids?

iii. What time periods are used in conjunction with the above formula?

iv. What is the Muir Barclay formula?

v. How does the Muir Barclay formula differ from crystalloid only resuscitation?

vi. Is crystalloid resuscitation superior to colloid resuscitation after burns?

vii. Is invasive cardiac monitoring recommended to aid fluid management of burn patients?

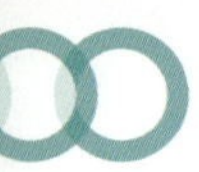

Answer 220

220

Measure	1 point	2 points	3 points
Total bilirubin (μmol/l [mg/dl])	<34 (<2)	34–50 (2–3)	>50 (>3)
Serum albumin (g/l)	>35	28–35	<28
Prothrombin time/INR	<1.7	1.71–2.30	>2.30
Ascites	None	Mild	Moderate to severe
Hepatic encephalopathy	None	Grade I–II (or suppressed with medication)	Grade III–IV (or refractory)

Points	Class	One-year survival	Two-year survival
5–6	A	100%	85%
7–9	B	81%	57%
10–15	C	45%	35%

Answer 221

221i. This is the Parkland formula and is for crystalloid resuscitation using Hartmann's solution (similar to lactated Ringers solution).

ii. It does not include the insensible losses but gives only the additional fluids required after the burn.

iii. Estimated fluid requirements from the time of the burn must be included. Half of the Parkland formula fluid should be given in the first 8 hours after the burn, the remainder over the remaining 16 hours.

iv. The Muir Barclay formula is:

$$\frac{\text{body weight (kg)} \times \text{\% BSA}}{2} = \frac{\text{volume (ml)}}{\text{time increment}}$$

v. The Muir Barclay formula uses plasma protein fraction (human albumin) as the fluid of choice. Each volume is given in 3 × 4-hour time increments for the first 12 hours then 2 × 6-hour increments and finally one 12 hour increment.

vi. There is no advantage to colloid over crystalloid resuscitation and albumin is considerably more expensive.

vii. Fluid resuscitation formulae should be regularly adjusted, principally according to urine output. Invasive cardiac monitoring may be required as a supplementary guide but there are no established targets for cardiac output that have been verified in burns patients.

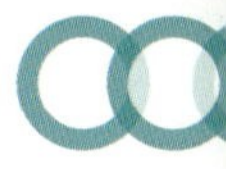

QUESTION 222

222 A 64-year-old male, 1.83 m (6 feet) tall, weighing 90 kg (198 lb) and with severe osteoarthritis of the right hip presents to the anaesthetic preassessment clinic for proposed total hip replacement. He is inactive secondary to hip pain and is wheelchair bound. He has no other complaints and denies any cardiac symptoms. He has chronic hypertension, which is being treated with an ACE inhibitor, and insulin-dependent diabetes mellitus (IDDM) for 20 years. His resting ECG (**222**), with no other ECG available for comparison, is shown. Other routine laboratory studies are within normal limits.

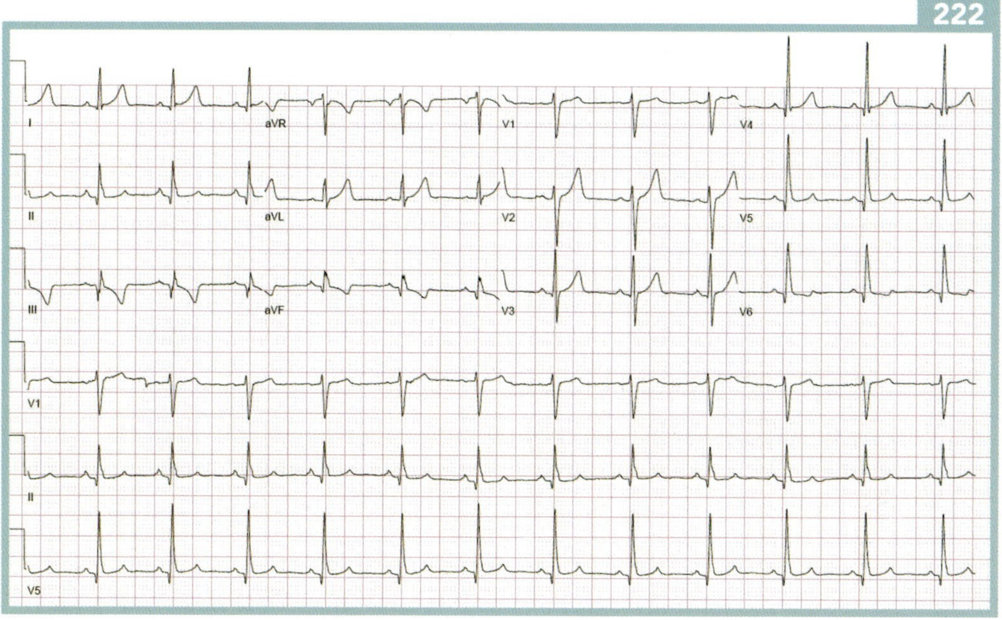

i. What does the ECG show?

ii. What further cardiac testing is required?

iii. Does the choice of anaesthetic technique influence outcome?

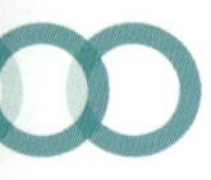

Answer 222

222i. An old inferior infarct. Note the Q waves in leads II, III and aVF. There are no acute changes (ST elevation, T wave inversion).

ii. Although the patient is asymptomatic, further cardiac investigation is needed. Absence of symptoms when sedentary does not equate to the situation during surgery, where considerable cardiovascular stress regularly occurs. The patient also has long-standing IDDM, associated with autonomic neuropathy. Cardiovascular reflexes are less active and haemodynamic instability may occur. Autonomic denervation may also eliminate the symptoms associated with acute myocardial ischaemia (MI) and 'silent ischaemia' can result. Although ECG criteria for MI are not 100% accurate, the possibility of a silent event must be considered.

Ventricular and valvular function should be assessed by transthoracic echocardiogram with a dobutamine stress test (as treadmill stress testing cannot be performed). By measuring regional wall motion the efficacy of the test is validated by the heart rate achieved. If inducible ischaemia (shown by abnormal wall motion) is found, cardiological intervention is required with pharmacological treatment, invasive cardiology (angioplasty, stenting, permanent antiplatelet drugs) or coronary artery bypass. Stenting and antiplatelet drugs pose problems, however. If antiplatelet medication is suspended for surgery, non-drug eluting stents may block, but if continued, intraoperative coagulopathy during surgery may occur. Whether to suspend antiplatelet medication is controversial and should be a joint decision between cardiologist, surgeon and anaesthesiologist. Heparin use around the time of surgery may help to reduce the risks of stent blockage and is more controllable during surgery.

iii. In this patient, several issues may be altered by anaesthetic technique and a regional technique may be preferable. Regional anaesthesia is associated with reduced thromboembolic events, may reduce perioperative blood loss, reduces the risk and amount of heterologous transfusion, and may be associated with less acute confusion.

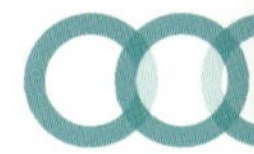

QUESTION 223

223 An X-ray of a 28-year-old, 1.88 m (6'2"), 80 kg (176 lb) skier who has sustained a bad fall is shown (**223**). He was completely healthy prior to his accident.

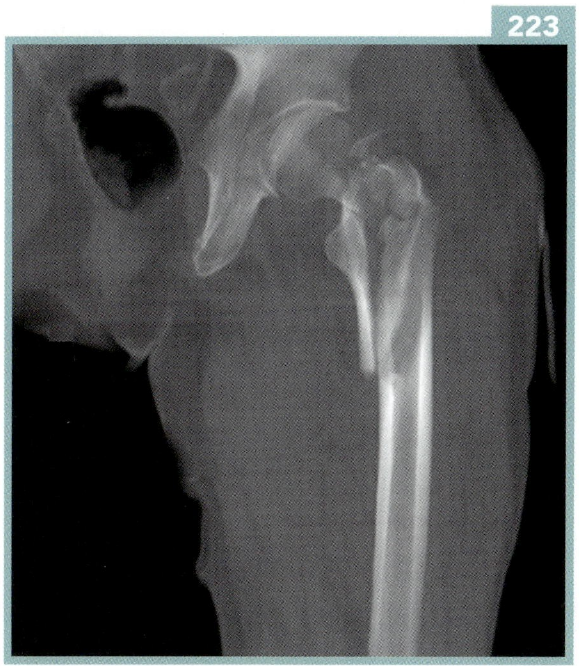

i. What does this X-ray show?

The patient was admitted for internal fixation. In the operating room, an epidural catheter was placed at L3/4 and dosed with 20 ml of premixed 2% mepivacaine/ epinephrine 1/200,000, in incremental doses, resulting in complete sensory anaesthesia to T8. The patient was placed supine on the fracture table and the fracture was then aligned, with some difficulty, under fluoroscopic control with the patient alert, unsedated and conversant. After 40 minutes, instrumentation of the femoral canal on both sides of the fracture occurred. Over a 10-minute interval, the patient became extremely anxious with a respiratory rate of 30 breaths per minute. Oxygen saturation declined to 90% despite increasing nasal cannula to 5 liters/minute. BP was 90/60 and pulse 90 bpm, and 5 minutes later was 80/50 with pulse 104 bpm. At this time the patient identified truncal itching and a fine rash was noted on the anterior chest.

ii. What pathology could explain this symptom complex?

iii. How should this be managed?

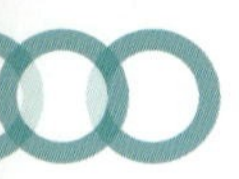

Answer 223

223i. A young athlete injured in a high velocity accident is at-risk for fat embolism syndrome (FES). With all long bone fractures some embolism of fat occurs, but not all develop FES and some elements of FES are unknown. The total fat embolised increases the risk of FES. The physical mobilisation of fat causes some of the elements of FES and various adverse effects are seen both from physical obstruction of vessels and activation of tissue lipase enzymes that cause destruction of adjacent normal tissues.

ii. Cardiac dysfunction can occur from fat accumulating in the proximal pulmonary circulation, which both increases pulmonary smooth muscle tone and may obstruct pulmonary vessels and cause an increase in pulmonary artery pressure. Petechial haemorrhage typically occurs in the skin, with itching a sign of histamine release with haemodynamic consequences. Lipase activity in the lungs causes alveolar destruction and progressive V-Q mismatching. CNS lipase activity causes intracerebral inflammation and can lead to cerebral oedema.

iii. Successful management requires recognition of FES, termination of causative actions and supportive management. Continued manipulation of the fracture should be minimised but completion of the operation is important as both actions will reduce further fat mobilisation. A decision by the surgeon in conjunction with the anesthaesiologist must occur. Aggressive support of the haemodynamic and respiratory consequences is a priority. Antihistamine and vasopressors should be used and titrated to maintain normal haemodynamics. If deoxygenation or agitation is progressive, it may be necessary to electively secure the airway. The patient will need close observation or treatment in the ICU. Mechanical ventilation with PEEP may be needed for an interval until pulmonary healing occurs. Aggressive management of cerebral oedema and increased intracranial pressure is necessary to avoid permanent CNS devastation.

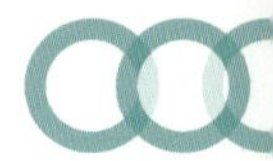

QUESTION 224

224 An X-ray of the hip of an elderly patient undergoing total hip replacement for osteoarthritis is shown (**224**). He has hypertension, which is controlled with a diuretic and an ACE inhibitor. Regional anaesthesia with combined spinal/epidural anaesthetic was commenced and the patient placed in the lateral position. The sensory level rose to T8 and the incision was pain free. Minimal sedation was required. Evidence of osteoporosis caused the surgeons to use methyl methacrylate for the femoral component. During the mixing of the double-batch, the patient was alert and BP 100/60, pulse rate 70, respiratory rate (RR) 16 breaths per minute and O_2 sats 99% on 2 liters/minute oxygen via nasal cannula. During pressurised placement of the methylmethacrylate, the patient became agitated. His haemodynamics changed to BP 70/40, pulse rate 120, RR 30 and O_2 sats of 88%.

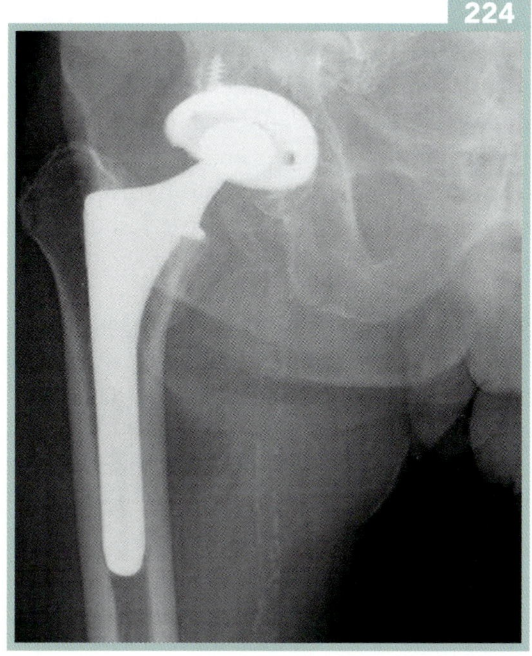
224

i. Give a differential diagnosis for this event.

ii. What is the mechanism of methylmethacrylate causing hypotension?

iii. Why did this event occur in this patient specifically?

iv. How should this patient be managed, and what is the prognosis?

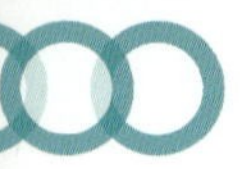

Answer 224

224i. A reaction to methylmethacrylate could be a cause of the onset of agitation, hypotension, tachycardia and decreased oxygen saturation. Alternatively, an embolism of air, fat or clot is possible as is an anaphylactic reaction to drugs or colloid solutions.

ii. Methylmethacrylate achieves tensile strength by multiple polymerisation of the basic molecule (monomeric form). If the monomer enters the circulation from medullary bone, it is a potent vasodilator and degranulates mast cells, releasing histamine. A significant amount of the monomer in the circulation can mimic an anaphylactoid reaction.

iii. Chronic hypertension results in intravascular volume contraction, exaggerated by chronic diuretic therapy, and ACE inhibitors reduce the reactivity of peripheral circulation. Vasodilation and attenuation of vasoconstrictor response results, which augments the effects of a large dose (double-batch) and pressurised application of methylmethacrylate. With pressurised application, the cement can be liquid and, although more effective, more monomer enters the circulation. The combination of intravascular volume reduction, sympathectomy from the epidural, diminished vasoconstriction reflexes and bolus exposure to a vasodilator (the monomer and histamine) makes haemodynamic deterioration likely.

iv. Hypoperfusion of the brainstem and decreased oxygen saturation must be treated promptly with enhanced oxygenation and measures to normalise haemodynamics. Application of a mask with high flow oxygen is the first step. Haemodynamic management should also be aggressive, with vasopressor infusions (e.g. adrenaline or noradrenaline) to restore BP. Mental status should improve with reduced agitation and may obviate the need to secure the airway by intubation. The haemodynamic effects of the monomer are dramatic but have a finite duration and are terminated by metabolism.

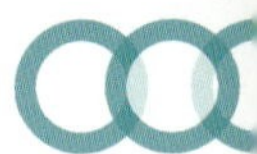

QUESTION 225

225 Compare the two lung function results A and B. Why do the two results differ so greatly, and which patient is at most risk of respiratory complications?

Patient A				
Spirometry	(BTPS)	Pred	Best	%Pred
FVC	Litres	2.54	2.45	96
FEV1	Litres	1.92	1.88	98
FEV1/FVC	%	76	77	101
FEF25–75%	L/sec	1.70	1.58	93
PEF		L/sec	5.61	
FIVC	Litres	2.54	2.34	92
PIF	L/sec		3.87	
FEF50/FIF50	Unitless			0.68
MVV	L/min			89
Lung volumes	(BTPS)	Pred	Avg	%Pred
VC	Litres	2.54	2.45	96
TLC	Litres	4.75	4.15	87
RV	Litres	2.17	1.70	78
RV/TLC	%		45	41
FRC He	Litres	2.72	2.61	96
ERV	Litres		0.91	
IC	Litres		1.31	
Vt	Litres		0.60	

Patient B				
Spirometry	(BTPS)	Pred	Best	%Pred
FVC	Litres	3.15	1.09 #	35*
FEV1	Litres	2.33	0.81 #	35*
FEV1/FVC	%	73	74	101
FEF25–75%	L/sec	1.85	0.63	34*
PEF	L/sec	2.13		
FIVC	Litres	3.15	1.11 #	35*
PIF	L/sec	1.74		
FEF50/FIF50	Unitless		0.49	
MVV	L/min		21	
Lung volumes	(BTPS)	Pred	Avg	%Pred
VC	Litres	3.15	1.22 #	39*
TLC	Litres	5.50	2.33 #	42*
RV	Litres	2.44	1.11 #	46*
RV/TLC	% 46	48		
FRC He	Litres	3.18	1.23 #	39*
ERV	Litres			0.12
IC	Litres			1.05
Vt	Litres			0.70

= outside 95% confidence interval; * = outside normal range; BTPS, body temperature and pressure standard; Pred, predicted.

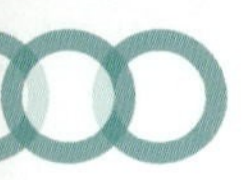

Answer 225

225 Patient A shows normal spirometric lung volumes (see **225a**). Patient B has a restrictive pattern with significantly reduced lung volumes (**225b**). There was no significant improvement after bronchodilators in patient B. While standard preoperative assessments are still applied, patient B (with scoliosis with the more restrictive pattern, and fixed chest) will need more careful monitoring. Positioning during surgery for best ventilation/perfusion matching is paramount. Postoperative pain control and methods to improve lung expansion need to be applied.

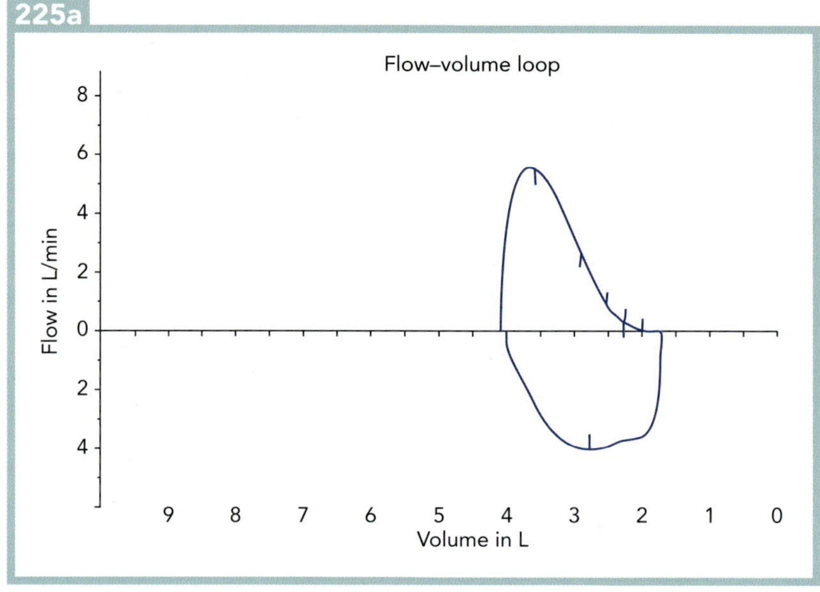

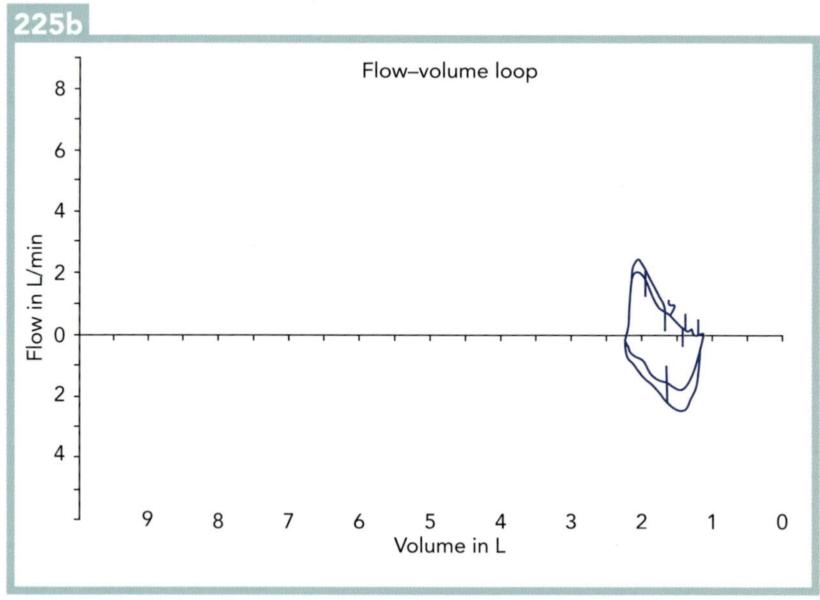

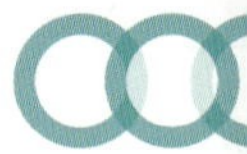

QUESTION 226

226 A 3-hour-old neonate presents with tachypnoea, cyanosis, a scaphoid abdomen and decreased breath sounds on the left side of the chest. The CXR is shown (**226**).

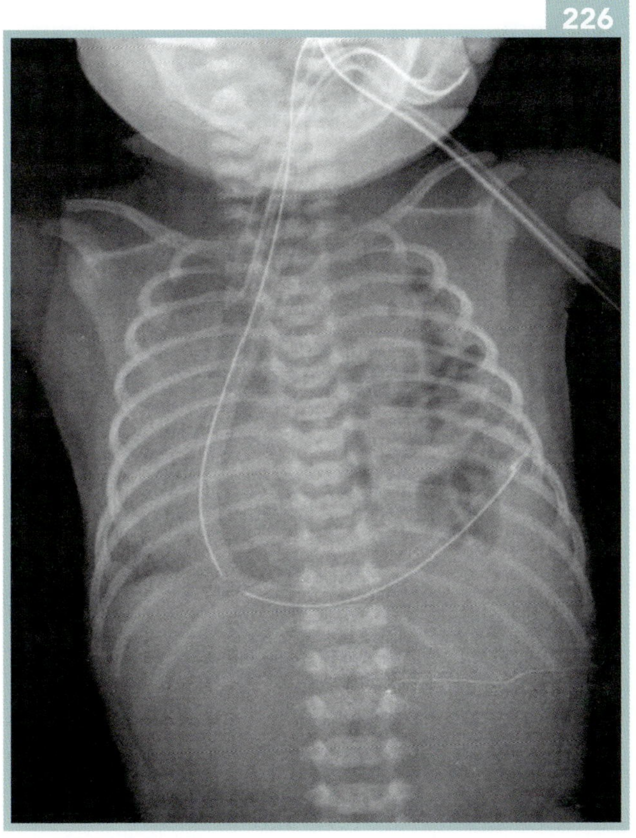
226

i. What is this patient's diagnosis?

ii. Describe the embryology.

iii. How does this affect the infant's physiology?

iv. What happens at birth?

v. What is seen on examination?

vi. What are the anaesthetic considerations, and why is surgery necessary?

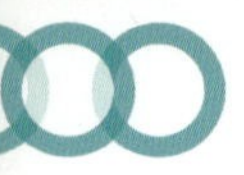

Answer 226

226i. Congenital diaphragmatic hernia.

ii. The pleuroperitoneal folds fail to separate the abdominal cavity from the pleural cavity during the fourth to ninth week of gestation. With the return of the gut from the yolk sac, the intestine herniates into the thoracic cavity, stunting lung growth with ipsilateral pulmonary hypoplasia proportional to the defect size and the amount of herniation. Pulmonary hypoplasia can be bilateral. Approximately 80–90% of the herniations are posterolateral defects through the foramen of Bochdalek, affecting the left side five times more than the right.

iii. Increased pulmonary vascular resistance, increased right-to-left shunting, hypoxemia, acidosis and right heart failure result.

iv. At birth cyanosis occurs soon after clamping the umbilical cord. A barrel-shaped thorax, scaphoid abdomen, dyspnoea and sternal and intercostal retractions are seen.

v. Heart sounds are often on the unaffected hemithorax. Peristaltic sounds can be heard on the affected side. The CXR shows herniated bowel on the affected hemithorax and a shift of mediastinal contents. Blood gases show a mixed metabolic and respiratory acidosis. Twenty-five percent of patients have associated neurological, cardiovascular and gastrointestinal anomalies.

vi. Surgery returns the gut to the abdomen and closes the diaphragmatic defect. IV access in an upper extremity is important as increased intra-abdominal pressure (after reduction of the thoracic hernia) decreases venous return from the lower extremities. A nasogastric tube should decompress bowel in the thoracic cavity. Positive pressure ventilation by bag mask should be avoided prior to intubation to limit insufflation of intragastric air. Awake, or deep inhalational, intubation with spontaneous respiration are recommended. Once intubated, a high respiratory rate with low tidal volumes and low peak pressures is desirable. High volumes or airway pressures can cause a tension pneumothorax and prophylactic placement of a chest tube on the unaffected hemithorax can help. If cardiovascular status remains poor after intubation, extracorporeal membrane oxygenation can relieve the stress on the heart and maintain ventilation until the defect is repaired and the pulmonary vasculature normalises.

Bowel relocation and diaphragmatic closure dramatically increase intra-abdominal pressure, sometimes causing impaired ventilation and decreased perfusion to abdominal organs or lower extremities. If this happens, a staged procedure is carried out with the bowels placed in a Silon pouch and reduced over a period of several days.

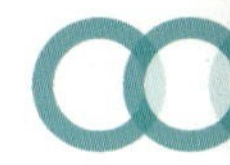

QUESTION 227

227i. What does this CXR show (**227a**)?

ii. What action is needed?

iii. What measurement is shown in **227b**, and why is this important?

iv. What precautions must be carried out prior to using the device shown for feeding?

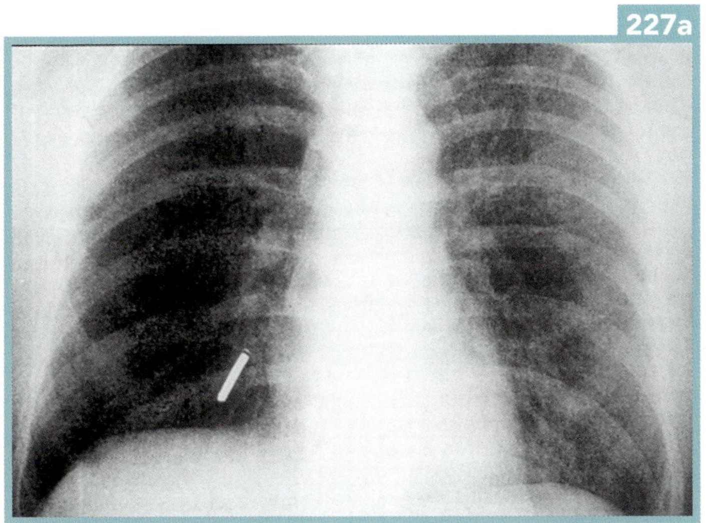

227a

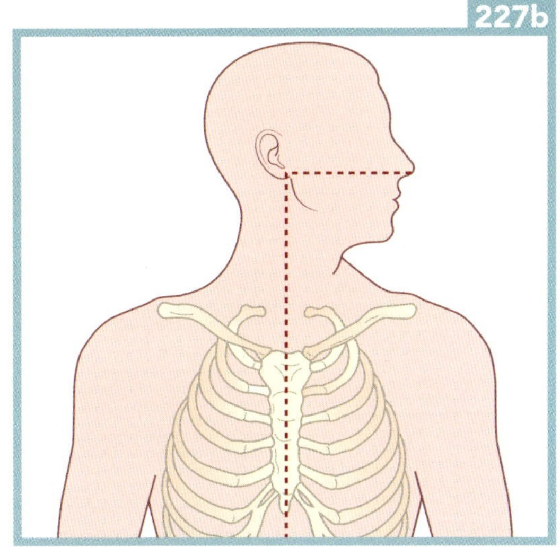

227b

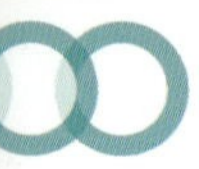

Answer 227

227i. It demonstrates a nasogastric (NG) tube positioned in the right mainstem bronchus.

ii. The NG tube must be removed and replaced.

iii. It shows the NEX (nose-earlobe-xiphisternum) measurement and is used to estimate whether an NG tube is of the correct length prior to insertion. If the exit port of the tube is at the tip of the nose and the tube is then extended to the earlobe and then to the xiphisternum, the tube is of an appropriate length. Once inserted, the external tube length should be recorded and confirmed before each feed.

iv. A decision tree from the National Patient Safety Agency (England and Wales) is shown (**227c**). NG tubes should never be used for feeding without following these guidelines.

227c

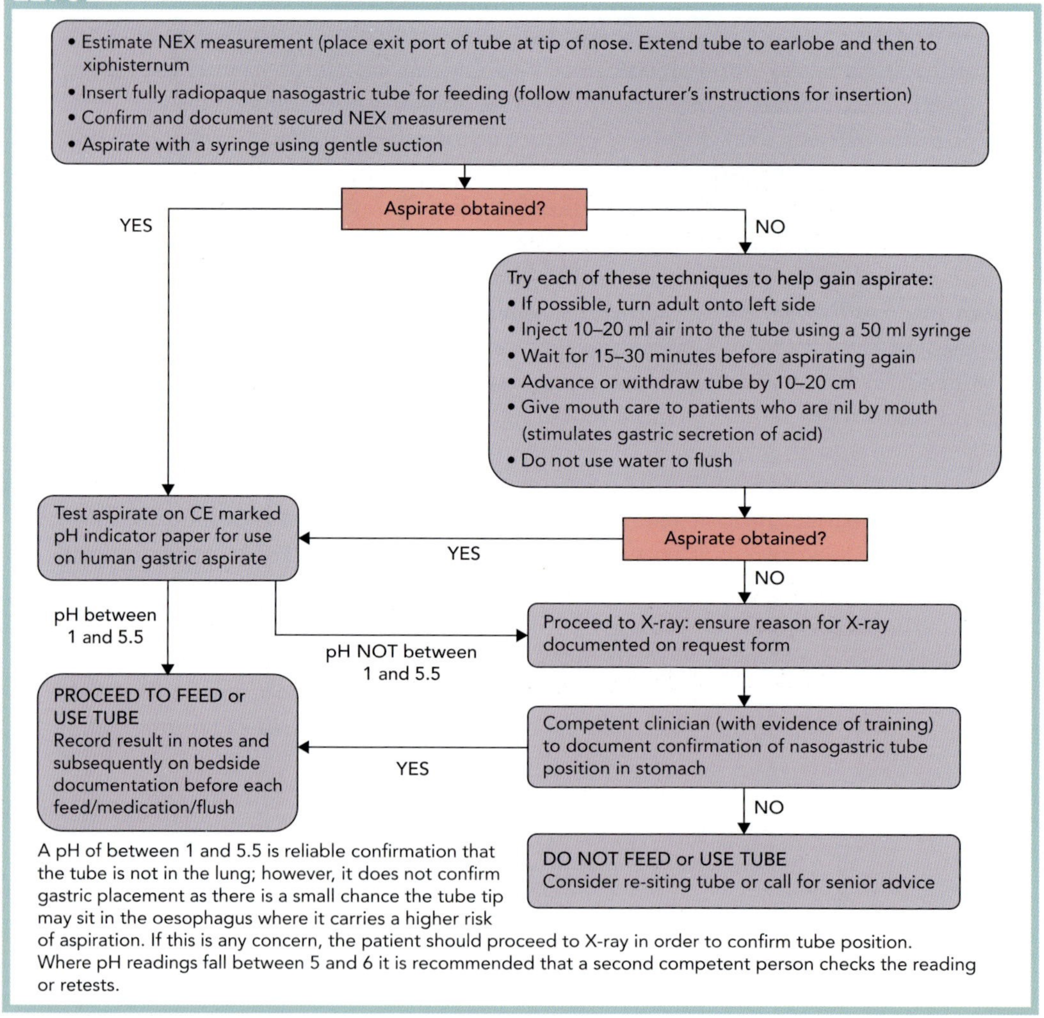

- Estimate NEX measurement (place exit port of tube at tip of nose. Extend tube to earlobe and then to xiphisternum
- Insert fully radiopaque nasogastric tube for feeding (follow manufacturer's instructions for insertion)
- Confirm and document secured NEX measurement
- Aspirate with a syringe using gentle suction

Aspirate obtained?

YES → Test aspirate on CE marked pH indicator paper for use on human gastric aspirate

NO → Try each of these techniques to help gain aspirate:
- If possible, turn adult onto left side
- Inject 10–20 ml air into the tube using a 50 ml syringe
- Wait for 15–30 minutes before aspirating again
- Advance or withdraw tube by 10–20 cm
- Give mouth care to patients who are nil by mouth (stimulates gastric secretion of acid)
- Do not use water to flush

Aspirate obtained?

YES → Test aspirate on CE marked pH indicator paper for use on human gastric aspirate

NO → Proceed to X-ray: ensure reason for X-ray documented on request form

Test aspirate: pH between 1 and 5.5 → PROCEED TO FEED or USE TUBE
Record result in notes and subsequently on bedside documentation before each feed/medication/flush

Test aspirate: pH NOT between 1 and 5.5 → Proceed to X-ray: ensure reason for X-ray documented on request form

Proceed to X-ray → Competent clinician (with evidence of training) to document confirmation of nasogastric tube position in stomach

YES → PROCEED TO FEED or USE TUBE

NO → DO NOT FEED or USE TUBE
Consider re-siting tube or call for senior advice

A pH of between 1 and 5.5 is reliable confirmation that the tube is not in the lung; however, it does not confirm gastric placement as there is a small chance the tube tip may sit in the oesophagus where it carries a higher risk of aspiration. If this is any concern, the patient should proceed to X-ray in order to confirm tube position. Where pH readings fall between 5 and 6 it is recommended that a second competent person checks the reading or retests.

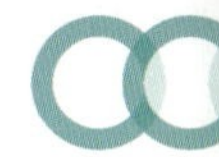

QUESTION 228

228 A bronchoscopic view of the upper respiratory tract of a newborn infant who coughs and chokes with feeding is shown (**228**). The green structure is a Fogarty catheter placed by the anaesthesiologist.

i. What is the diagnosis?

ii. What is the embryological origin of this pathology?

iii. What is the VACTERL association?

iv. How does an affected infant present?

v. What are the anaesthetic considerations?

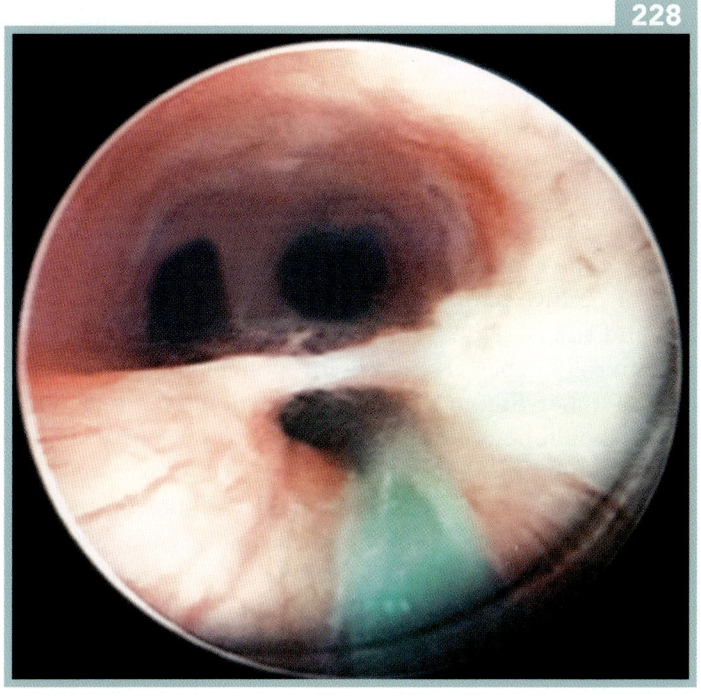

228

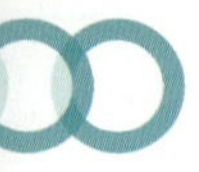

Answer 228

228i. Tracheoesophageal fistula (TOF). Shown is the typical carina with the left and right main bronchi (upper two openings) and a third opening (lower opening), the TOF, with the green catheter passing from the trachea into the oesophagus.

ii. In TOF the trachea fails to separate from the foregut during the fourth to fifth week of gestation. Several variants exist. The commonest (85%) consists of a dilated, blind, proximal oesophageal pouch and a fistula connecting the distal oesophagus to the trachea at a point just above the carina.

iii. TOF has a high association with other congenital anomalies. Vertebral, Anal (imperforate anus), Cardiac (septal defects), TOF, Esophageal atresia, Renal abnormalities and Limb (radial aplasia) have been referred to as VACTERL (previously VATER) association.

iv. With maternal polyhydramnios, excessive oral secretions, coughing, choking, cyanosis (especially with feeding) and a tympanitic abdomen. Diagnosis is confirmed by the inability to pass an oral or nasogastric tube or radiographic evidence of a blind pouch by either air or dye contrast.

v. Anaesthetic management includes:

- Positioning in a semi-upright position to reduce gastric reflux into the trachea. A nasogastric tube is inserted into the blind pouch to remove secretions.
- Avoidance of positive pressure mask ventilation, which increases gastric distension and risk of reflux. Intubation should be either awake or, if haemodynamically stable, via mask with spontaneous respiration.
- Ideally, an ET tube without a 'Murphy eye' should be used, otherwise the Murphy eye should be positioned anteriorly to prevent air entering the fistula.
- ET tube positioning is achieved by deliberate right mainstem intubation followed by withdrawal of the tube until bilateral breath sounds are heard. This positions the ET tube just above the carina and hopefully below the fistula. Positioning should be confirmed by fibreoptic endoscopy.
- Surgery is through a lateral thoracotomy opposite the aortic arch and can be either complete or staged. Prolonged ventilation with high airway pressures should be avoided postoperatively as this may unduly stress the tracheal closure and result in pneumomediastinum.

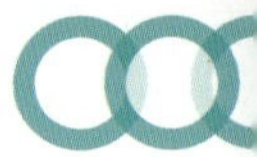

QUESTION 229

229 This arterial waveform (**229a**) is the result of combining the waveforms in **229b** and **229c**, as shown on the lower half of **229a**. Consider the sine wave forms in **229b** and **229c** (the time scale [x-axis] and the amplitude [y-axis] are the same for both figures):

i. How many cycles (fractions of a cycle) are depicted in **229b**?

ii. How many cycles are depicted in **229c**?

iii. Are the wave forms 'in phase'? Explain your answer.

iv. Are the amplitudes of each wave form as depicted in **229b** and **229c** the same?

v. What is the term given (person's name) to the building up of complex sinus wave forms from the constituent parts? Is this mathematical technique valid when constructing complex waveforms?

vi. What is the name given to the frequency depicted in **229b**? Given that the frequency of the sinus wave form in **229c** is exactly twice as fast, and the period half as long, as the frequency in **229b**, what is the name of the frequency depicted in **229c**?

vii. Give five examples of physiological signals that can be analysed using this technique. (To further understand the reason why it is important that anaesthesiologists understand these principles, see case **157**.)

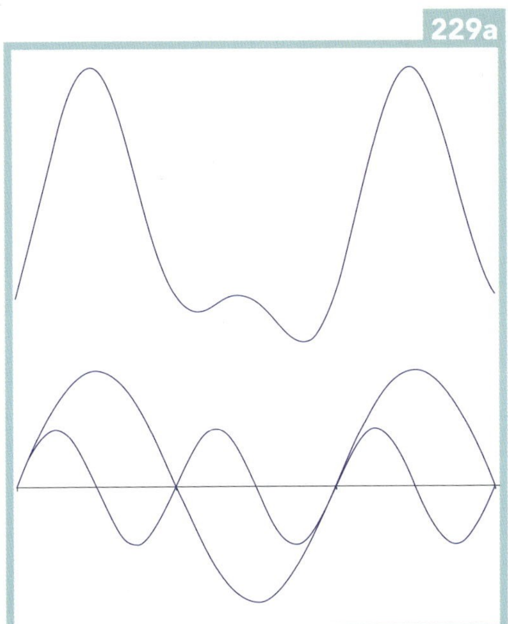

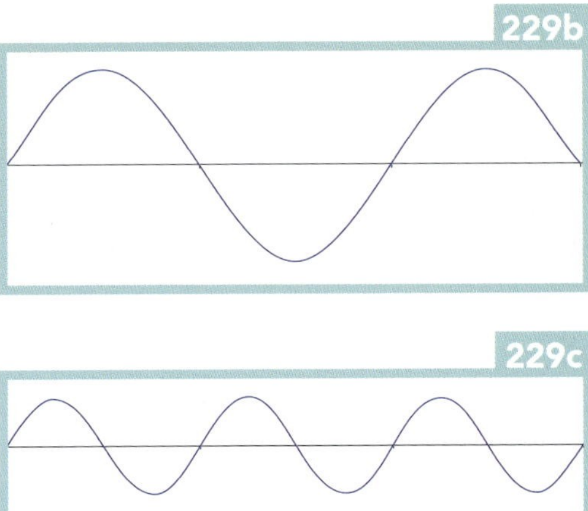

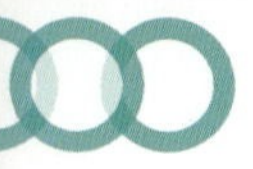

Answer 229

229i. One full sinus cycle, plus another half cycle.

ii. Three full cycles in the same time period as **229b**.

iii. The two sine waves are in phase. They both start at the same time point and they both cross the zero line at the same time point (see **229a**).

iv. The amplitude ('excursion', 'top to bottom') of the sine wave form in **229b** is larger than the amplitude in **229c**.

v. The technique of describing a repeating wave form by calculating its constituent components is called a 'Fourier Analysis'. The mathematical summation of the sine wave forms in **229b** and **229c** form 'represent', for instance, the arterial pressure wave form illustrated in **229a**. This is a valid way of analysing and constructing complex waveforms.

vi. The simplest single sinus wave that forms the basis of the Fourier analysis is called the fundamental waveform. Subsequent waveforms are built on to the fundamental and are named 'harmonics'. The sine wave form that is exactly twice as fast as the fundamental wave form is called the first harmonic. Subsequent waveforms are called second, third harmonics, etc. In an arterial line system, the number of harmonics must be sufficient to correctly display the BP.

vii. Any regularly repeating physiological signal can be represented using a Fourier transformation technique. Examples of wave forms that can be analyzed using the Fourier technique include: EEG, ECG, SpO_2, pressure wave forms (e.g. arterial, venous, ICP). A newer signal includes the pulse pressure variation used to dynamically determine intravascular fluid status.

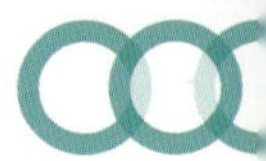

QUESTION 230

230 A patient presents with a mild flu-like illness with shortness of breath, no cough, but some aches. She has a normal BP, normal temperature and good urine output.

i. What derangement is shown on these data?

ii. Calculate the anion gap.

iii. What could be the cause of her metabolic derangement?

iv. Give causes of her hypoxia?

Na^+	140 mmol/l (140 mEq/l)
K^+	2.8 mmol/l (2.8 mEq/l)
Cl^-	108 mmol/l (108 mEq/l)
HCO_3^-	11 mmol/l (11 mEq/l)
Urea (BUN)	3.6 mmol/l (22 mg/dl)
Creatinine	70 mmol/l (0.8 mg/dl)
Glucose	7.3 mmol/l (132 mg/dl)
Acetone/ketones	NEG
pH	7.40
pCO_2	2.23 kPa (16.8 mmHg)
pO_2	10.3 kPa (77.4 mmHg)
FiO_2	Room air
Lactate	1.6 mmol/l (1.6 mEq/l)
Osmolarity	286 mmol/l

QUESTION 231

231i. What is this test (**231**) called?

ii. What is measured by the parameters indicated as R, K and MA?

iii. What other tests are available to measure these parameters?

iv. Is this a normal test result?

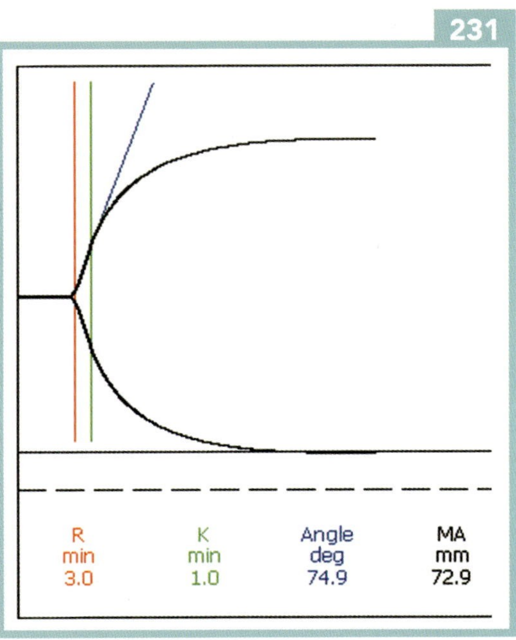

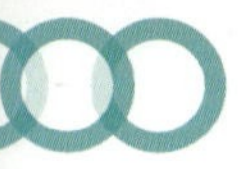

Answer 230

230i. The patient has a metabolic acidosis with an increased anion gap. Explanation of the anion gap allows understanding of what is wrong with this patient.

ii. The anion gap = $(Na^+ + K^+) - (Cl^- + HCO_3^-)$; in this case: (140 + 2.8) – (108 + 11) = 23.8. This is a raised anion gap as the normal range should be <11 mmol/l (11 mEq/l).

iii. MUDPALES is an acronym used to list the main causes of metabolic acidosis with an increased anion gap and stands for **M**ethanol, **U**remia, **D**iabetic ketoacidosis, **P**araldehyde, **A**lcoholic ketoacidosis (from ethanol), **L**actic acidosis, **E**thylene glycol and **S**alicylates. Without a serum osmolar gap, methanol, ethanol and ethylene glycol are excluded. The patient is not diabetic, has no ketones in her serum and is not in renal failure. Her toxicology screen was positive for salicylates. She had been taking home remedies and aspirin for her symptoms for over a week in higher than recommended dosages.

iv. Her hypoxia is unusual and a CXR should be ordered to exclude pneumonia or other acute respiratory pathology. Her chronic salicylate ingestion caused pulmonary oedema, which quickly improved once the aspirin was stopped.

Answer 231

231i. A thromboelastogram (TEG); also known as a thrombelastogram.

ii. R is the clotting time, which indicates the time from the start of the test until clotting starts. This time is influenced by platelet function and clotting factors. K is the angle or rate of clot formation, which is influenced by platelet function, clotting factors and fibrinogen concentration. MA is the maximum amplitude, which measures the strength of the clot and is influenced by platelet function and fibrinogen concentration.

iii. Skin 'bleeding time' was used extensively, but has been found to have a poor sensitivity and a poor specificity for clotting and platelet function. The platelet function assay measures the function of platelets and can be used to determine the residual effects of aspirin-like compounds on the clotting cascade in a patient.

iv. It is a normal test result.

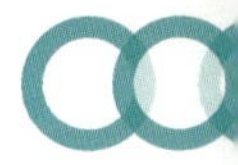

QUESTION 232

232 At a small, outlying outpatient surgical centre, a 50-year-old patient presents for colonoscopy. He is obese (BMI 35 kg/m^2), on medication for hypertension and sedentary. He was diagnosed with type 2 diabetes mellitus 10 years ago with poor control. He denies any heart problems. His ECG at the preoperative visit is shown (**232a**). Preoperatively, the patient complains of sudden chest tightness and his ECG is shown (**232b**). It will take at least 2 hours for an ambulance to transport the patient to the nearest cardiology centre (a helicopter cannot be used due to bad weather).

i. Comment on his suitability for day-case colonoscopy in a remote hospital.

ii. What are the changes noted in the ECG (describe: heart rate, P-R interval, specific leads with changes)? What diagnosis do these changes indicate?

iii. What is the definitive therapy for such patients?

iv. Mention four treatment modalities that should be considered while waiting for the transport. What are the contraindications for each?

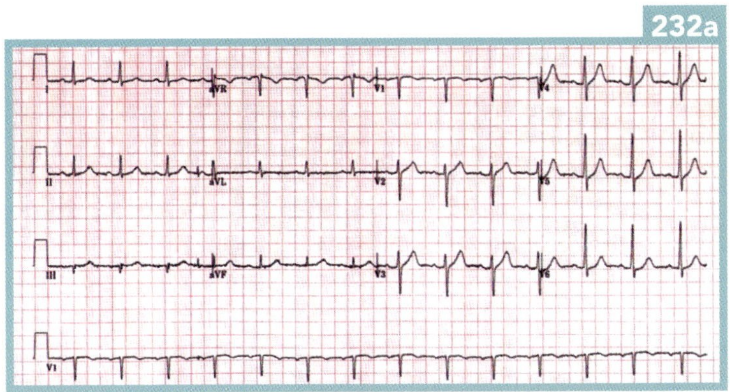

232a

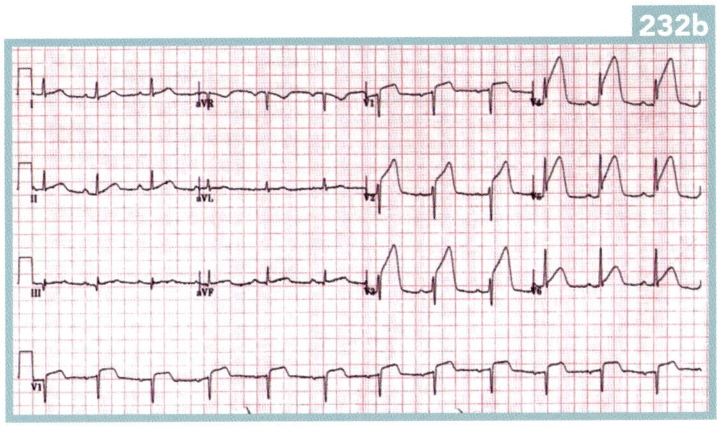

232b

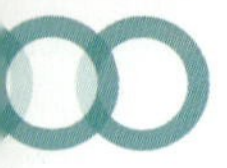

Answer 232

232i. This man has multiple co-morbidities and is obese (ASA 2). He would have been better managed in a major hospital with acute medical facilities. If his BMI had been 39 or above, this would be morbid obesity and ASA 3.

ii. The ventricular rate is 71 bpm; the P-R interval 184 msec; the anterolateral leads (V1–V5) show marked ST elevation. The diagnosis is an acute anterolateral infarct: an ST elevation myocardial infarct (STEMI).

iii. Definitive therapy is early percutaneous coronary intervention (PCI). Compared with fibrinolysis, PCI results in less re-occlusion, improved left ventricular function and improved overall outcome (including reduced risk of stroke). PCI should be performed within 90 minutes of the onset of pain (may show benefit even if performed within 12 hours). When access to PCI is not possible within 90 minutes, coronary artery reperfusion with thrombolysis (i.e. fibrinolytics) may help, but this should be discussed with a cardiologist.

iv. After placing monitors and establishing IV access, the immediate treatment includes:

- Morphine for chest discomfort that does not respond to nitroglycerine (glyceryl trinitrate, GTN). Use with caution in patients who are dependent on preload. Always administer an antiemetic concurrently.
- Oxygen for oxygen saturations <94%. Supplemental oxygen may be harmful if the saturation is >94% as oxygen free radicals and oxygen-induced vasoconstriction are postulated to worsen outcome.
- GTN can be administered sublingually as 'spray dosing'. This should be avoided if the patient is haemodynamically unstable and used with care if right ventricular infarction complicates an inferior myocardial infarct, as a sudden drop in cardiac output may occur due to decreased venous return. GTN should also be avoided if recent use of a phosphodiesterase inhibitor for erectile dysfunction has occurred (sildanefil, vardenafil or tadafil.)
- Aspirin (160–325 mg, US: 300 mg, UK) to chew. Avoid if aspirin allergy or history of recent GI bleeding.
- The mnemonic 'MONA' is sometimes used.

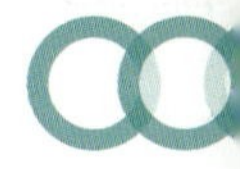

QUESTION 233

233 A schematic diagram of a bronchial tree as visualised by an endoscopist from the trachea is shown (**233a**).

i. Identify the bronchial branches marked and state whether they are secondary (lobar) or tertiary (segmental) bronchi.

ii. What is the anatomical and surgical significance of the tertiary subdivisions?

iii. Draw a schematic of the lobes and segments of the lung (a) as surface markings and (b) as viewed from the mediastinum.

iv. What factor in the anatomy of the bronchial tree must be taken into consideration when using a double-lumen ET tube for one-lung ventilation?

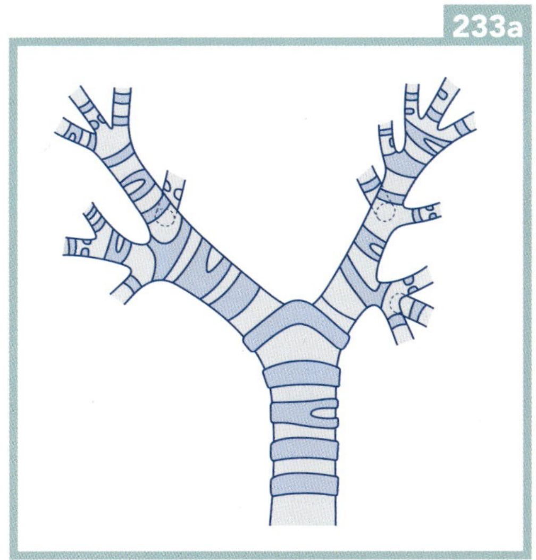

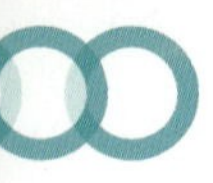

Answer 233

233i. There are 10 tertiary bronchial subdivisions in each lung, each of which supplies a segment of lung tissue called a bronchopulmonary segment with its own discrete vascular supply and lymphatic drainage (**233b**).

ii. Tumours or abscesses localised in a bronchopulmonary segment may be surgically removed without seriously disrupting the surrounding lung tissue.

iii. The anatomy of the lobes and segments is shown in **233c**. The top illustrations show the surface markings of the lungs as viewed from outside the chest; the lower diagrams show the lobes and segments as if viewed from the mediastinum out. This anatomy is important to understand both for pneumonectomy and how to place a double-lumen ET tube for one-lung ventilation

iv. The right upper lobe orifice arises early in the course of the right main bronchus (about 2.5 cm from the carina) and may be occluded by the cuff or tip of a right-sided double lumen (D/L) tube placed in the right mainstem bronchus. Right-sided D/L tubes are designed with a ventilation slot at their tip (usually incorporated into the endobronchial cuff). Considerable variation occurs in the origin of the right upper lobe bronchus (including anomalous origin from the trachea) and even with the modifications described above, a left-sided ET tube is preferable for most cases requiring one-lung ventilation.

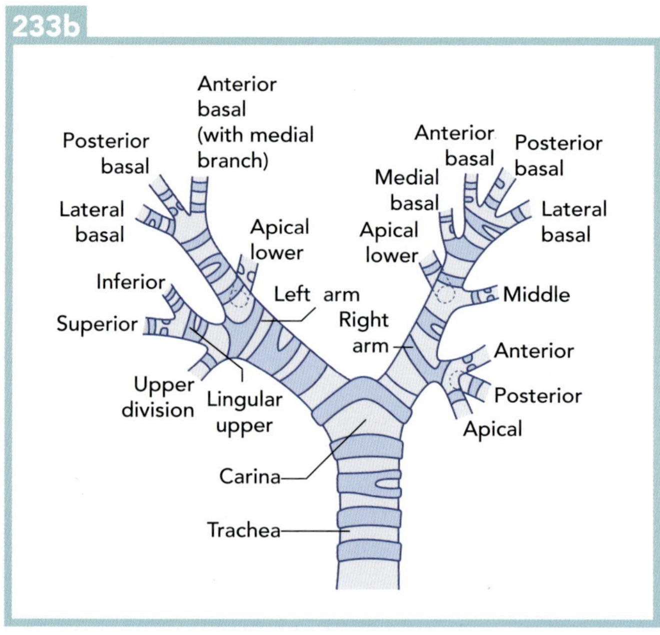

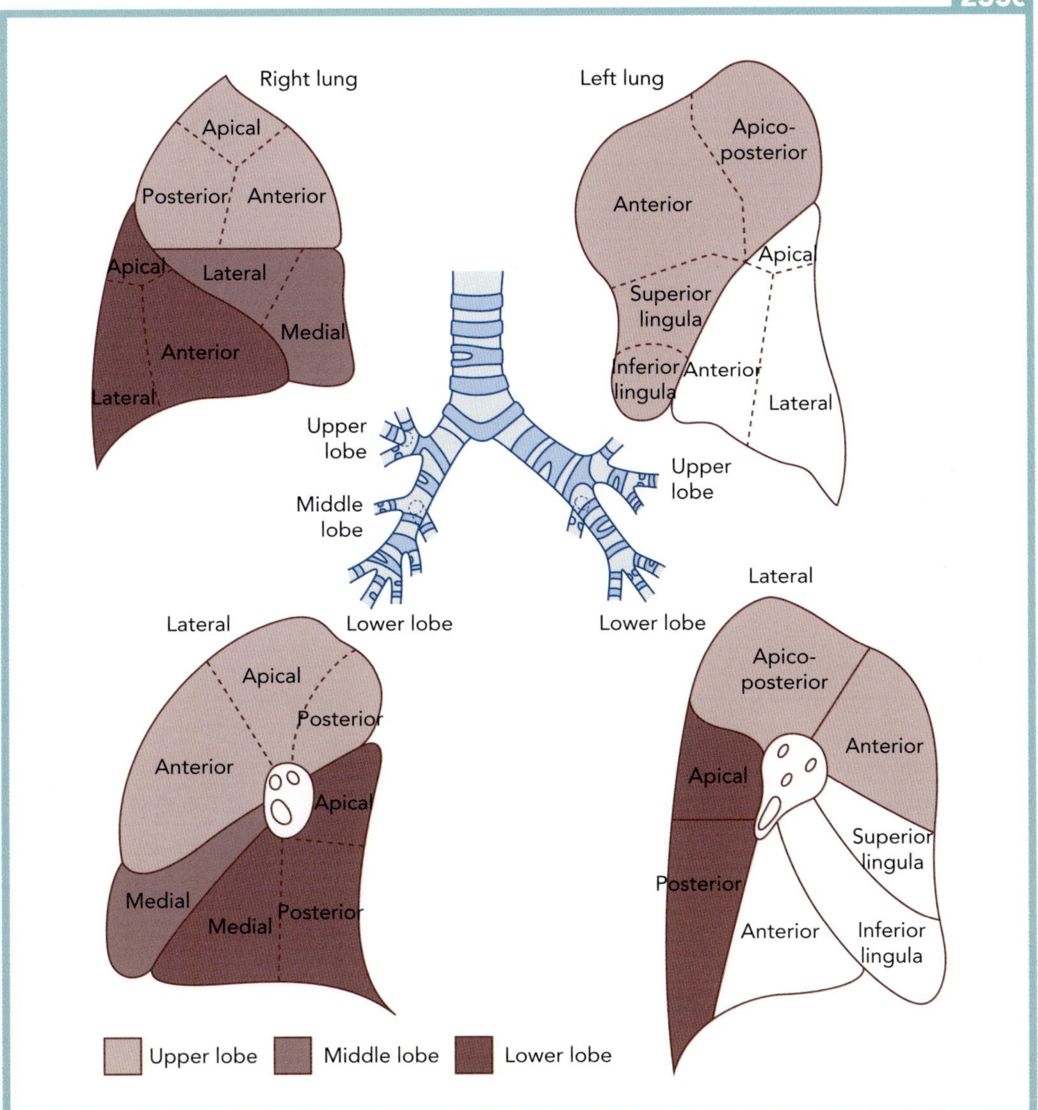
Right lung
Apical
Posterior
Anterior
Apical
Lateral
Medial
Anterior
Lateral
Left lung
Apico-
posterior
Anterior
Apical
Superior
lingula
Inferior
lingula
Anterior
Lateral
Upper
lobe
Middle
lobe
Upper
lobe
Lower lobe
Lower lobe
Lateral
Apical
Posterior
Anterior
Apical
Medial
Medial
Posterior
Lateral
Apico-
posterior
Anterior
Apical
Superior
lingula
Posterior
Anterior
Inferior
lingula
Upper lobe
Middle lobe
Lower lobe

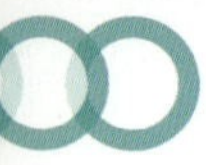

Appendix – Answer 93ii, page 118

Drug	Time to peak effect	Elimination half-life	Acceptable time after drug for block performance
		Heparins	
UFH s.c. prophylactic	<30 min	1–2 h	4 h and normal APTT
UFH i.v. treatment	<5 min	1–2 h	4 h and normal APTT
LMWH s.c. prophylactic	3–4 h	3–7 h	12 h
LMWH s.c. treatment	3–4 h	3–7 h	24 h
		Heparin alternatives	
Lepirudin	0.5–2 h	2–3 h	10 h
Desirudin	0.5–2 h	2–3 h	10 h
Bivalirudin	5 min	25 min	10 h
Argatroban	<30 min	30–35 min	4 h
Fondaparinux*	1–2 h	17–20 h	>36 h
		Antiplatelet drugs	
NSAIDs	1–2 h	1–12 h	No additional precautions
Aspirin	12–24 h	Not relevant	No additional precautions
Clopidogrel	12–24 h	Irreversible effect	7 days
Ticlopidine	8–11 days	24–32 h but 90 h in chronic use	10 days
Tirofiban	<5 min	4–8 h	8 h
Eptifibatide	<5 min	4–8 h	8 h
Abciximab	<5 min	24–48 h	48 h
Dipyridamole	75 min	10 h	No additional precautions
		Oral anticoagulants	
Warfarin	3–5 days	4–5 days	INR ≤1.4
Rivaroxaban*	3 h	7–9 h	21 h
Dabigatran†	0.5–2.0 h	12–17 h	36 h
		Thrombolytic drugs	
Alteplase, anistreplase reteplase, streptokinase	<5 min	4–24 min	Contraindicated

Notes: The data used to populate this table are derived from the German guidelines adopted by ESRA [2], the ASRA guidelines [1] and data presented by drug manufacturers. Ticlopidine no longer has a UK licence. These recommendations relate primarily to neuraxial blocks.

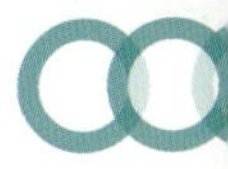

Acceptable time for next drug dose after block	Acceptable time after drug for catheter removal	Acceptable time af ter catheter removal for next drug dose
Heparins		
1 h	4 h and normal APTT	1 h
4 h	4 h and normal APTT	4 h
4 h	12 h	4 h
4 h	24 h	4 h
Heparin alternatives		
4 h	10 h	4 h
4 h	10 h	4 h
4 h	10 h	4 h
2 h	4 h	2 h
12 h	42 h	12 h
Antiplatelet drugs		
No additional precautions		
No additional precautions 6 h		
After block performance	7 days	6 h
After block performance	10 days	6 h
After block performance	8 h	After catheter removal
After block performance	8 h	After catheter removal
After blcok performance	48 h	After catheter removal
No additional precautions	6 h	
Oral anticoagulants		
After catheter removal	INR ≤1.4	1 h
5 h	*	*
6 h	†	†
Thrombolytic drugs		
Contraindicated	Not applicable	10 days

Abbreviations: UFH = unfractionated heparin; APTT = activated partial thromboplastin time; LMWH = low molecular weight heparin; s.c. = subcutaneous; i.v. = intravenous; NSAIDs = non-steroidal anti-inflammatory drugs; INR = international normalised ratio.

* Manufacturer recommends caution with use of neuraxial catheters.

† Manufacturer recommends that neuraxial catheters are not used.

Index

Note: references are to case numbers

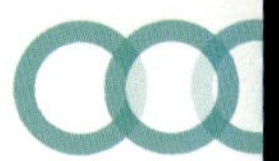

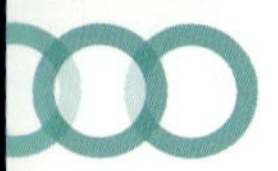

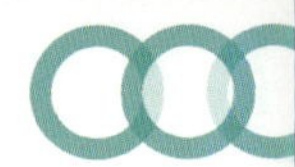

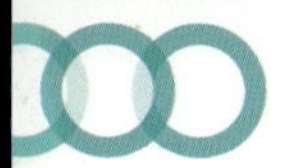

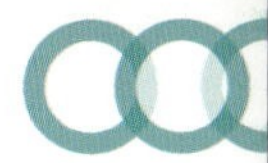

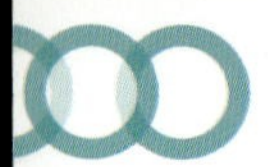

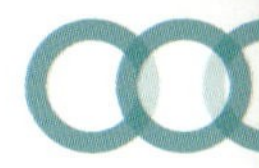

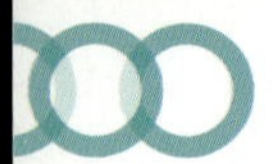